International Perspectives on Aging

Volume 36

Series Editors
Jason L. Powell, Department of Social and Political Science, University of Chester, Chester, UK
Sheying Chen, Department of Public Administration, Pace University, New York, NY, USA

The study of aging is continuing to increase rapidly across multiple disciplines. This wide-ranging series on International Perspectives on Aging provides readers with much-needed comprehensive texts and critical perspectives on the latest research, policy, and practical developments. Both aging and globalization have become a reality of our times, yet a systematic effort of a global magnitude to address aging is yet to be seen. The series bridges the gaps in the literature and provides cutting-edge debate on new and traditional areas of comparative aging, all from an international perspective. More specifically, this book series on International Perspectives on Aging puts the spotlight on international and comparative studies of aging.

Raya Elfadel Kheirbek • Maria D. Llorente
Editors

Current Perspectives on Centenarians

Introduction to Lifespan and Healthspan

Springer

Editors
Raya Elfadel Kheirbek
University of Maryland School of Medicine
Baltimore, MD, USA

Maria D. Llorente
Department of Veterans Affairs
Washington, DC, USA

Department of Psychiatry
Georgetown University School of Medicine
Washington, DC, USA

ISSN 2197-5841 ISSN 2197-585X (electronic)
International Perspectives on Aging
ISBN 978-3-031-30914-4 ISBN 978-3-031-30915-1 (eBook)
https://doi.org/10.1007/978-3-031-30915-1

This Springer imprint is published by the registered company Springer Nature Switzerland AG
The registered company address is: Gewerbestrasse 11, 6330 Cham, Switzerland

Paper in this product is recyclable.

Preface

The study of centenarians and the factors that contribute to a long and healthy life is a fascinating and important field of research. As the global population continues to age, the number of centenarians is on the rise. According to the United Nations, the number of centenarians worldwide is projected to increase from around 562,000 in 2019 to more than three million by 2050. This increase in longevity presents both challenges and opportunities for individuals, families, communities, and societies.

This book aims to provide a comprehensive look at the various factors that not only contribute to longevity, but also can contribute to long lived quality of life, including nutrition, physical activity, genetics, and whole health. We also delve into unique aspects of longevity seen in underserved and minority populations, such as the "Hispanic paradox" and the Black-White mortality crossover seen among African Americans. Additionally, we examine the role of dental care in overall health and the unique experiences of supercentenarians, those individuals who have lived to 110 years or older.

One of the most important factors to maintain independent function in longevity is regular physical activity. Studies have shown that regular exercise can help to reduce the risk of chronic diseases, such as heart disease, diabetes, and cancer, which are common causes of death among older adults. It also helps to improve overall cardiovascular health and boost the immune system. However, many older adults face barriers to physical activity, such as mobility limitations or lack of access to appropriate facilities and programs. It is important to address these barriers in order to promote wholistic and individual centered system of care.

Nutrition also plays a crucial role in longevity. A balanced diet that includes a variety of fruits, vegetables, whole grains, beans, and lean proteins can help to promote good health and reduce the risk of chronic diseases. However, older adults may face challenges in accessing healthy food options or may have difficulty preparing meals due to physical limitations. Additionally, many older adults may have specific dietary needs, such as a need for more protein or calcium, that should be considered.

Genetics plays a crucial role in the study of centenarians, as it helps to understand the underlying biological mechanisms that contribute to exceptional longevity. Researchers have identified specific genetic variations that are associated with increased lifespan, such as mutations in the FOXO3A gene. Additionally, studying the genetics of centenarians can also provide insight into the development of age-related diseases and how to potentially prevent or delay their onset. Understanding the genetic factors that contribute to exceptional longevity can also lead to the development of new therapies and interventions to improve health and extend lifespan for the general population. This book explores the concept of ageism, discrimination specifically aimed against people solely because of their age. Ageism is a pervasive costly problem that can have a negative impact on older adults' physical and mental health, as well as their social and economic well-being. It is important to raise awareness about ageism and its harmful effects, and to work to promote positive attitudes towards aging.

In addition to the aforementioned topics, we also examine the phenomenon of the "Hispanic paradox," in which Latino individuals have been found to have a higher life expectancy despite having similar or higher prevalence of diseases associated with mortality, as well as experiencing multiple adverse social determinants of health. We explore the potential reasons for this paradox, such as cultural and familial support, and the role of community in promoting healthy aging. Similarly, the phenomenon of Black-White mortality crossover is observed among older African Americans.. This crossover effect is observed at about age 85 years, after which African Americans exhibit lower mortality compared to same age Whites. Proposed hypotheses are discussed and include select survivor cohort, poor data quality, cohort effects, and self-reported quality of life.

Furthermore, we explore the role of dental care in overall health. Dental health is an often overlooked aspect of overall health, but it plays an important role in maintaining a healthy body. Poor oral health can lead to a host of health issues, including diabetes and heart disease, and poor oral health can also contribute to malnourishment.

In closing, we would like to express our deepest gratitude to all the authors who have contributed their expertise and insights to this book. The breadth of knowledge and experience represented in these chapters is truly impressive and has greatly enriched the content of this book. We would like to thank each and every one of them for their hard work and dedication in making this book a reality. We hope that this book will serve as a valuable resource for researchers, healthcare professionals, policymakers, and the general public as we all strive to understand aging and add quality years for our patients, our relatives and friends, and ourselves.

Baltimore, MD, USA Raya Elfadel Kheirbek

Washington, DC, USA Maria D. Llorente

Contents

Chapter 1
Ageism Revolution and Human Longivity Beyond Age 100

Diane Blazejewski Martin, Nadia Ijaz, and Raya Elfadel Kheirbek

> *A process of systematic stereotyping or discrimination against people because they are old, just as racism and sexism accomplish with skin color and gender. Ageism allows the younger generations to see older people as different than themselves; thus, they subtly cease to identify with their older adults as human beings.*
>
> ~Robert Butler, MD 1969

Key Take Away Points

1. Ageism is a detrimental practice that results in pervasive mistreatment of older adults, including physical and financial abuse, inappropriate public and medical services, and unequal treatment in employment.
2. Negative depiction of aging can lead to adverse outcomes in terms of the health and wellbeing of older adults.
3. Increasing public literacy and awareness along with educating health professionals about the realistic expectations of aging can help promote the concept of healthy aging and undermine the effects of ageism.

D. B. Martin
Baltimore Graduate School, University of Maryland, Baltimore, MD, USA
e-mail: Diane.Martin@umaryland.edu

N. Ijaz · R. E. Kheirbek (✉)
University of Maryland School of Medicine, Baltimore, MD, USA
e-mail: nijaz@som.ummaryland.edu; rkheirbek@som.umaryland.edu

R. E. Kheirbek, M. D. Llorente (eds.), *Current Perspectives on Centenarians*, International Perspectives on Aging 36,
https://doi.org/10.1007/978-3-031-30915-1_1

1.1 Introduction

Making a note of a person's age should not be considered negative. Many older adults proudly disclose their age. Acknowledging someone's age is not considered a transgression but the reaction to that chronological age and the connotation attached to it, is what makes people ageists. Ageism occurs when we no longer value a person and their individuality but rather focus on the minutiae of a group compartmentalized by a certain number defined as age. Ageism is prevalent in our society. It is considered the third greatest -ism (behind racism and sexism) and many researchers believe that it is the only -ism that still goes unnoticed and unchallenged. Ageism has become ingrained in our culture affecting several aspects of civil life including hiring practices, medical care, and social policy. As a society, we disparage older adults without fear of censure, and aging is viewed as something to be dreaded of, rather than the natural manifestation of life.

1.2 Illustrative Vignette

The small town in the Midwest had always been a tight-knit community. But as the population began to age, many of the older longtime residents felt like felt like outsiders.

The community center, which had always been a hub of activity, was focused on programs for younger families and children. The senior center, which had been the heart of the community for older residents, had been closed due to budget cuts. The older residents felt like their needs and interests were being ignored. Many older residents started to feel isolated and lonely, like they didn't belong in their own community anymore. They felt like their contributions and experiences were no longer valued, and they were being pushed out of the community.

The town's local government and community leaders realized that this was a problem. They organized a meeting with older residents to listen to their concerns and started making changes to be more inclusive and age friendly. They reopened the senior center that offered activities and programs tailored to the older residents' interests and abilities. They also started to involve them in the planning and decision-making process in the community, including establishing an intergenerational program where elders provided support and mentoring for the young.

The older residents felt like they were finally being heard and valued. They were no longer invisible in their own community. They started to participate more actively in their community and felt more connected to their town.

This case illustrates the reality of ageism in communities, where older residents can feel excluded and invisible. It also shows how the community and local government can take steps to be more inclusive and age-friendly, making sure that older residents feel valued and included in the community. This helps combat ageism and create a more equitable and inclusive community for all.

More than 80% of people over the age of 60 experience ageism, assuming they have memory or physical impairments simply because they were older, and almost 1/3 of older adults report being ignored or not taken seriously because of their age. (Palmore, 2001). This is an issue of importance in the oldest old group including centenarians. According to the United Nations and Pew Research Center, there were an estimated 573,000 centenarians worldwide in 2020. This number is expected to grow exponentially to nearly 3.7 million centenarians by 2050, an increase of almost 650%, therefore societal work to stop negative stereotypes against oldest generations is critical.

A recent cross-sectional study from University of Michigan illustrates US adults 50 to 80 years mentioned encountering ageism (prevalence of >90%), at various levels and was associated with poor physical and mental health. (Allen et al., 2022; Hu et al., 2021) There may not be a single clear-cut explanation for why ageism is prevalent. Perhaps, it is the lack of older adult role models, or because older adults are not as integrated into families as in previous generations. Much of what we perceive about aging comes from what we see and hear in pop culture. About 6% of characters on television and in films are older and those who are portrayed, are often depicted based on age stereotypes (Markov & Yoon, 2020). They are shown as conduits of comic relief or as feeble and decrepit individuals. The media promotes negative stereotypes and misconceptions about aging and older adults (Prieler, 2020).

Ageism can impact the quality of life in older individuals. Negative stereotypes can lead to demeaning of older adults whereas ageism in favor of older adults can be seen in numerous government programs, including Social Security benefits, Supplemental Security Income, Military Retirement and Veteran's Health Care, and the services provided through the Area Agencies on Aging (AAA). AAA are supported by local government and provide numerous programs for older adults through direct service, supplements to federal and state programs, and tax reductions. However, programs such as these may perpetuate negative stereotypes of older adults as being a homogenous at-risk vulnerable group (Palmore, 1999) and may find support from legislators holding negative stereotypes in which older adults are viewed as destitute, depressed, dependent, incompetent, lonely, frail, sick, and mentally slow (Lubomudrov, 1987).

The COVID-19 pandemic highlighted the prevalence of ageism. Although mortality rates are higher in older adults compared to other age groups, age seems to be conflated with frailty and co-morbidity, which are likely to be the more important factors associated with mortality rather than just age.

The pandemic also brought forth the idea that in case of medical equipment shortages, and hospital capacity scarcity, care providers may be faced with the ethical decisions about whose life takes priority and age may become a deciding factor.

Regardless of the cause and its effects, ageism needs to be carefully examined to be understood.

1.3 Defining Ageism

Ageism is defined as prejudice and discrimination against an individual based on age.

In 1969, the prominent gerontologist Robert N. Butler, introduced the term "ageism" to describe discrimination and prejudice against adults when they reach a certain age. Palmer defines ageism in his book, *Ageism: Negative and Positive* (1999) as "prejudice or discrimination against or in favor of an age group".

1.3.1 Three Levels of Ageism

Ageism can be seen at several different levels in society.

- Micro level: Interpersonal
- Mezo level: Within social networks
- Macro level: Through institutional policies or cultural traditions

1.3.2 Potential Causes of Ageism (Theoretical Level)

Stereotype Embodiment Theory (SET) SET explains a lifetime process by which age stereotypes are internalized by absorbing the social norms and cultural values surrounding individuals (Levy, 2009). SET has four tenets: (1) a lifelong exposure to age-stereotypes, (2) unconscious internalization, (3) facilitating by self-relevance, and (4) a wide range of impact.

Terror Management Theory A negative bias against older adults helps protect younger individuals from thinking about the negative aspects of aging. (ageism exists because older people are associated with imminent loss and death. Social distancing behaviors, then, serve to buffer us from threatening aspects of old age, thereby reducing anxiety).

Functional Approach Theory Stereotypes serve individuals in the cognitive realm by helping them increase efficiency through categorization and in the social realm by helping them identify with their social group.

Intergroup Contact Theory Building a positive view towards a target group can be achieved by having positive interactions with the group members. Lack of intergroup connection may lead to a negative view towards older adults.

Cognitive Economy Theory In order to deal with the enormous complexity that confronts us on a daily basis, we use cognitive short cuts or categories. Stereotypes are shortcuts for perceptual processing regarding categories of people. Under conditions of incomplete knowledge, stereotyping draws on generalizations about how characteristics or attributes go together, which may overshadow all other relevant characteristics of individuals.

Social Identity Theory This theory posits that humans use group identity to maintain positive self-identity, and this results in in-group/out-group distinctions. In order to achieve a greater positive distinction between groups, humans tend to look for "evidence" that confirms the superiority of their group (the in-group) and the inferiority of the other groups (out-group).

1.4 Evolution of Ageism

The industrial revolution seems to be the pivotal point in time when the notion of ageism surfaced. Prior to this, older adults were regarded as valuable and venerable members of society. They were viewed as wise, knowledgeable, and experienced. They held positions of authority in politics and the government, as well as in their church, synagogue, or mosques. It was "something special" if an individual lived to be old, as people aged 65 and above made up just 4% of the demographics. However, with the industrial revolution (and the discovery of Alzheimer's disease in 1901), negative stereotypes about older adults started to emerge. These stereotypes became commonplace through the middle of the twentieth century as social programs for older adults were developed, considering them as physically, mentally, socially, and economically impaired. The fastest growth in these programs occurred between the 1930s and the 1990s (Social security, Medicare). Slowly stereotypes have begun to shift toward a more positive view of older adults with focus on their financial and health needs.

1.5 Why Is Ageism Important?

The last decade has seen increasing life spans in the Western hemisphere due to better health care, drug development, and preventive practices. The aging American population has raised concerns among policy makers, health care providers, and economic analysts. This has resulted in several issues coming to the spotlight such as the financial and economic impact and health care costs of an aging demographic. Analysts with an interest in the ever-increasing federal debt have begun focusing their attention on social security payments and cost of care (especially in the last year of life). We have seen this play out recently with the health care debate.

It is important to remember that these debates are not new. In the past they have been resisted by older adults and organizations such as AARP, who claim that older adults are entitled to these programs. However, others see it as reverse discrimination against younger adults, who don't qualify for these programs and view them as a form of positive ageism.

The other side of the debate sees ageism like any –ism, which violates the basic democratic ideal that each person should be judged on merit rather than on group characteristics. It is considered unethical, oftentimes illegal, to discriminate based on characteristics, as with any –ism.

1.6 Age-Differentiated Behavior

Ageism is difficult to detect, and more research is necessary to understand the construct of ageism and how best to measure it. To do so, an understanding of normal and abnormal aging processes is needed as well as an understanding of age-differentiated behaviors.

An age-differentiated behavior is considered behavior that differs depending on the age of the person being involved in the interaction. Is showing such differences between groups ageist?

That can be a tricky question to answer. Ageism is a sub-set of age-differentiated behavior, either because it is caused by inaccurate attitudes and beliefs about aging or because it has a clear and harmful impact on older adults. So, how do you distinguish between the two?

Understanding some key facts about aging and older adults is a good place to start.

Health Status: There is more variability in the health of adults over 65 years of age than in any other age group. Therefore, age is a poor indicator of functional ability.

Sensory Changes: 8.5% of the 65+ age group experience significant visual impairment; 35% have significant hearing impairment; <2% speech impairment.

Independent and everyday functioning: 64% of the 65+ age group experience no major physical limitations. Only 2% require assistance with ADLs (bathing, grooming, feeding, toileting, ambulating). Of note, this increases to 26% over age 80 (about 1 in 4), but still not the majority of older adults.

Cognition: may decline but individual differences cannot be discerned as the magnitude of loss is influenced by the environment (i.e., stimulating environment = less loss, isolation = greater loss).

Language: age-related changes in expressive language are documented (simpler syntactical sentence structure). However, this is often viewed positively since the speech is often clearer and simpler to understand. Receptive vocabulary overall is intact, unless presented too quickly, or with complexity. Interestingly, story-telling improves with age, since older adults are not prone to rambling and irrelevancy of details.

Social and emotional functioning: There seems to be better emotional regulation with age, as people become more adaptive to changes.

What are the take-aways? No single age-related impairment affects most older adults. They are more different from one another than are younger adults. Therefore, age as a number is a poor indicator of competency. However, some developmental discontinuity occurs after age 65 to the end of life and warrants sensitivity to changes that may come later.

1.7 Distinguishing Between Ageism and Age-Differentiated Behavior

When trying to distinguish between ageism and age differentiated behavior, consider these three questions when evaluating the appropriateness of behavior while interacting with older adults:

What type of Behavior is Occurring? Behaviors are considered ageist when they distance, ignore, exclude, or under-represent older adults. For example, doctors often don't include older adults in care discussions, older adults are often under-represented in media, politics, etc. Additional red-flags of ageist behavior are those that are not protective, beneficial, positive, or compassionate and behaviors that are negative or overtly harmful to the person, such as negative images etc.

What is the Cause of the Behavior? Is the behavior linked to stereotypical beliefs such as uselessness or decreased competency? It is important to consider where the behavior is coming from and not just the interpretation of the behavior, since ageist behavior is not always linked to ageist attitudes.

What is the Appropriateness of the Behavior? Age related treatment results from an increased frequency of visits, as we learn the characteristics of the older adult with whom we interact (e.g., communication needs, health, work status, etc.). It is through this process that we get to know the person (bottom-up processing) and begin engaging based on individual needs, not group assumptions (top-down processing).

Ageism is a subset of age-differentiated behavior (behaviors that differs depending on the age of the person involved in the interaction) either because it is caused by inaccurate attitudes and beliefs about aging or because it has a clear and harmful impact on older adults.

Behaviors toward the aging adult and the corresponding impact on the older adult include:

1. Behaviors that distance, ignore, exclude or under-represent older adults (e.g., physicians spend less time with and show less receptivity to older patients, nursing home staff ignore and fail to reinforce independence, the under-representation in mass media, etc.).

2. Behaviors that are more positive or protective toward older adults than younger adults (e.g., legislative protections, Medicare in the US, positive stereotypes of aging in mass media such as warm and friendly individuals).
3. Behaviors that are negative or overtly harmful (e.g., negative images of aging in mass media; differential access to treatments, denial of access to jobs and housing despite equal qualifications, and older adult abuse).

> Ageism is the only –ism that is still on top of the table, not under it. Stereotypes are changing and older adults will continue to change them. People aged 60 to 100+ represent a huge age group – don't even try to stereotype them. (Trish Herbert, Journeywell: A Guide to Quality Aging)

1.8 Consequences of Ageism

> Older adults…have not been subjected to a history of purposeful and equal treatment…Old age also does not define a discrete and insular minority because all adults, if they live out their normal life, will experience it. (Supreme Court Justice Sandra Day O'Connor 1999)

Several consequences become evident when negative stereotyping and ageism is prevalent in society.

1. **Health care consequences:**

   Unidimensional thinking about age and its ramifications leads to denied opportunities and rights to medical care for elderly patients. The Ventilator Allocation Guidelines state, "age may be considered as a tie-breaking criterion in limited circumstances". This may lead people to believe that an older person's life may be less valuable than that of someone younger.
2. **Negative self-perceptions among older adults**

   Older adults can internalize these age-related stereotypes which become self-perceptions and have negative health consequences (self-ageism). Becca Levy, a leading researcher in gerontology, examined negative age stereotypes and the presence or absence of biomarkers for Alzheimer's Disease using data from the Baltimore Longitudinal Study on Aging (Levy et al., 2016a, b). The participants who were dementia free were assessed by MRI and brain autopsies. Those who held negative age stereotypes for over twenty years, had MRIs and autopsies showing significantly steeper reduction in hippocampal volume and greater accumulation of plaques.

   Levy observed that individuals enrolled in the Ohio Longitudinal Study of Aging and Retirement who reported more positive self-perceptions of aging had better overall functional health (Levy, 2009). In fact, people with positive self-perception of age live an average to 7.5 years longer than those who do not (Levy et al., 2002).

   Negative stereotyping was also associated with poorer functional health, delayed recovery from illness or myocardial infarction, greater memory decline, shakier handwriting, hearing loss, blood pressure, and heart rate, whereas the internalization of positive age stereotypes resulted in a heightened will to live, reduced cardiovascular response to stress, faster gait speed and better health outcomes (Levy, 2009).

3. **Decreasing autonomy**

   Undue concerns about diminished faculties in elderly has led to the concept of 'New Ageism' which refers to the view that important life-changing decisions such as health care, money management, and living arrangements, decisions that affect older adults' lives, should be made without consulting them i.e., daughters making living arrangements for their mother without her input or consent when she does not have any mental or physical ailment.

4. **Functional and mental decline**

   Negative misconceptions such as the idea that most older adults make inadequate employees or volunteers as they are less productive, less efficient, less motivated, or less innovative than younger workers or volunteers. The idea that older adults are mentally slower or more forgetful and unable to learn new things also limits opportunities available to older people.

5. **Issues with communication**

   The negative stereotypes about older adults contribute to a less effective style of communication. Older adults are often excluded from conversations, patronized, or treated disrespectfully. According to the Interaction Model (Harwood, 2007), a sequence of considerations made before interacting with an individual can result in over-accommodation with belittling of the older adult and encourages them to withdraw from the conversation while under accommodation does not provide them with enough input to be completely involved. On the other hand, some people are more patient and considerate with older adults. Boswell's study of variables leading to the issues with communication (aging, death, anxiety, compassion) were all significant factors predictive of ageism (Boswell, 2012).

1.8.1 Healthcare Professionals & Ageism

The healthcare community is not immune to the deleterious effects of ageism. It permeates the attitudes of medical providers, the mindset of older patients, and the structure of the healthcare system. It has a profound influence on the type and amount of care offered, requested, and received (Ouchida & Lachs, 2015). It puts older patients at risk for under-treatment and over-treatment. Pain is highly undertreated in elderly (Levi-Minz et al., 2013). Overall, there is a loss of billions of dollars in terms of revenue due to ineffective patient encounters.

Using Butler's original definition of ageism as "systematic stereotyping and discrimination against people because they are old," one could argue that the healthcare system discriminates against older adults in several ways. First, the number of doctors with advanced geriatrics training is declining. Second, more physicians are opting out of Medicare. Third, using data from clinical trials and the recommendations from clinical practice guidelines is problematic when caring for older adults with multiple chronic illnesses because they are often excluded from the study populations (Ouchida & Lachs, 2015).

Ageism biases the attitudes of those whose job it is to help others, specifically physicians and allied health professionals. While some physicians do acknowledge that they treat older adults differently from younger patients, they argue that what appears to be ageism on their part reflects a bias in their hospital budgeting priorities. The problem is made more complicated in that ageism is institutionalized in American culture, so that prejudice and stereotypes about aging and older people tend to be recognized not as serious problems, but more as 'amusing truths' (Nelson, 2016).

1.9 How to Avoid and Prevent Ageism

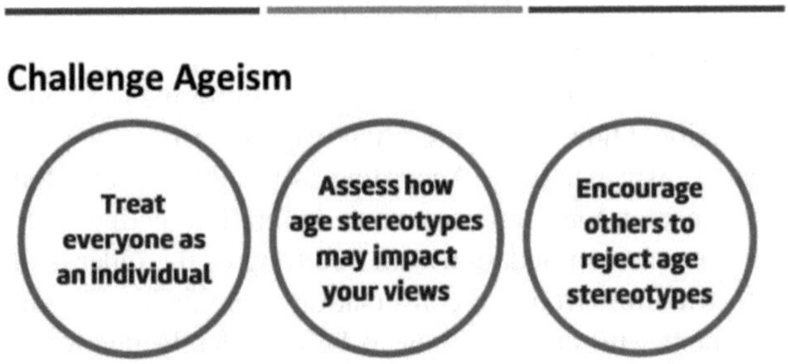

Educating society in general and health care professionals in particular is essential to help change mindsets in the community, and the change in narrative will follow.

Older adults reside at all points along the spectrum from independent and healthy to frail and dependent on others for care. All deserve respect, dignity, and advocacy. Discussion of "affirmative aging", which "promotes an acceptance of age in all of its diversity and does not covet agelessness." It accepts the differences among aging bodies, from sedentary to dynamic, from sexually active to indifferent. It affirms an individual's pain and vulnerability as experiences of aging without perceiving them as diseased. "Only when the aged are allowed to be frail and wrinkled, to not have to be exceptional or young, will age no longer have stigma attached" (Sandberg, 2013, p. 35).

In top-down processing, having the knowledge of one's chronological age or viewing the physical characteristics of later life, such as gray hair, wrinkles, or even a stooped posture, can trigger stereotypical beliefs about the person and lead to false assumptions about older adults and our future selves. These are usually negative beliefs that are applied to older adult as a group that dehumanize the individual and limits opportunities to continue to engage in meaningful activity.

Promoting healthy aging among older adults is a key component to combat ageism. Strategies for reducing ageism will require targeted educational and media campaigns like the successful AARP campaign to increase physical activity among older adults, which included an intensive consumer market research plan based on data combined from three national surveys, focus groups, and in-depth one-on-one interviews to identify opportunities and barriers to change behaviors at the individual and community levels (Ory et al., 2003).

The use of e-health for personalized tailored information can educate older adult patients about their health (Kopera-Frye, 2017). In addition, promoting changes in the health care system that improve health information, partnerships, and local efforts, dissemination of evidence-based health literacy and training health care professionals in geriatric medicine will help tackle the bias of age.

1.10 Chapter Summary

Ageism is defined as a prejudice directed against someone based on his or her age. The negative stereotype perpetuated in society about age impacts the mental and physical well-being of older adults. Myths and stereotypes about older adults and the aging process are pervasive in today's culture. Like any form of bias, ageism can lead people to make false assumptions about older adults, stereotyping them as disabled, demented, and dependent. People over the age of 85 including centenarians are the fastest growing segment of our population and are the most affected group by ageism.

Reducing ageism begins with becoming age educated. It allows us to consider the aging processes that we will all experience on relatively the same timetable. Age differentiated behavior encourages us to register and process information about the person rather than his or her known or perceived age-group membership. It helps us understand the uniqueness and the diversity found in the older adult population.

Additional Resources

Health Professional knowledge and attitudes toward older people (2017)
Assessing Medical Students' Attitudes toward older adults (2018)
Ageism in mental health assessment and treatment of older adults (2018)
Ageism in medicine is a pressing problem (2019)
Ageism in home care quality and retention (2022)
Ageism among doctors and nurses (2021)
Measuring Ageism Based on Knowledge, Attitudes and Behavior: Findings from an Israeli Pilot Study (2016)
Global Report on Ageism: Executive Summary (2021)

Multiple Choice Questions

1. Older adults who believe in negative stereotypes about ageism tend to:
   (a) Internalize these stereotypes
   (b) Project these stereotypes on others
   (c) Do not care about these stereotypes
   (d) Make fun of these stereotypes
   Correct answer: **a**
2. Ageism became prevalent during which period in history?
   (a) In the Middle Ages
   (b) after the Classical Era
   (c) during the Modern Era
   (d) after the Industrial Revolution
   Correct answer: **d**
3. Positive ageist attitudes lead to:
   (a) lower retirement age
   (b) social programs for aging adults
   (c) high health care costs
   (d) isolation
   Correct answer: **b**

References

Allen, J. O., Solway, E., Kirch, M., Singer, D., Kullgren, J. T., Moïse, V., & Malani, P. N. (2022). Experiences of everyday ageism and the health of older US adults. *JAMA Network Open, 5*(6), e2217240–e2217240. https://doi.org/10.1001/jamanetworkopen.2022.17240

Boswell, S. S. (2012). Predicting trainee ageism using knowledge, anxiety, compassion, and contact with older adults. *Educational Gerontology, 38*(11), 733–741. https://doi.org/10.1080/03601277.2012.695997

Butler, R. N. (1969). Age-ism: Another form of bigotry. *The Gerontologist, 9*, 243–246. https://www.romolocapuano.com/wp-content/uploads/2017/03/Butler_Age-ism.pdf

Hu, R. X., Luo, M., Zhang, A., & Li, L. W. (2021). Associations of ageism and health: A systematic review of quantitative observational studies. *Research on Aging, 43*(7–8), 311–322. https://doi.org/10.1177/0164027520980

Kopera-Frye, K. (2017). *Health literacy among older adults*. Springer Publishing Company.

Levi-Minzi, M. A., Surratt, H. L., Kurtz, S. P., & Buttram, M. E. (2013). Under treatment of pain: A prescription for opioid misuse among the elderly? *Pain Medicine (Malden, Mass.), 14*(11), 1719–1729. https://doi.org/10.1111/pme.12189

Levy, B. (2009). Stereotype embodiment: A psychosocial approach to aging. *Current Directions in Psychological Science., 18*(6), 332–336. https://journals.sagepub.com/doi/pdf/10.1111/j.1467-8721.2009.01662.x?casa_token=qUvTTGDGBCwAAAAA:qhxnzKj9vvb87BIU3fQMVaTbrE5On6anyJ3cPzjIx4CoQFWeG3z8awWmcp1O7qdiTcOF8TYiFoQTlg

Levy, B. R., Slade, M. D., Kunkel, S. R., & Kasl, S. V. (2002). Longevity increased by positive self-perceptions of aging. *Journal of Personality and Social Psychology, 83*(2), 261–270. https://doi.org/10.1037//0022-3514.83.2.261

Levy, B. R., Ferrucci, L., Zonderman, A. B., Slade, M. D., Troncoso, J., & Resnick, S. M. (2016a). A culture–brain link: Negative age stereotypes predict Alzheimer's disease biomarkers. *Psychology and Aging, 31*(1), 82–88. https://doi.org/10.1037/pag0000062

Levy, B., Moffat, S., Resnick, S. M., Slade, M. D., & Ferrucci, L. (2016b). Buffer against cumulative stress. *GeroPsych, 29*(3), 141–146. https://doi.org/10.1024/1662-9647/a000149

Lubomudrov, S. (1987). Congressional perceptions of the elderly: The use of stereotypes in the legislative process. *The Gerontologist, 27*(1), 77–81. https://doi.org/10.1093/geront/27.1.77

Markov, Č., & Yoon, Y. (2020). Diversity and age stereotypes in portrayals of older adults in popular American primetime television series. *Ageing and Society, 41*, 2747–2767.

Nelson, T. D. (2016). Promoting healthy aging by confronting ageism. *American Psychologist, 71*(4), 276–282. https://doi.org/10.1037/a0040221

Ory, M., Kinney Hoffman, M., Hawkins, M., Sanner, B., & Mockenhaupt, R. (2003). Challenging aging stereotypes: Strategies for creating a more active society. *American Journal of Preventive Medicine, 25*(3 Suppl 2), 164–171. https://doi.org/10.1016/s0749-3797(03)00181-8

Ouchida, K. M., & Lachs, M. S. (2015). Not for doctors only: Ageism in healthcare. *Generations: Journal of the American Society on Aging, 39*(3), 46–57. https://www.jstor.org/stable/26556135

Palmore, E. (1999). *Ageism: Positive and negative* (2nd ed.). Springer.

Palmore, E. (2001). The ageism survey: First findings. *The Gerontologist, 41*(5), 572–575. https://doi.org/10.1093/geront/41.5.572

Prieler, M. (2020). Gender representations of older people in the media: What do we know and where do we go from here? *Asian Women, 36*(2), 73–95. (SSCI).

Sandberg, L. (2013). Affirmative old age-the ageing body and feminist theories on difference. *International Journal of Aging and Later Life, 8*(1), 11–40. https://doi.org/10.3384/ijal.1652-8670.12197

Chapter 2
Demography of Centenarians

Emily Zagorski and Conrad May

Key Take Away Points

1. The number of centenarians is on the rise globally, faster than the growth of the general population.
2. Areas called "Blue Zones" are geographic hot spots where high volumes of centenarians reside. Multiple factors including diet, lower overall prevalence of chronic disease, strong family bonds and physical activity are amongst possible contributions to longevity in these regions.
3. Japan has the highest life expectancy and the greatest number of centenarians per capita of all nations.
4. There are many more female than male centenarians throughout the world, although this gender gap is projected to narrow in the future.
5. There are important limitations to consider in the analysis of studies of centenarians.

2.1 Introduction

The existence of communities of exceptionally long-lived individuals has long captured the popular imagination, perhaps with the hope of identifying some mystery factor that would prolong lives in general. This concept was exploited to great effect

E. Zagorski
The Fleming Memory Center, Lehigh Valley Health Network, Allentown, PA, USA
e-mail: EMILY.ZAGORSKI@lvhn.org

C. May (✉)
University of Maryland School of Medicine, Baltimore, MD, USA
e-mail: cmay@som.umaryland.edu

R. E. Kheirbek, M. D. Llorente (eds.), *Current Perspectives on Centenarians*, International Perspectives on Aging 36,
https://doi.org/10.1007/978-3-031-30915-1_2

by the Dannon Yogurt Company in their classic television commercial that aired in 1977 (video available on YouTube). It featured several centenarians from a village in Abkhazia (then part of the Soviet Republic of Georgia) whose diet included large amounts of yogurt, performing various vigorous tasks—farming, chopping wood and riding a horse. The highlight was a clip of an 89-year-old man cheerfully spooning down two cups of Dannon Yogurt, while his 114-year-old mother looked on adoringly. The implication was clear—eating yogurt promoted longevity. The campaign was a spectacular success, and the sales of Dannon Yogurt skyrocketed (https://georgianjournal.ge/discover-georgia/30231-in-soviet-georgia-the-story-behind-the-cult-yogurt-ad.html). However, subsequent investigations revealed that the advanced ages of the Abkhazian villagers had likely been exaggerated or misrepresented (Palmore, 1984).

According to the United Nations and Pew Research Center, there were an estimated 573,000 centenarians worldwide in 2020. This number is expected to grow exponentially to nearly 3.7 million centenarians by 2050 (Stepler, 2016), an increase of almost 650% (Fig. 2.1). Although the United States has the largest total number of centenarians, Japan and Italy have more centenarians per 10,000 people, followed by the United States and China, respectively.

While the global population continues to grow, the increase in number of centenarians is disproportionally rapid. Since the end of World War II, the growth of

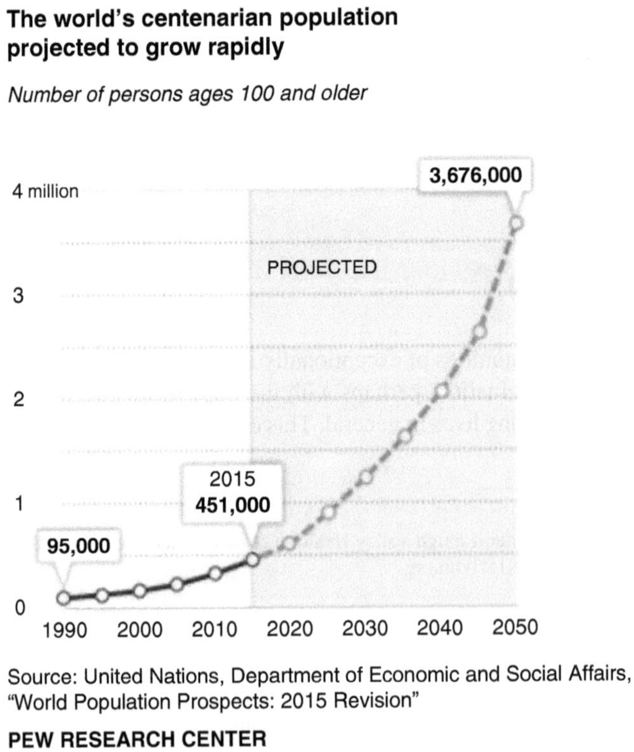

Fig. 2.1 Projected number of centenarians by 2050

centenarians has been almost exponential, roughly doubling every decade. This is due to not only more people surviving to the 100-year milestone but also a decrease in the mortality rate of centenarians (Robine & Cubaynes, 2017). This rate of increase is expected to slow and will eventually plateau as the population life expectancy abuts against the limits of the human lifespan.

Many reasons have been proposed for the global aging trends including improved public health measures and sanitation. They do not, however, completely explain the specific observations noted in the oldest old.

2.2 International Studies on Centenarians

The Japanese are known to have the world's longest life expectancy, at 88 years for women and 82 years for men. In 2020, Japan was noted to have over 80,000 centenarians in the country, which is the largest number of centenarians per capita (Spary, 2020). It has been projected that 7.2% of newborn girls in Japan will become centenarians (Robine & Cubaynes, 2017). The country has long been known to not only respect but celebrate its aged population. This includes an annual day of respect for the aged. New centenarians also receive a silver cup and a letter of congratulations from the Japanese prime minister (McCurry, 2012). This element of reverence for their fellow countrymen may indeed contribute to an overall lifestyle that promotes the possibility of reaching extremes of aging.

While the Eastern world reports its highest per capita of centenarians in Japan, Western countries with the highest volume of centenarians include France, Italy and Greece as of 2011 (Teixeira et al., 2017). A composite of census data from over 30 countries in Europe found that the ratio of centenarians to those under 80 years is exponentially increasing over time. In 2011, there were 89,156 centenarians residing within 32 European countries, representing 17.3 centenarians per 100,000 people. This review aimed to see if common trends amongst European centenarians could be established; however, data varied widely. For example, per census data, those without any education amongst centenarians varied from 0.0% in Iceland, Finland and the United Kingdom to 61.6% in Portugal (Teixeira et al., 2017). Although it was challenging for this study to find consistency amongst these populations of centenarians, it did advocate for heightened awareness of this fast-growing group in the European Union.

2.3 Geographic Clusters of Centenarians

Community clusters of centenarians have become more prominently recognized throughout the world. Studying the centenarians in these communities will hopefully shed light on the genetic and environmental influences on longevity. The specific geographic locations where the clusters of older adults live are commonly

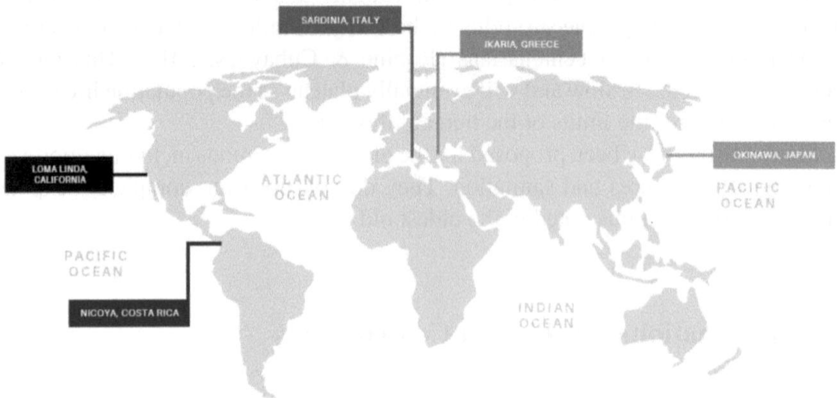

Fig. 2.2 Global distribution of "Blue Zones" (Blue Zones, 2008)

referred to as "Blue Zones" (Fig. 2.2). There may be genetic similarities amongst these individuals; environment, lifestyle, diet and habits are also important considerations and likely contributors to longevity. Some examples of these international Blue Zone communities are described below.

The Nicoya Peninsula of Costa Rica has been reported for many years as a "hot spot" of centenarians. According to the 2011 census, among a population of 161,000 inhabitants there, 32 were centenarians (Rosero-Bixby et al., 2013). As of 2020, 43 centenarians were living on this 80-mile long Peninsula. A 60-year-old Nicoyan male had a probability of living to 100 years that was 7 times that of a Japanese male. However, this survival advantage was not found among Nicoyan women (Rosero-Bixby et al., 2013). In a study conducted by the National Geriatric and Gerontology Hospital in Costa Rica, the overall health status, laboratory tests and electrocardiograms of these individuals were reviewed. These centenarians were found to have a low prevalence of diabetes, ischemic heart disease, chronic obstructive pulmonary disease and polypharmacy (Madrigal-Leer et al., 2019).

Another study of the Nicoyan centenarians investigated the residents' genetics and ancestral heritage (Azofeifa et al., 2018). They compared 20 Nicoyan centenarians with 20 Nicoyan adults aged 65–99 years and reviewed their genetic profiles. It was noted that each 10% increase in Amerindian ancestry was associated with more than two-fold chance of living to become a centenarian. Another study examined the telomere length of leukocytes of Nicoyan centenarians. Longer telomeres are thought to be associated with longevity (Rosero-Bixby et al., 2013). After controlling for age, rainy season, gender, potential dietary social mediators and rurality, they found that telomere lengths in the Nicoyan centenarians were significantly longer compared to those residing in other regions of Costa Rica.

Their lifestyle may also contribute to the Nicoyan's longevity. *Plan de vida*, meaning a reason to live, has been cited by Nicoyan centenarians as something that keeps them active and happy (Blue Zones website). Many attributed a sense of community with neighbors, families and friends to be a major contributing factor to their longevity. However, the lower mortality rates are not found in Nicoyan men who migrate from the area, supporting the importance of environmental factors (Rosero-Bixby et al., 2013).

The natives of Okinawa are the longest lived of all Japanese, with the highest prevalence of centenarians among Japan's prefectures. In 2005, there were 54.37 centenarians per 100,000 people in Okinawa. The number of centenarians in Okinawa has continued to increase over time (Willcox et al., 2008). This is explained by the low mortality rates of those over the age of 65 years from cardiovascular disease and certain cancers. The Okinawa Centenarian Study, started in 1975, and is the oldest of its kind. This study suggested that diet was a major influence in successful aging. The Okinawan diet is termed "naturally calorically restricted" and is highly made up of root vegetables, specifically sweet potatoes, other vegetables, as well as fish and lean meats, with use of various spices and garnishes and even moderate consumption of alcohol (Willcox et al., 2014). Another identified factor that contributes to longevity in this population has been the temperate climate of this region, with average temperatures around 17.2 °C. This temperate environment may have promoted food supply availability especially in the early to mid-twentieth Century, which, in turn, may have increased longevity (Robine et al., 2012).

Another region of interest is Sardinia, Italy. Several areas within Sardinia have been highlighted as Blue Zones, specifically Ogliastra, a mountainous region of Eastern Sardinia. Here, many cite close family ties, diet, and physical activity as the secret to their longevity. In a study of movement and activity of these Sardinians, portable movement devices were used to monitor total energy expenditure. It concluded that older adults who continued to be active and have high total energy expenditure into their 90 s were more likely to survive to ultra-advanced age (Pes & Dore, 2021). It has also been suggested that this increase in physical activity may be associated with better cognitive ability. Mental health through standardized questionnaires of these centenarians were reviewed. These questionnaires revealed a higher sense of personal well-being than the national average in Italy amongst centenarians who were more physically active (Fastame et al., 2018).

Diet has been explored as a possible link amongst Blue Zone centenarians. Nicoyans specifically were found to have a traditional Mesoamerican diet consisting of 26% whole grains, 24% dairy, 14% vegetables with the rest of this diet consisting of meats, eggs and fruits. Dinners were light and earlier in the evening (around 4 pm), to promote a prolonged fast (Blue Zones website). In one recent study, 210 older adults (aged 80–109 years) from Nicoya and Ogliastra had their diets reviewed (Nieddu et al., 2020). It showed that diet was predominantly plant-based, while also containing some amount of animal products, especially milk/dairy products.

2.4 Studies in the United States

The dramatic increase in probability of survival to advanced ages during the past century has led to the "greying of America." The longer life expectancy of Americans is attributed primarily to reductions in the mortality rates of adults. This

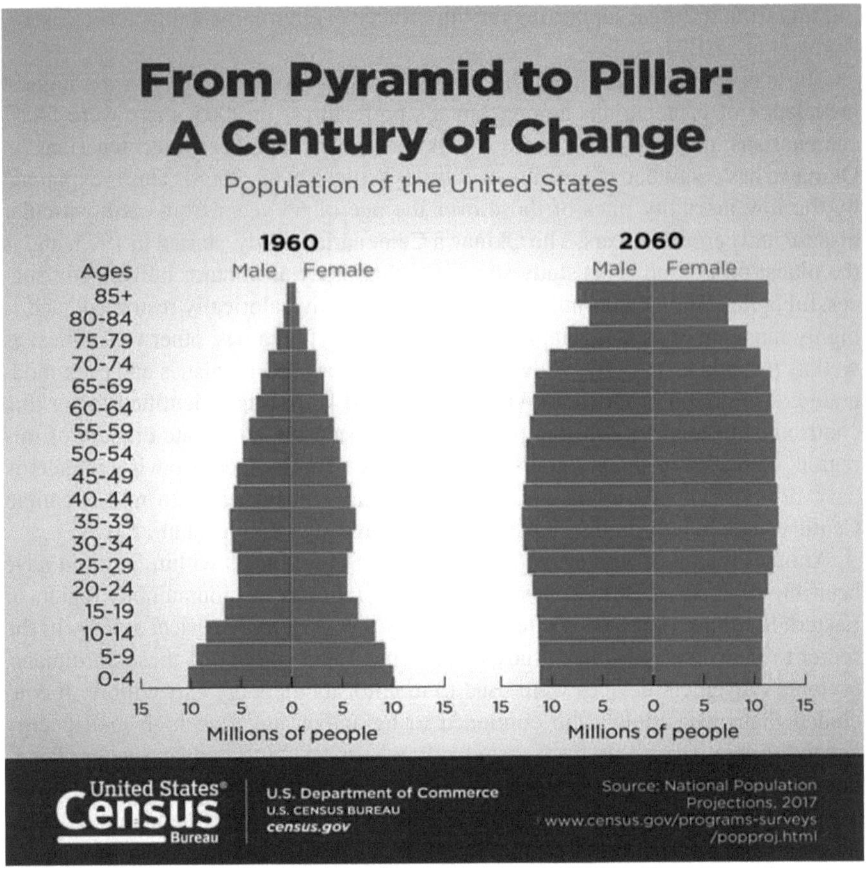

Fig. 2.3 Changing trends of the oldest old from 1960–2060 according to the United States Census Bureau

phenomenon is reflected in the transformation of the age pyramid to a more cylindrical configuration (Fig. 2.3), of which centenarians are included in the uppermost tier.

Although centenarians in the United States are relatively rare (approximately one in 5–6000 people), they are an expanding segment both in terms of absolute numbers and percentage of the total population. There were approximately 32,000 centenarians in 1980 (.00142% of the population) which had grown to more than 53,000 by 2010 (.00173% of the population), an increase of 65.8% (Fig. 2.4). During the same period, the total population of the United States rose by 36.3% (U.S. Census Bureau, 2012). In 2020, an estimated 92,000 centenarians lived in the United States; if the current trends continue, that number could rise to nearly 600,000 centenarians by 2060 (U.S. Census Bureau projection).

Among the 50 states, the distribution of centenarians roughly mirrors that of the general population, that is, the greatest number of centenarians are found in the most populous states such as California, New York, Florida and Texas. On a per

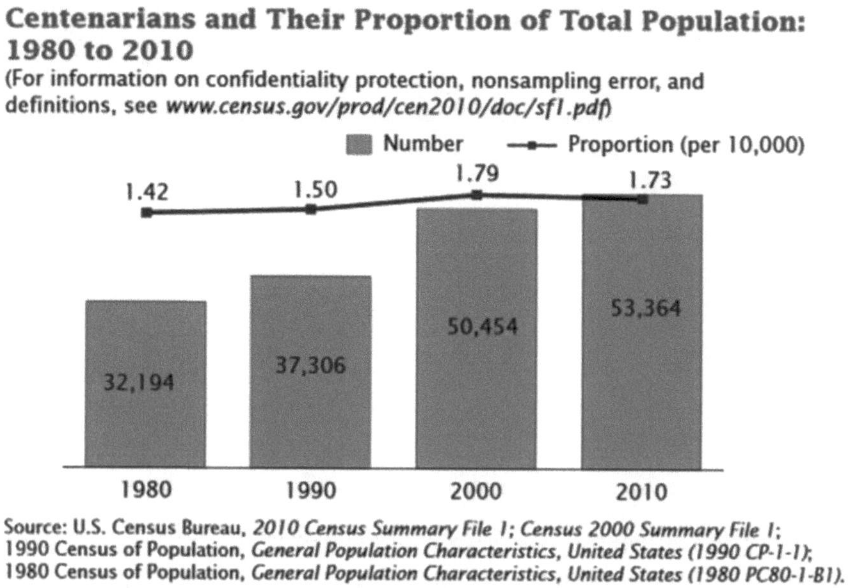

Fig. 2.4 Changes in the total population from 1980 to 2010

capita basis, the Midwestern states have the most centenarians: North Dakota, followed by South Dakota, Iowa and Nebraska. Within the states, centenarians tend to gravitate towards urban centers, presumably drawn by the availability of support services. In the 2010 census, 85.7% of centenarians resided in an urban setting, as compared with 76.6% of those in their 70's (U.S. Census Bureau, 2012).

Several studies have been conducted in the United States to characterize the physical, psychological and social function of centenarians. The largest and most extensive of these is the New England Centenarian Study, which was initiated in 1994 and continues to the present day. Population-based studies have also been performed in northern Georgia (Davey et al., 2010) and New York City (Jopp et al., 2016).

2.5 Gender

As the mortality rate in the United States is higher for men than women at nearly every age bracket, centenarians are predominantly female. This "gender gap" increases with advancing age (Fig. 2.5). In 2010, 82.8% of centenarians were women. Put another way, for every 100 centenarian women, there were only 20.7 centenarian men (U.S. Census Bureau, 2012). This is consistent with the demographic data from the Georgia Centenarian Study where 85% of the participants were women (Davey et al., 2010) and the Fordham Centenarian Study where 78% were women (Jopp et al., 2016). Similarly, in a composite of European census

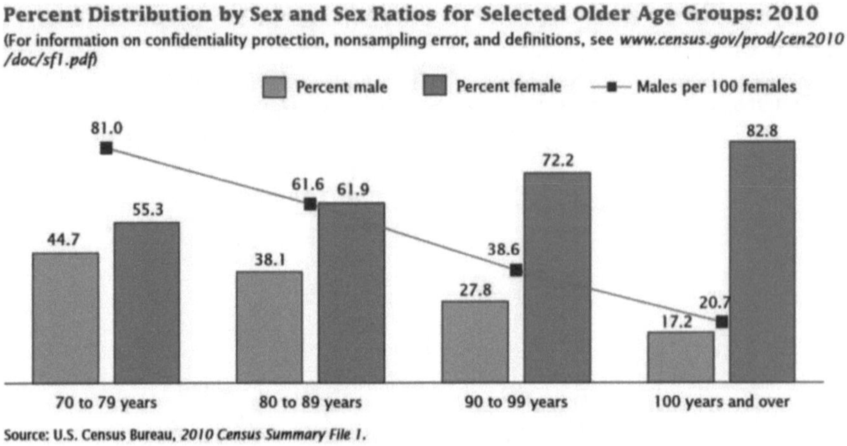

Fig. 2.5 Gender demographics among older adults. U.S. Census Bureau, 2010 Census Special Reports, Centenarians: 2010, C2010SR-03, U.S. Government Printing Office, Washington, D.C., 2012

reports, on average only 16.5% of centenarians were male, ranging from 13% in Germany, Latvia and Belgium to 37% in Hungary (Teixeira et al., 2017). Within countries, there may be significant gender differences. In Italy, there is a north-south gradient in the female:male ratio of centenarians with a lower ratio in the south due to a decreased mortality rate of men from cardiovascular disease (Montesanto et al., 2017), In the Chinese Longitudinal Health and Longevity Study (CLHLS), in 2008 only 20% of their sample of centenarians were men (Zeng et al., 2017).

This gender gap is anticipated to narrow in the years to come. Internationally, the female:male advantage in centenarians is predicted to decrease by nearly 50% between 2015 and 2100 (Fig. 2.6) (Robine & Cubaynes, 2017). In the United States, the percentage of male centenarians relative to females is projected to gradually increase in more recent birth cohorts as the effect of secular factors, such as the disparity in the prevalence of smoking between men and women, diminishes over time (Perls, 2017). A notable exception to the gender gap is found in Nicoya, Costa Rica where extreme longevity is found in men but not women. There may be unique longevity factors among the Nicoyans that differ from other parts of the world (Rosero-Bixby et al., 2013).

Corresponding to the greater numbers of women than men in the older age groups, widowhood is more common. Of women at or over the age of 85 years in the U.S., 70% were widowed as compared with 15% who were married. Men at or over the age of 85 years were more likely to be married (54%) than single (Roberts et al., 2018). Among female centenarians, this trend is magnified. In the 1990 census, 79% of centenarians were widowed, including 84% of women and 58% of men. Of the male centenarians, nearly 25% were still married (Krach & Velkoff, 1999). In the CLHLS, 87.7% of the Chinese male and 98.1% of the female centenarians were widowed. However, the men were more than 8 times as likely to be married as the women (Zeng et al., 2017). The predominance of single female centenarians is more likely due to the longer female life expectancy in general than some deleterious effect of marriage on women.

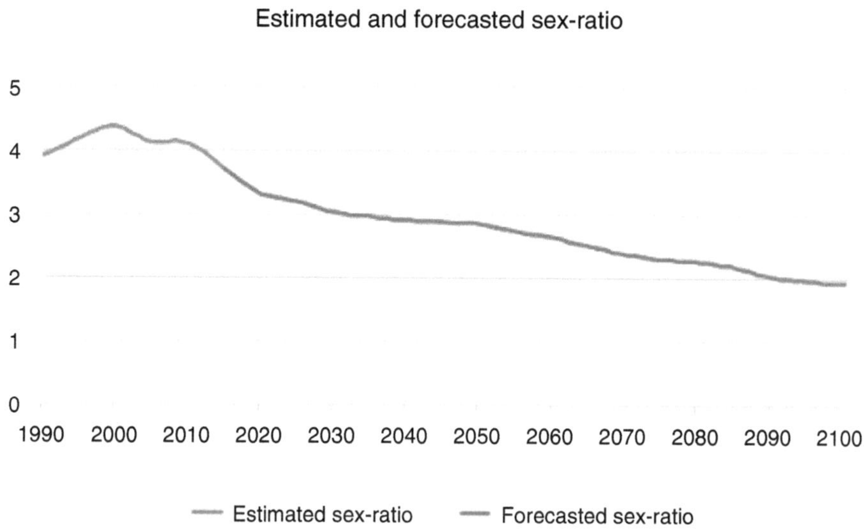

Fig. 2.6 Estimated and forecasted numbers of centenarians worldwide by sex-ratio from 1990 to 2100. (Source: 2015 Revision of the World Population Prospects, Robine & Cubaynes, 2017)

2.6 Race

The racial composition of centenarians as reported in the 2010 U.S. Census was 82.5% White, 12.2% African American, 2.5% Asian, 0.5% American Indian or Alaskan Native, 0.1% Hawaiian and Other Pacific Islander and 1.3% Other. The percentage of African American centenarians (12.2%) is comparable to that of all African Americans in the total U.S. population (12.6%) (U.S. Census Bureau, 2012). An even higher percentage (16%) of African American centenarians was found in the 1990 census (Krach & Velkoff, 1999). However, these findings are surprising in light of higher mortality rates for African Americans than Whites in all of the preceding decades. It is unclear whether this represents a true lower mortality rate for African American than White centenarians, referred to as a crossover event, or is due to errors in reporting.

2.7 Socioeconomic Factors

The importance of socioeconomic status is underscored by the finding that the vast majority of centenarians are found in high- and middle-income countries (Fig. 2.7). The percentage of centenarians residing in low-income countries is less than 1% (Robine & Cubaynes, 2017). On the other hand, the extreme longevity of the Nicoyan men is reported to be independent of socioeconomic factors (Rosero-Bixby et al., 2013). According to the 1990 U.S. census, the likelihood of older Americans living below the poverty level increased with advancing age. For centenarians,

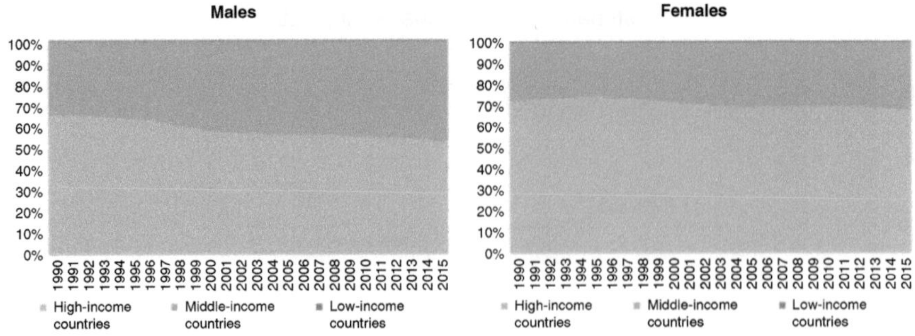

Fig. 2.7 Proportion of centenarians living in high-, middle-, and low-income countries, in percentage, by sex, from 1990 to 2015. (Source: 2015 Revision of the World Population Prospects, Robine & Cubaynes, 2017)

25.9% of women and 21.1% of men were considered to be living in poverty. Women were more likely than men to be poor at all ages. However, nursing home residents were not considered in this analysis (Krach & Velkoff, 1999).

Likewise, older Americans tend to be less well-educated than younger ones. Whereas 80% of 65 to 69-year-olds had some high school education, only half of centenarians did so. African American centenarians were even less likely to have entered high school (Krach & Velkoff, 1999). In both the Georgia Centenarian Study (Davey et al., 2010) and the Fordham Centenarian Study (Jopp et al., 2016), the subjects were relatively better educated; half of the participants in the Georgia study and two-thirds of the Fordham cohort had completed at least high school; one third of the latter group also attained a college or higher degree.

A higher socioeconomic status is generally associated with a lower mortality rate. Interestingly, one study from the U.S. reported that neighborhood walkability was predictive of becoming a centenarian. It is probable that living in a more walkable neighborhood is a surrogate marker for a higher socioeconomic status. Conversely, people who lived where there was a high area deprivation index, a measure of socioeconomic disadvantage, were less likely to reach the century mark (Bhardwaj et al., 2020). However, that same study found a negative correlation between educational level and the likelihood of becoming a centenarian. This seems to be a contradictory finding as educational level is often tied to socioeconomic status. In Italy, the majority of female centenarians were illiterate; however, later birth cohorts had higher levels of education (Montesanto et al., 2017). In the CLHLS, there was a striking gender difference in education. Among the female centenarians, the mean years of schooling was 0.29 and 93.4% had no schooling at all; for the male centenarians, the mean years of schooling was 2.2 and 57% had no schooling. This disparity in education among men and women were found in both rural and urban areas. The majority of both female and male centenarians had earned their living in agriculture. However, 27.7% of the male centenarians had been professionals, technicians, managers or clerks as compared with only 3.9% of the female centenarians, corresponding to their educational attainments (Zeng et al.,

2017). The Chinese male centenarians had a clear advantage in socioeconomic status as compared with the women, but that did not seem to confer a survival benefit.

The living arrangements of centenarians are likely influenced by their functional abilities and family support, including marital status and financial means. In the 1990 U.S. census, slightly less than 20% of centenarians reported no self-care or mobility limitations, and 15% were living alone (Krach & Velkoff, 1999). Not surprisingly, with advancing age as disabilities become more common, the percentage residing in nursing homes increases. In 2010, slightly more women centenarians were in nursing homes (35.2%) than living alone at home (34.0%) or at home with others (28.5%) (U.S. Census Bureau, 2012). On the other hand, men centenarians were most likely to be living with others in a household (43.5%), perhaps reflecting their higher percentage of still being married (U.S. Census Bureau, 2012). In population-based studies, the places of residence can reflect recruitment strategies. For example, 63% of the Georgia Centenarian Study participants were living in nursing or personal care homes, as they were primarily recruited from these sites (Davey et al., 2010), whereas 74% in the Fordham Centenarian Study were community-dwelling, initially identified through the voter registry (Jopp et al., 2016). In contrast, in the CLHLS, the vast majority of Chinese centenarians were living at home with family (88.98%) while only 3.14% were residing in an institution. The remainder of the centenarians (7.88%) were living alone (Zeng et al., 2017). In the European study, the percentage of centenarians residing in the community varied widely, from over 90% in Romania, Bulgaria, Lithuania, Greece and Latvia to about 11% in Iceland (Teixeira et al., 2017).

2.8 Limitations in the Study of Centenarians

While the study of such clusters of centenarians has led to a multitude of interesting findings, it should be noted that controversies do exist. It remains challenging to quantify exact numbers of persons aged over 100 years. Reasons include the difficulty in verifying birth records and data misreporting censuses of individual countries (Heshmati, 2021). In 2010, Young et al. called an attention to "false claims of longevity" (Young et al., 2010). Comparison data from the American Social Security Death Index and the Gerontology Research Group in New England showed that the rate of falsification of records in persons over 110 years of age was approximately 65% between 1980 and 2009. Researchers cited a belief in religious/spiritual wealth at extreme ages, individual and family notoriety, and nationalism as major causes of falsification of greater age. Simple administrative errors in transcription of important documents such as birth certificates and military records were also listed as reasons for false representation of extreme age. Unreported deaths with malicious intent such as pension or social security fraud were also noted in this study (Young et al., 2010). Therefore, in interpreting the results of centenarian studies, it is important to consider the reliability of the reports of advanced ages.

The prevalence of centenarians in a particular location is determined not only by the resident centenarian population but also the fertility rate and immigration patterns. For example, the departure of large numbers of younger people, a falling fertility rate or an influx of retirees can create an apparent community cluster of centenarians. Two indices have been proposed to mitigate the influence of these confounders, the Centenarian Rate (CR) and the Extreme Longevity Index (ELI). The CR is the ratio of centenarians with respect to the same cohort 40 years earlier, which eliminates the factor of infant mortality; however, it does not account for the effects of migration. The ELI is the number of centenarians compared with the newborns of the same area 100 years earlier (Montesanto et al., 2017). However, it is often difficult to obtain birth records. Neither index is yet widely applied.

There is an obvious source of bias in attempting to study individual centenarians. Such studies are necessarily confined to people who can participate in a meaningful way. For example, as a part of the New England Centenarian Study, neuropsychologic testing was performed in 34 centenarians; seven had no signs of dementia (Clinical Dementia Rating Scale score of 0) and another four had an indeterminate CDR score of 0.5 (Silver et al., 2001). In the Fordham Study, 93% of participants were found to have little or no cognitive limitations and 72% were found to have few or no depressive symptoms. The subjective perception of better health was associated with lower scores on the Geriatric Depression Scale and greater life satisfaction. (Jopp et al., 2016). However, many centenarians were unable to participate because of cognitive or physical conditions. Fewer than one-third of the eligible centenarians were interviewed in the Fordham Centenarian Study (Jopp et al., 2016), and only 19% of an estimated 1244 centenarians in the region were included in the Georgia Centenarian Study (Davey et al., 2010). Therefore, the findings may not be representative of centenarians in general. Nonetheless, it is encouraging to note that declines are not inevitable and a significant number of centenarians were able to maintain a high level of physical and cognitive function.

2.9 Conclusion

The rapid worldwide growth in numbers of centenarians, outpacing that of the general population, has significant social and economic implications. The great majority of centenarians are women, reflecting the higher mortality rate in men in preceding age groups; however, this gender disparity is anticipated to lessen over time. The demography of centenarians can give important clues to the contributors of longevity. While these elements are likely to be multiple, interacting and variable from country to country, there are factors such as diet, lifestyle and socioeconomic conditions that tie together these communities of the oldest old and merit further study. There are several important caveats to consider in interpreting studies of centenarians including the reliability of reported ages, migration patterns and selection biases.

Demography of Centenarians Review Questions

1. Compared to the current worldwide population growth, the increase in numbers of centenarians is:

   A. Slightly higher
   B. Significantly higher
   C. About the same
   D. Less

2. The numerical predominance of female centenarians over male centenarians is projected to:

   A. Increase over time
   B. Decrease slowly over time
   C. Decrease rapidly over time
   D. Stay about the same

3. The largest demographic group of centenarians is comprised of:

   A. Widowed women
   B. Women who are divorced or who have never married
   C. Married men
   D. Single men

4. Geographic clusters of centenarians are referred to as:

   A. Hot spots
   B. Blue zones
   C. Islands of longevity
   D. Shangri-la

5. The country with the longest life expectancy is currently:

   A. The United States
   B. Sweden
   C. France
   D. Japan

Demography of Centenarians Review Questions: Answers

1. Correct Answer: B- Significantly higher. According to the United Nations and Pew Research Center, there is expected to be an eight fold increase in the number of centenarians globally by 2050.
2. Correct answer: B- Decrease slowly over time. The "gender gap" decreases over time (see Fig. 2.6).

3. Correct answer: A- Widowed women. Corresponding to the greater numbers of women than men in the older age groups, widowhood is more common. Of women at or over the age of 85 years, 70% were widowed as compared with 15% who were married.
4. Correct answer: B- Blue Zones. 5 major Blue Zones have been studied in attempts to determine the etiology behind the region's citizens' advanced age.
5. Correct answer: D- Japan. The Japanese are known to have the world's longest life expectancy, at 88 years for women and 82 years for men.

References

Azofeifa, J., Ruiz-Navaez E. A., Leal, A., et al. (2018). Amerindian ancestry and extended longevity in Nicoya, Costa Rica. *American Journal of Human Biology, 30*.

Bhardwaj, R., Amiri, S., Buchwald, D., & Amram, O. (2020). Environmental correlates of reaching a centenarian age: Analysis of 144,665 deaths in Washington state for 2011–2015. *International Journal of Environmental Research and Public Health, 17*, 2828.

Blue Zones. (2008). Nicoya, Costa Rica: A Latin American Blue Zone. Retrieved from https://www.bluezones.com/explorations/nicoya-costa-rica/

Davey, A., Elias, M. F., Siegler, I. C., et al. (2010). Cognitive function, physical performance, health and disease: Norms from the Georgia centenarian study. *Experimental Aging Research, 36*, 394–425.

Fastame, M. C., Hitchcott, P. K., Mulas, I., et al. (2018). Resilience in elders of the Sardinian Blue Zone: An explorative study. *Behavioral Sciences (Basel), 8*(3), 30.

Heshmati, H. (2021). The centenarians: An emerging population. In *Update in Geriatrics,* edited by Somchai Amornyotin, IntechOpen, 2021.

Jopp, D. S., Park M-K, S., Lehrfield, J., & Paggi, M. E. (2016). Physical, cognitive, social and mental health in near-centenarians and centenarians living in New York City: Findings from the Fordham centenarian study. *BMC Geriatrics, 16*, 1.

Krach, C. A., & Velkoff, V. A. (1999). *U.S. Bureau of the Census, Current Population Reports, Series P23-199RV "Centenarians in the United States"*. U.S. Government Printing Office.

Madrigal-Leer, F., Martinez-Montandon, A., Solis-Umana, M., et al. (2019). Clinical, functional, mental and social profile of the Nicoya peninsula centenarians, Costa Rica, 2017. *Aging Clinical Experimental Research*, 313–321.

McCurry, J. (2012, September 14). Japan's centenarian population reaches more than 50,000. *The Guardian.*

Montesanto, A., De Rango, F., Pirazzini, C., et al. (2017). Demographic, genetic and phenotypic characteristics of centenarians in Italy: Focus on gender differences. *Mechanisms of Ageing and Development, 165*(Pt B), 68–74.

Nieddu, A., Vindas, L., Errigo, A., et al. (2020). Dietary habits, anthropometric features and daily performance in two independent long-lived populations from Nicoya peninsula (Costa Rica) and Ogliastra (Sardinia). *Nutrients, 12*.

Palmore, E. B. (1984). Longevity in Abkhazia: A reevaluation. *Gerontologist, 24*, 95–96.

Perls, T. T. (2017). Male centenarians: How and why are they different from their female counterparts? *Journal of the American Geriatrics Society, 65*, 1904–1906.

Pes, G. M., Dore, M. P. (2021). Understanding the impact of motor activity on the mental well-being of older people. *International Psychogeriatrics., 33*, 1237–1239.

Roberts, A. W., Ogunwole, S. U., Blakeslee, L., & Rabe, M. A. (2018). *The population 65 years and older in the United States: 2016, American Community Survey Reports*. ACS-38, U.S. Dept of Commerce, U.S. Census Bureau.

Robine, J.-M., & Cubaynes, S. (2017). Worldwide demography of centenarians. *Mechanisms of Ageing and Development, 165*(Pt B), 59–67.

Robine, J.-M., Herrmann, F. R., Arai, Y., et al. (2012). Exploring the impact of climate on human longevity. *Experimental Gerontology, 47*(9), 660–671. https://doi.org/10.1016/j.exger.2012.05.009. Epub 2012 May 18.

Rosero-Bixby, L., Dow, W. H., & Rehkopf, D. H. (2013). The Nicoya region of Costa Rica: A high longevity island for elderly males. *Vienna Yearbook of Population Research, 11*, 109–136.

Silver, M. H., Jilinskaia, E., & Perls, T. T. (2001). Cognitive functional status of age-confirmed centenarians in a population-based study. *The Journals of Gerontology. Series B, 56*, 134–140.

Spary, S. (2020, September 18). *A record one person in every 1,500 in Japan is aged at least 100—and they're probably a woman*. Retrieved from CNN: https://www.cnn.com/2020/09/18/asia/japanese-centenarians-scli-intl/index.html

Stepler, R. (2016, April 2016). World's centenarian population projected to grow eightfold by 2050. Retrieved from Pew Research Center: https://www.pewresearch.org/fact-tank/2016/04/21/worlds-centenarian-population-projected-to-grow-eightfold-by-2050/

Teixeira, L., Araújo, L., Jopp, D., & Ribeiro, O. (2017). Centenarians in Europe. *Maturitas, 104*, 90–95. https://doi.org/10.1016/j.maturitas.2017.08.005. Epub 2017 Aug 12.

U.S. Census Bureau. (2012). *Special reports, centenarians 2010, C2010SR-03*. U.S. Government Printing Office.

Willcox, D. C., Willcox, B. J., He, Q., Wang, N.-C., & Suzuki, M. (2008). They really are that old: A validation study of centenarian prevalence in Okinawa. *Journal of Gerontology, 63*, 338–349.

Willcox, D. C., Scapagnini, G., & Willcox, B. J. (2014). Healthy aging diets other than the Mediterranean: A focus on the Okinawan diet. *Mechanisms of Ageing and Development, 136–137*, 148–162, ISSN 0047-6374. https://doi.org/10.1016/j.mad.2014.01.002

Young, R. D., Desjardins, B., McLaughlin, K., Poulain, M., & Perls, T. (2010). Typologies of extreme longevity myths. *Current Gerontology and Geriatrics Research, 2010*, 423087.

Zeng, Y., Feng, O., Deng, G., & Vaupel, J. (2017). Demographics, phenotypic health characteristics and genetic analysis of centenarians in China. *Mechanisms of Ageing and Development, 165*(Pt B), 86–97.

Chapter 3
The Genetics of Exceptional Longevity in Humans and Relevance to Healthy Aging

Braxton D. Mitchell

Key Take Away Points

1. Although there is a strong familial component to exceptional longevity, the genetic component to this phenotype is complex and not attributable to a small number of large effect genetic variants.
2. Single gene mutations associated with human progeroid syndromes of accelerated aging and animal models of pronounced lifespan extension have revealed biological mechanisms and pathways that are potential therapeutic targets for healthy aging and lifespan extension in humans.
3. Caloric restriction represents one of the most robust interventions available to extend lifespan. It likely exerts anti-aging effects through some of the same signaling and nutrient sensors of growth and development pathways that are apparent in model organisms.

3.1 Introduction

Mean lifespan in the US is 77 years, but there is substantial variability in the age at which people die. This large variability in lifespan prompts important questions about the aging process and its determinants. Among these questions are: "Why do we age? What are the cellular and molecular mechanisms underlying aging? Can we delay aging? And can we maintain productivity even late in life?"

B. D. Mitchell (✉)
Departments of Medicine and Epidemiology and Public Health, University of Maryland School of Medicine, Baltimore, MD, USA
e-mail: bmitchel@som.umaryland.edu

R. E. Kheirbek, M. D. Llorente (eds.), *Current Perspectives on Centenarians*, International Perspectives on Aging 36,
https://doi.org/10.1007/978-3-031-30915-1_3

In this chapter, we discuss how genetics can inform discussion of these issues. Specifically, we address the following topics:

- What is the evidence that extreme lifespan aggregates in families?
- What can clinical syndromes of premature aging in humans teach us about the aging process?
- What is the relevance of animal studies of aging to humans?
- Are there longevity enhancing genes in humans?

Lifespan Vs Extreme Longevity It has not been firmly established if extreme longevity (e.g., being a centenarian, or living to the age of 100 years) should be considered merely as the extreme tail of the distribution of lifespan or whether it represents a separate phenotype that has overlapping but distinct determinants. On one hand, individuals living to a very old age might be viewed as those with a relative lack of disease-associated risk factors, including a relative absence of genetic variants associated with common age-related diseases, such as heart disease and cancer. To the degree that genetic risk to these common disorders shorten lifespan, these might be considered longevity-associated variants. On the other hand, extreme longevity might also be viewed as a distinct phenotype that includes more than just a relative absence of detrimental disease-causing variants, but also an enrichment of protective anti-aging genetic variants. Our focus in this chapter is on genetic influences on extreme longevity per se, and not on the much broader topic of genetic determinants of lifespan.

Environmental Contributions to Lifespan While the focus of this chapter on the genetic contribution to lifespan, this should not be taken in any way to downplay the overwhelming contribution of environmental factors to lifespan. Numerous observations point to a massive effect of environmental and lifestyle factors. Life expectancy has increased steadily over the last 100 years. It is longer for women than for it is for men, it is longer for whites than it is for blacks, and these trends are not limited to the United States. Additionally, there is wide variation in life expectancy worldwide, with life expectancy much lower in Africa than it is in Australia, Western Europe, and Canada (Galvani-Townsend et al., 2022). Environmental influences on lifespan are numerous and include water and air quality, diet, physical activity levels, lifestyle, and multiple other factors, many related to socioeconomic status.

3.2 Extreme Longevity and Families

Precise estimates of the numbers of centenarians in the population are difficult because many centenarians lack birth records to confirm their age. With this caveat, it is estimated that there were 548,000 documented centenarians worldwide in 2020 with this number projected to increase to 3,117,000 by 2050 (Statistica Research Department, 2022). In the United States, the number of centenarians in 2020 is 97,000. The overall number of centenarians doubles every 10 years, mostly as a consequence of a growing population with increasing life expectancy. The vast majority of centenarians are women and nearly all are capable of functioning independently until at least the age of 90. The oldest, confirmed living centenarian was Jeanne Calment of Arles, France (1875–1997), who lived to the ripe old age of 122 years and 164 days. There are numerous reports in the lay literature of individuals living even longer than Ms. Calment, and of regions of the world where the number of centenarians is unusually high. However, these reports are largely unsubstantiated, and current limits to human lifespan appear to be in the range of 110 years, with a small number of individuals, Ms. Calment being the most extreme, living beyond this age.

Multiple lines of evidence point also to a genetic contribution to human lifespan. Twin and family studies have consistently estimated lifespan heritability in the 15–30% range (Herskind et al., 1996; Iachine et al., 1998; Ljungquist et al., 1998; Mitchell et al., 2001). However, more recent studies leveraging very large datasets comprised of millions of individuals obtained from online ancestry databases have cast doubts on these estimates, reporting instead heritabilities of 16% and < 10% (Kaplanis et al., 2018; Ruby et al., 2018). For example, using pedigrees constructed from *Ancestry.com* that included hundreds of millions of people, Ruby et al. estimated a heritability of lifespan of <10% after accounting for unexpectedly high correlations in lifespan among spouse pairs and among nongenetic (in-law) relatives. The higher-than- expected correlations among these relative pairs were interpreted as evidence of assortative mating, or a familial, but nongenetic, source of resemblance in lifespan leading to a tendency for people from similar backgrounds to marry each other. (Ruby et al., 2018)

Regardless of the actual estimate of heritability, evidence of a heritable component for lifespan per se does not inform what genes are involved nor do these estimates necessarily apply to the genetic contribution to exceptional lifespan. Studies focusing on long-lived individuals have provided evidence that exceptional longevity is also heritable. The New England Centenarian Study identified one family in which six of the eight siblings lived to age 90 or older. In a second family that included 20 grandchildren, 13 reached the age of 90, and seven of these lived to 100. Using age-specific mortality rates, the probability of observing this many long-lived individuals within the same family occurring solely by chance was estimated at approximately 1 in 10^9 in the first family, and 1 in 10^{18} in the second family. Since the total number of families in the world is less than 1 in a billion (i.e., 10^9 (Perls & Terry, 2003)), the researchers concluded that this was strong evidence for familial aggregation of exceptional longevity. (Perls & Terry, 2003)

Additional evidence of familial clustering of living to an exceptional age, also from the New England Centenarian Study, comes from a 1998 comparison of survival between siblings of centenarians (n = 456) and siblings of 73 year-old controls (n = 240). At younger ages, survival rates were similar between the two groups of siblings, but at older ages survival rates were 3–4 times higher among siblings of the centenarians. (Perls et al., 1998) Hypothesizing that centenarians might be more likely to pass down 'healthy' genes to their children, Terry et al. compared health profiles between offspring of centenarians and offspring of controls and found that the offspring of centenarians had lower rates of all-cause, cardiovascular, and cancer mortality compared to controls (Terry et al., 2004a) and were less likely to suffer from hypertension, cardiovascular disease, diabetes, and stroke. (Terry et al., 2004b)

3.3 The Biology of Aging

In this section we describe lessons learned from clinical syndromes of premature aging in humans and animal models of exceptional longevity.

Clinical Syndromes of Premature Aging Progeroid syndromes are a group of rare genetic disorders that lead to premature aging. These disorders are monogenic, that is, they are caused by mutations in a single gene, and they typically occur either as 'de novo' mutations or as autosomal recessive disorders because affected individuals do not typically have children. Most progeroid syndromes are due to mutations that lead to defects in DNA repair or in lamin A/C, an important protein in the cell nucleus. Because these disorders mimic physiological aging, they have provided unique opportunities for understanding the normal process of aging. We describe briefly below three progeroid syndromes, highlighting how the genetic defects in each relate to the biology of aging (see Table 3.1).

Hutchinson-Gilford progeria is a progressive genetic disorder that causes children to age rapidly, generally beginning within the first 2 years of life. Clinical features include growth delay, short height, and small face and large head. Patients with Hutchinson-Gilford progeria are genetically predisposed to early heart disease. The genetic cause of Hutchinson-Gilford progeria was discovered in 2003 with the identification of a sporadic mutation in the lamin A (*LMNA*) gene. (Eriksson et al., 2003) The mutation causes the production of an abnormal lamin A, or progerin. Since lamin A protein constitutes the scaffolding that holds the cell nucleus together, the defective lamin A protein is believed to make the nucleus unstable, leading to a diverse set of premature aging-associated phenotypes. Hutchinson-Gilford progeria

Table 3.1 Three progeroid syndromes illustrating how single gene mutations can give rise to accelerated aging phenotypes

Syndrome	Inheritance	Gene	Clinical features	Defect
Hutchinson-Gilford progeria	Sporadic	*LMNA*	Growth delay, short height, and small face and large head	Cell integrity
Werner syndrome	Autosomal recessive	*WRN*	Onset at puberty. Wrinkled, ulcerated skin, subcutaneous fat loss, cataracts, diabetes, atherosclerosis, osteoporosis, and malignancies	DNA repair
Cockayne syndrome	Autosomal recessive	*ERCC8*, *ERCC6*	Microcephaly, failure to thrive, and delayed development	DNA repair

is extremely rare. It Is not generally passed down in families but rather occurs as a result of sporadic mutations occurring in *LMNA* since affected individuals generally die young and do not have children.

Werner syndrome is inherited as an autosomal recessive disorder. First manifesting at puberty, the phenotype is characterized by wrinkled, ulcerated skin, subcutaneous fat loss, cataracts, diabetes, atherosclerosis, osteoporosis, and malignancies. (Oshima et al., 2017) In 1992, the gene responsible for Werner syndrome was localized to chromosome 8 through linkage analysis (Goto et al., 1992) and the responsible gene finally identified 5 years later (Yu et al., 1997). The *WRN* gene encodes the WRN protein, an enzyme in a family of DNA helicases that unwind and separate double stranded DNA. These enzymes are essential for transcription and play a pivotal role in DNA repair. To date, over 70 different mutations have been found in the *WRN* gene in Werner syndrome patients (Oshima et al., 2017). While the prevalence of Werner syndrome is rare worldwide, its frequency is relatively higher in Japan, likely due to a founder effect (Satoh et al., 1999).

Cockayne Syndrome is a neurogenerative disorder, also inherited as an autosomal recessive. It is a form of leukodystrophy, a class of disorders characterized by degradation of white matter. Key clinical features include microcephaly, failure to thrive, and delayed development, and hypersensitivity to sunlight. The underlying defect in Cockayne syndrome is a DNA repair mechanism that is caused by mutations in either the *ERCC8* or *ERCC6* gene that lead to defects in the nucleotide excision DNA repair pathway, a complex system that eliminates structural DNA lesions (Karikkineth et al., 2017).

These three syndromes all involve single gene defects affecting either integrity of the cell or DNA replication or repair. They share in common the end result that affected individuals experience a wide panel of phenotypes that mimic accelerated aging. These discoveries prompt the question as to whether genetic variation favoring efficient DNA repair might favor longevity and healthy aging in human populations (Kim et al., 2018) as well as the potential of stimulating DNA repair mechanisms as a therapeutic strategy to prolong lifespan (Qian et al., 2018; Tian et al., 2019).

Animal Models of Lifespan Extension While human progerion syndromes have demonstrated how single gene mutations can accelerate the process of physiologic aging, studies carried out in animals (principally, nematodes, drosophila, yeast, and mice) have revealed the presence of single mutations that can extend lifespan. Specifically, mutations discovered in these organisms have revealed that the aging process is regulated by classical signalling pathways and transcription factors. The first of these mutations was identified in 1993 in *C elegans*, a type of nematode (worm), and led to a two-fold increase in lifespan. (Kenyon et al., 1993) This mutation occurred in the gene, *daf-2*, which encodes a hormone receptor similar to the insulin and IGF-1 receptor. The mutation causes a decrease in insulin and IGF-1 signalling activity, which, in turn, leads to changes in expression of a host of downstream genes. Among the genes down-regulated as a result of decreased insulin and IGF-1 signalling activity are many involved in stress-response and nutrient sensing.

It is thought that reducing these activities promotes lifespan extension in these organisms by redirecting physiologic resources away from growth and towards cell maintenance.

Many other lifespan extending mutations have been discovered in worms, flies, yeast, and mice, some in the insulin and IGF-1 signalling pathway, but many occurring in other signalling pathways, including the kinase target of rapamycin (TOR), AMP kinase, and sirtuin pathways. Like the insulin and IGF-1 signalling pathways, these pathways also mediate response to stress and nutrient sensing with down-regulation associated with lifespan extension. Excellent reviews of the nutrient sensing pathways and their relevance to aging have been published by Kenyon (2010) and Fontana et al. (2010)

Because these signalling pathways are highly conserved across animals, including humans, there is great interest in researching the therapeutic potential of inhibiting insulin and IGF-1 signalling (and activities of related signalling pathways) to extend lifespan (e.g., see Campisi (Campisi et al., 2019)). Moreover, since these pathways have downstream effects on nutrient sensing and stress response, dietary approaches are considered potential attractive therapeutic strategies to promote healthy aging and extend lifespan. We describe in the next section the connection between caloric restriction and lifespan extension in humans.

Caloric Restriction Many environmental and physiological factors can influence stress-response and nutrient sensors that mediate lifespan. The best known of these is caloric restriction, which has been shown experimentally to increase lifespan in a variety of organisms, including drosophila, yeast, rotifers, spiders, worms, fish, mice, rats, and non-human primates. Across a wide range of organisms, caloric restriction not only increases lifespan, but decreases the incidence of multiple aging-related disorders. For example, caloric-restricted rhesus monkeys have a lower incidence of neoplasia, cardiovascular disease, and glucose regulatory impairment. (Colman et al., 2009)

Direct evidence that caloric restriction increases human lifespan is lacking because long-terms trials of caloric restriction in humans are not feasible. Nonetheless, there seems little reason to think that the experience of humans would differ from that of other animals, including non-human primates. Moreover, as in non-human primates, available evidence suggests that humans who voluntarily decrease their caloric allotment experience wide improvements in metabolic health that are consistent with longer lifespan.

To examine long term effects of caloric restriction on cardiovascular health in human, Fontana et al. studied 18 members from the Caloric Restriction Society who had been practicing caloric restriction for an average of 6 years. (Fontana et al., 2004) These individuals consumed between 1112 to 1958 calories per day, with 46% of caloric intake coming from complex carbohydrates. Metabolic parameters were captured at baseline and 6 years later. At baseline, mean age of these 18 individuals was 50.3 years. After 6 years, body mass index decreased from 20.5 kg/m^2 to 19.5 kg/m^2, and total cholesterol dropped from 194 mg/dl to 157 mg/dl. This was accompanied by an increase of HDL cholesterol and a decrease in LDL cholesterol. Systolic blood pressure decreased from 132 mmHg to 97 mmHg, and diastolic blood pressure decreased from 80 mmHg to 59 mmHg. The baseline parameters of these subjects were very similar to those recorded for a control set of 18 individuals.

A further piece of evidence comes from the "natural" experiment associated with the Biosphere 2 experiment. In 1991, eight volunteers were sealed inside a 3-acre closed ecological space ('Biosphere 2') for 2 years and due to an unanticipated decrease in food availability their caloric consumption decreased from 2500 calories per day to 1784 calories per day. (Walford et al., 2002) All volunteers experienced a marked and sustained weight loss of ~17% and significant decreases in blood pressure, cholesterol, and insulin and glucose, among other parameters, resembling changes seen in rodents and monkeys on such diets. Although this and the previous study were based on highly selective volunteer populations, these observations are nonetheless compelling.

Caloric restriction represents one of the most robust interventions available to extend lifespan. While the exact mechanisms involved are as yet unknown, caloric restriction likely exerts anti-aging effects through some of the same signaling and nutrient sensors of growth and development pathways as apparent in model organisms. (Fontana et al., 2010) Whether these pathways can be manipulated to promote lifespan extension and healthy aging in ways other than caloric restriction (say through pharmacologic means) is an area of intense interest.

Summary Single genes can have dramatic effects on their aging process as demonstrated by rare syndromes of premature aging in humans. Multiple animal models have identified mutations in growth and development pathways that have illuminated new biology relevant to human aging.

Genes influencing human aging in regulatory pathways are regulated by nutrient and stress sensors. These sensors may mediate health promoting effects associated with caloric restriction. A challenge is determining whether these observations can lead to the development of new therapeutic targets to promote healthy aging.

3.4 Longevity-Enhancing Genes in Humans

Genetic Association Studies Identifying genetic variants that influence exceptional longevity human is challenging because of the complexity of the phenotype. Numerous factors, both genetic and environmental, influence mortality. Moreover, the genetics of exceptional longevity undoubtedly includes an enrichment of variants that delay physiological aging as well as a relative absence of risk variants that are associated with common aging-related diseases. Genetic variants contributing to exceptional longevity likely include numerous common variants, each having very small effect sizes, as well as rare variants, some that may even have relatively large effect sizes. Experience with other complex traits indicates that very large sample sizes will be required to detect robust associations.

Case-control study designs are commonly used to map genes for complex traits. For exceptional longevity, one might test for enrichment of genetic variants in centenarians (cases) compared to a control group of non-centenarians who are matched for sex and genetic ancestry. For exceptional longevity, a major challenge has been to accrue large numbers of subjects to provide sufficient statistical power. Numerous candidate gene studies, many restricted to relatively small sample sizes, have employed the case-control design to test for association of exceptional longevity with variants in candidate genes that have been selected for their known role in relevant biologic processes. Although many positive findings have been reported, the only association from these studies that has been consistently replicated is at the *APOE* locus, where the *APOE* E4 allele is underrepresented in centenarians (Gerdes et al., 2000; Wright et al. 2019). APOE is an apolipoprotein that has a prominent role in cholesterol metabolism, including transport of cholesterol to peripheral tissues and the brain. The *APOE* E4 allele has been associated with dyslipidemia, risk of early onset Alzheimer's disease, and higher rate of heart disease, while conversely the E2 allele is protective against these disorders.

In recent years, several genome-wide association studies (GWAS) of extreme longevity have been carried out. (Sebastiani et al., 2017; Broer et al., 2015; Deelen et al., 2019) While confirming the association of *APOE* with exceptional longevity, these studies generally remain underpowered to detect variants having smaller effect sizes given the importance in GWAS of accounting for the large numbers of variants tested. One recent study combined existing GWAS summary results for exceptional longevity and two other related phenotypes, healthspan and parental lifespan, to markedly increase sample size (to >1.3 million individuals). This study reported associations of 24 different loci influencing one or more of these traits. (Timmers et al., 2020) Interestingly, one of these loci mapped to *FOX03*, a gene encoding a transcription factor and downstream target of insulin/IGF-1 signalling that has previously been linked to multiple aging and age-related phenotype, including with lifespan itself (reviewed in Sanese et al. (2019)), albeit not consistently. Particularly relevant, this gene plays an important function in modulating survival in response to caloric restriction. (Kenyon, 2010)

Biomarkers of Aging Numerous biomarkers of aging have been proposed, which include a vast array of biochemical measures and indices of frailty, among others. Such markers have been very useful in distinguishing among individuals of the same chronological age who have very different trajectories of health and lifespan. It is tempting to consider whether genetic studies of these 'intermediate' traits might provide insights into the biology of aging, and by extension, lifespan expansion. In this context, we discuss one class of aging biomarkers, biological clocks.

Telomere length has been widely studied for its relation to aging. Telomeres are regions of repetitive DNA sequences at the end of a chromosome whose function is to protect the chromosomes from the shortening that occurs each time a cell divides. With normal aging, telomeres become gradually shorter until at some point the cell can no longer divide successfully and it dies. Telomere length has been associated with a large number of disease outcomes, although its association with overall mortality is controversial (reviewed in Lohman (Lohman et al., 2021)). A large GWAS of telomere length has recently been carried out in over 109,000 individuals, identifying variants at 36 different loci (Taub et al., 2022). The relevance of any of these variants to extreme longevity remains to be determined.

Biological clocks based on DNA methylation and proteomics have also become widely used in the aging literature. DNA methylation entails a form of chemical modification of nucleotide bases in the DNA that does not alter the DNA sequence. DNA methylation sites are spread throughout the genome, where they play a key role in regulating gene expression. DNA methylation, or epigenetic, clocks are based on a small subset of these sites that have been shown to correlate with a wide variety of health-related outcomes. These clocks, in fact, predict overall mortality better than telomere length (Porter et al., 2021). Similarly, proteomic clocks, which are based a curated set of proteins typically measured in blood, have also been shown to correlate strongly with a variety of health-related outcomes and overall mortality. It is important to appreciate, however, that while these clocks do correlate with current and future health outcomes, which makes them useful as predictive tools, their utility for making causal inferences about healthy aging is limited. One problem is that a huge fraction of the genome (epigenetic clocks) and large number of proteins (proteomic clocks) is used to make the prediction, making it difficult to assign a precise biological connection that underlies the prediction. But even more fundamentally, the associations of these clocks to aging are only correlative. It is not known whether changes in DNA methylation or proteins drive the associations with health, whether underlying disease drives changes in the methylome and proteome, or even whether age-associated changes in DNA methylation and proteome are passive by-standers that occur along with changes in health but are not causally related with each other (Field et al., 2018). Thus, at least at the present time, aging biomarkers have not proven useful targets for unraveling the genetics of exceptional lifespan.

3.5 Chapter Summary

There is a clear familial heritable component to lifespan. Human progeroid syndromes have shown that single gene mutations affecting DNA repair and cell stability lead to accelerated aging. Moreover, single gene mutations in worms, flies, yeast, and mice have illustrated the importance of growth and development pathways in aging, and these pathways are likely to have relevance to humans. These same pathways also appear to be relevant to lifespan extension associated with caloric restriction. Targeting some of these pathways offers promise as a therapeutic approach for promoting healthy aging and extending lifespan. Identifying genes for exceptional longevity in humans is a work in progress.

Multiple Choice Questions

1. The most robust lifespan enhancing intervention is:
   A. Exercise
   B. Meditation
   C. Caloric restriction
   D. Vegetarian diet
   CORRECT RESPONSE: C
2. The insights most relevant to exceptional lifespan in humans that have been provided by animal models of extreme longevity pertain to:
   A. DNA repair
   B. Nutrition sensors and signaling pathways
   C. Disease resistance
   CORRECT RESPONSE: B
3. Human progerion syndromes are mostly due to:
   A. Mutations in genes related to DNA repair and cell instability
   B. Mutations in genes related to signaling pathways related to nutrition sensing
   C. Chromosome abnormalities
   D. Autosomal dominant disorders
   CORRECT RESPONSE: A

References

Broer, L., Buchman, A. S., Deelen, J., Evans, D. S., Faul, J. D., Lunetta, K. L., Sebastiani, P., Smith, J. A., Smith, A. V., Tanaka, T., et al. (2015). GWAS of longevity in CHARGE consortium confirms APOE and FOXO3 candidacy. *The Journals of Gerontology. Series A, Biological Sciences and Medical Sciences, 70*, 110–118.

Campisi, J., Kapahi, P., Lithgow, G. J., Melov, S., Newman, J. C., & Verdin, E. (2019). From discoveries in ageing research to therapeutics for healthy ageing. *Nature, 571*, 183–192.

Colman, R. J., Anderson, R. M., Johnson, S. C., Kastman, E. K., Kosmatka, K. J., Beasley, T. M., Allison, D. B., Cruzen, C., Simmons, H. A., Kemnitz, J. W., et al. (2009). Caloric restriction delays disease onset and mortality in rhesus monkeys. *Science, 325*, 201–204.

Deelen, J., Evans, D. S., Arking, D. E., Tesi, N., Nygaard, M., Liu, X., Wojczynski, M. K., Biggs, M. L., van der Spek, A., Atzmon, G., et al. (2019). A meta-analysis of genome-wide association studies identifies multiple longevity genes. *Nature Communications, 10*, 3669.

Eriksson, M., Brown, W. T., Gordon, L. B., Glynn, M. W., Singer, J., Scott, L., Erdos, M. R., Robbins, C. M., Moses, T. Y., Berglund, P., et al. (2003). Recurrent de novo point mutations in Lamin A cause Hutchinson-Gilford progeria syndrome. *Nature, 423*, 293–298.

Field, A. E., Robertson, N. A., Wang, T., Havas, A., Ideker, T., & Adams, P. D. (2018). DNA methylation clocks in aging: Categories, causes, and consequences. *Molecular Cell, 71*, 882–895.

Fontana, L., Meyer, T. E., Klein, S., & Holloszy, J. O. (2004). Long-term calorie restriction is highly effective in reducing the risk for atherosclerosis in humans. *Proceedings of the National Academy of Sciences of the United States of America, 101*, 6659–6663.

Fontana, L., Partridge, L., & Longo, V. D. (2010). Extending healthy life span—From yeast to humans. *Science, 328*, 321–326.

Galvani-Townsend, S., Martinez, I., & Pandey, A. (2022). Is life expectancy higher in countries and territories with publicly funded health care? Global analysis of health care access and the social determinants of health. *Journal of Global Health, 12*, 04091.

Gerdes, L. U., Jeune, B., Ranberg, K. A., Nybo, H., & Vaupel, J. W. (2000). Estimation of apolipoprotein E genotype-specific relative mortality risks from the distribution of genotypes in centenarians and middle- aged men: Apolipoprotein E gene is a "frailty gene," not a "longevity gene". *Genetic Epidemiology, 19*, 202–210.

Goto, M., Rubenstein, M., Weber, J., Woods, K., & Drayna, D. (1992). Genetic linkage of Werner's syndrome to five markers on chromosome 8. *Nature, 355*, 735–738.

Herskind, A. M., McGue, M., Holm, N. V., Sorensen, T. I., Harvald, B., & Vaupel, J. W. (1996). The heritability of human longevity: A population-based study of 2872 Danish twin pairs born 1870–1900. *Human Genetics, 97*, 319–323.

Iachine, I. A., Holm, N. V., Harris, J. R., Begun, A. Z., Iachina, M. K., Laitinen, M., Kaprio, J., & Yashin, A. I. (1998). How heritable is individual susceptibility to death? The results of an analysis of survival data on Danish, Swedish and Finnish twins. *Twin Research, 1*, 196–205.

Kaplanis, J., Gordon, A., Shor, T., Weissbrod, O., Geiger, D., Wahl, M., Gershovits, M., Markus, B., Sheikh, M., Gymrek, M., et al. (2018). Quantitative analysis of population-scale family trees with millions of relatives. *Science, 360*, 171–175.

Karikkineth, A. C., Scheibye-Knudsen, M., Fivenson, E., Croteau, D. L., & Bohr, V. A. (2017). Cockayne syndrome: Clinical features, model systems and pathways. *Ageing Research Reviews, 33*, 3–17.

Kenyon, C. J. (2010). The genetics of ageing. *Nature, 464*, 504–512.

Kenyon, C., Chang, J., Gensch, E., Rudner, A., & Tabtiang, R. (1993). A C. elegans mutant that lives twice as long as wild type. *Nature, 366*, 461–464.

Kim, Y. J., Kim, H. S., & Seo, Y. R. (2018). Genomic approach to understand the association of DNA repair with longevity and healthy aging using genomic databases of oldest-old population. *Oxidative Medicine and Cellular Longevity, 2018*, 2984730–2984712.

Ljungquist, B., Berg, S., Lanke, J., McClearn, G. E., & Pedersen, N. L. (1998). The effect of genetic factors for longevity: A comparison of identical and fraternal twins in the Swedish twin registry. *The Journals of Gerontology. Series A, Biological Sciences and Medical Sciences, 53*, M441–M446.

Lohman, T., Bains, G., Berk, L., & Lohman, E. (2021). Predictors of biological age: The implications for wellness and aging research. *Gerontol Geriatr Med, 7*, 23337214211046419.

Mitchell, B. D., Hsueh, W. C., King, T. M., Pollin, T. I., Sorkin, J., Agarwala, R., Schäffer, A. A., & Shuldiner, A. R. (2001). Heritability of life span in the old order Amish. *American Journal of Medical Genetics, 102*, 346–352.

Oshima, J., Sidorova, J. M., & Monnat, R. J., Jr. (2017). Werner syndrome: Clinical features, pathogenesis and potential therapeutic interventions. *Ageing Research Reviews, 33*, 105–114.

Perls, T., & Terry, D. (2003). Genetics of exceptional longevity. *ExpGerontol, 38*, 725–730.

Perls, T. T., Bubrick, E., Wager, C. G., Vijg, J., & Kruglyak, L. (1998). Siblings of centenarians live longer. *Lancet, 351*, 1560.

Porter, H. L., Brown, C. A., Roopnarinesingh, X., Giles, C. B., Georgescu, C., Freeman, W. M., & Wren, J. D. (2021). Many chronological aging clocks can be found throughout the epigenome: Implications for quantifying biological aging. *Aging Cell, 20*, e13492.

Qian, M., Liu, Z., Peng, L., Tang, X., Meng, F., Ao, Y., Zhou, M., Wang, M., Cao, X., Qin, B., et al. (2018). Boosting ATM activity alleviates aging and extends lifespan in a mouse model of progeria. *eLife, 7*, e34836.

Ruby, J. G., Wright, K. M., Rand, K. A., Kermany, A., Noto, K., Curtis, D., Varner, N., Garrigan, D., Slinkov, D., Dorfman, I., et al. (2018). Estimates of the heritability of human longevity are substantially inflated due to assortative mating. *Genetics, 210*, 1109–1124.

Sanese, P., Forte, G., Disciglio, V., Grossi, V., & Simone, C. (2019). FOXO3 on the road to longevity: Lessons from SNPs and chromatin hubs. *Computational and Structural Biotechnology Journal, 17*, 737–745.

Satoh, M., Imai, M., Sugimoto, M., Goto, M., & Furuichi, Y. (1999). Prevalence of Werner's syndrome heterozygotes in Japan. *Lancet, 353*, 1766.

Sebastiani, P., Gurinovich, A., Bae, H., Andersen, S., Malovini, A., Atzmon, G., Villa, F., Kraja, A. T., Ben-Avraham, D., Barzilai, N., et al. (2017). Four genome-wide association studies identify new extreme longevity variants. *The Journals of Gerontology. Series A, Biological Sciences and Medical Sciences, 72*, 1453–1464.

Statistica Research Department. (2022). Number of centenarians worldwide 2000–2100. Available from www.statista.com/statistics/996597/number-centenarians-worldwide/. Accessed on 1/7/2023.

Taub, M. A., Conomos, M. P., Keener, R., Iyer, K. R., Weinstock, J. S., Yanek, L. R., Lane, J., Miller-Fleming, T. W., Brody, J. A., Raffield, L. M., et al. (2022). Genetic determinants of telomere length from 109,122 ancestrally diverse whole-genome sequences in TOPMed. *Cell Genom, 2*, 100084.

Terry, D. F., Wilcox, M. A., McCormick, M. A., Pennington, J. Y., Schoenhofen, E. A., Andersen, S. L., & Perls, T. T. (2004a). Lower all-cause, cardiovascular, and cancer mortality in centenarians' offspring. *Journal of the American Geriatrics Society, 52*, 2074–2076.

Terry, D. F., Wilcox, M. A., McCormick, M. A., & Perls, T. T. (2004b). Cardiovascular disease delay in centenarian offspring. *The Journals of Gerontology. Series A, Biological Sciences and Medical Sciences, 59*, 385–389.

Tian, X., Firsanov, D., Zhang, Z., Cheng, Y., Luo, L., Tombline, G., Tan, R., Simon, M., Henderson, S., Steffan, J., et al. (2019). SIRT6 is responsible for more efficient DNA double-strand break repair in long-lived species. *Cell, 177*, 622–638.e622.

Timmers, P., Wilson, J. F., Joshi, P. K., & Deelen, J. (2020). Multivariate genomic scan implicates novel loci and haem metabolism in human ageing. *Nature Communications, 11*, 3570.

Walford, R. L., Mock, D., Verdery, R., & MacCallum, T. (2002). Calorie restriction in biosphere 2: Alterations in physiologic, hematologic, hormonal, and biochemical parameters in humans restricted for a 2-year period. *The Journals of Gerontology. Series A, Biological Sciences and Medical Sciences, 57*, B211–B224.

Wright, K. M., Rand, K. A., Kermany, A., Noto, K., Curtis, D., Garrigan, D., Slinkov, D., Dorfman, I., Granka, J. M., Byrnes, J., et al. (2019). A prospective analysis of genetic variants associated with human lifespan. *G3 (Bethesda), 9*, 2863–2878.

Yu, C. E., Oshima, J., Wijsman, E. M., Nakura, J., Miki, T., Piussan, C., Matthews, S., Fu, Y. H., Mulligan, J., Martin, G. M., et al. (1997). Mutations in the consensus helicase domains of the Werner syndrome gene. Werner's Syndrome Collaborative Group. *American Journal of Human Genetics, 60*, 330–341.

Chapter 4
Cardiovascular Risk Factors in Centenarians

Amanda Lange, Michael A. Silverman, and Adam G. Golden

Key Take Away Points

1. Although prevalence of heart disease among centenarians is lower than other geriatric age groups, it remains the most common cause of mortality for this group.
2. No evidence-based clinical treatment guidelines exist to manage hypertension, hyperlipidemia or congestive heart failure among centenarians.
3. Providing medical care to centenarians is a careful balance between the benefits of improved function and lower morbidity with the risk of adverse events.
4. Shared decision-making discussions between patients, families, and health care professionals must include values and preferences of patient/family units.

4.1 Introduction

Cardiovascular disease is a leading cause of mortality among middle-aged and older adults. The prevalence of cardiovascular disease is lower among the predominantly female centenarian population than among younger geriatric populations. For

A. Lange
Private Practice, Orlando, FL, USA

M. A. Silverman
West Palm Beach VA Healthcare System, West Palm Beach, FL, USA
e-mail: Michael.Silverman@va.gov

A. G. Golden (✉)
Orlando VA Healthcare Sytem, University of Central Florida College of Medicine, Orlando, FL, USA
e-mail: Adam.Golden@va.gov

R. E. Kheirbek, M. D. Llorente (eds.), *Current Perspectives on Centenarians*, International Perspectives on Aging 36,
https://doi.org/10.1007/978-3-031-30915-1_4

successful aging. Centenarian research may therefore provide insights into cardiovascular pathophysiology with implications for the care of middle aged and younger older adults. Observational research has shown that a "healthy" lifestyle is associated with extreme longevity. At the present time, however, there are no evidence-based recommendations for medical interventions that increase the likelihood that an individual older adult will live to be 100 years of age.

Lack of obesity and a personal history that does not include heavy tobacco use are common among Chinese centenarians as well as participants of the New England Centenarian Study (NE Centenarian Study; Liu et al., 2021). Compared with younger geriatric patients, centenarians have a lower prevalence of diabetes (Hirata et al., 2020; Andersen et al., 2012). A study of dietary habits of Portuguese centenarians identified a lower consumption of red meat and a higher consumption of fruits and vegetables than younger aged controls (da Silva et al., 2018).

4.4 Difficulties and Limitations Studying Centenarians

Research involving centenarians often involves identifying a cohort of elderly individuals living in a defined geographic area. As a result, there is a degree of homogeneity with regards to race, ethnicity, and culture among the centenarian cohort under study. This homogeneity may play a role in the prevalence of specific genetic alleles among the study population. Comparison of different centenarian cohorts must also take into account variations in diet, social determinants, and environmental factors that vary geographically and culturally. With changing diets, increased migration, new environmental exposures, social upheaval, and medical therapy innovations, centenarian cohorts may also differ over time. Thus, a cohort that was studied even 10 – 20 years ago may now have different genetics, diets, chronic illness prevalences, and environmental exposures.

Measuring the prevalence of cardiovascular diseases and cardiac risk factors may not be uniform across studies. Many studies list the risk factors of hypertension, diabetes mellitus, congestive heart failure, coronary artery disease, hyperlipidemia as categorial variables (i.e., grouping). However, all of these variables are heterogeneous interrelated continuous variables whose severity may vary greatly across a wide range of values. Further complicating efforts to accurately estimate risk factor prevalence is that many centenarians who are "free" of the clinical signs and symptoms of a specific illness may have subclinical diseases. Differences may also exist based on whether information is self-reported by the patient, obtained from chart review, or prospectively obtained through a structured clinical evaluation. In a Danish study of centenarians, the self-reporting of coronary artery disease, heart failure, and hypertension is likely underreported compared to clinical evaluation (Andersen-Ranberg et al., 2013). The high prevalence of cognitive and sensory impairments would further hamper the ability to utilize self-reported data.

The enrollment of large numbers of centenarians in clinical studies continues to be a challenge due to the relatively low percentage of advanced aged individuals in the general population. For example, a review of the Society of Thoracic Surgeons National Database of 662,033 patients who underwent cardiac surgery only included five centenarians (Bridges et al., 2003). Limited life expectancy and the presence of advanced comorbid illness(es) are common exclusion criteria for many cardiovascular research studies. With a high prevalence of dementia and sensory (i.e., hearing and vision) impairment, the inability to obtain an informed consent represents an important real-world selection bias for the enrollment of the oldest-old into prospective clinical trials. Geographic isolation (i.e., lack of transportation) and functional impairments may further hamper efforts to enroll a broad spectrum of nonagenarians and centenarians for studies based at tertiary medical centers. Similarly, centenarians with impairments in instrumental activities of daily living may not be able to participate in clinical trials that use technology-based equipment. As a result, most centenarian studies are limited to retrospective analysis or survey-based data.

4.5 The Aging Heart and Blood Vessels

Normal aging is associated with heart and blood vessel changes that impact organ performance and functional reserve. On a molecular and cellular level, a variety of changes are associated with the aging process (Table 4.1). Age-related mitochondria dysfunction has been well studied in heart muscle. These complex changes affect how the cell utilizes energy and distributes calcium intracellularly. Multiple intracellular signaling pathways and transcription alterations occur in aging cardiac muscle. The role of cell senescence is another area of keen research interest. Senescent cells are unable to further divide, are resistant to apoptosis, and have a pro-inflammatory impact on their surrounding microenvironment.

At the tissue and organ level, there is a decrease in blood vessel elasticity that is often accompanied by calcium and cholesterol deposition in the arterial wall. As a result, the arteries become harder and stiffer. Other age-related cardiovascular physiologic changes are listed in Table 4.2. These changes increase the risk of developing cardiovascular diseases and decrease the reserve capacity of the heart to withstand environmental and disease-related stressors. The rate of decline in organ and tissue function may vary considerably among older adults and may be impacted by comorbid illnesses and lifestyle behaviors.

Table 4.1 Molecular and Cellular Changes with Aging

• Telomere shortening
• Increase glycation end-products
• Increase DNA damage
• Increase errors in RNA transcription and protein translation
• Increase mitochondria dysfunction
• Increase cellular senescence

Table 4.2 Cardiovascular Physiologic Changes with Aging

• Decrease arterial elasticity
• Increase endothelial dysfunction
• Increase left ventricular wall thickness (hypertrophy)
• Increase myocardial stiffness
• Decrease responsiveness of beta-adrenergic receptors
• Decrease responsiveness of baroreceptors
• Increase levels of catecholamines
• Decrease number of pacemaker cells

Surprisingly, for some centenarians the amount of age-related cardiovascular changes is less than what would be expected based on an age-based extrapolation of observations seen in younger geriatric populations. Clinically, the development of cardiovascular disease in centenarians likely follows a heterogenous pattern. In a large retrospective review of the New England Centenarian Study survey data, the authors eloquently identified three somewhat overlapping groups of centenarians (Evert et al., 2003) based on their affliction with age-related illnesses. "Survivors" are those who have been living with long-term advanced illnesses. Improved medical care allows patients to live longer with more advanced cardiovascular disease and may dampen the pathophysiological effects of hypertension, hyperlipidemia, and diabetes. "Delayers" are centenarians whose chronic illnesses did not arise clinically until later in life (i.e., after 80 years of age). "Escapers" are the individuals who become centenarians without the clinical affliction of common age-associated illnesses.

4.6 Genetics Biomarkers

Genetics is presumed to play an important, yet undefined, role and may increase the chances that an individual will live long enough to become a centenarian. A family history of relatives with advanced age may be associated with extreme longevity. Similarly, the children of centenarians often have similar cardiovascular risk factor profiles as their parents.

Much effort has been channeled to identify genetic alleles to explain the frequent observation that extreme longevity seems to occur across family generations. These genetic polymorphisms would act to dampen pro-inflammatory processes and result in a lower atherosclerotic burden. Lower levels of inflammatory markers, such as N-terminal pro B-type natriuretic peptide (NT-proBNP) and interleukin-6 may play a role in the delayed onset of cardiovascular mortality (Hirata et al., 2020). Among participants 105 years of age and older in the Tokyo Centenarian Study an elevated

NT-proBNP (a biomarker of myocyte stress) was associated with increased mortality (Hirata et al., 2020).

There is evidence to suggest that there may be a genetic contribution to the delayed onset of cardiovascular disease, stroke, diabetes, and hypertension in centenarians. (Ismail et al., 2016; Galioto et al., 2008). Variations in the forkhead box O3 (FOXO3A) gene that are associated with a lower risk of diabetes mellitus and heart disease may be more prevalent in some centenarian cohorts (Santos-Lozano et al., 2016). Angiotensin-converting enzyme (ACE) plays an important role in the conversion of angiotensin I into angiotensin II which serves as a vasoconstrictor and stimulant of smooth and cardiac muscle growth. Both ACE insertion and deletion alleles have been observed more frequently in some centenarian cohorts but not in other studies (Santos-Lozano et al., 2016).

Other genes, such as glutathione peroxidase-1 (rs1050450), adiponectine, and paraoxonase 1 (PON1) may have a theoretical role in lipid metabolism and atherogenesis (Santos-Lozano et al., 2016). However, at this time, genetic polymorphisms that are definitively associated with extreme longevity remain unclear. More importantly, there is currently no proven clinical utility for the testing of any specific genetic mutation that can predict individuals who are more likely to live to be centenarians.

4.7 Clinical Management Considerations for Cardiovascular Disease

Many cardiovascular disease guideline recommendations may not be applicable for centenarian patients. Without specific evidence-based recommendations, health care professionals must not base treatment options on age alone. Health care professionals should take into account important geriatric assessment issues, such as multimorbid illnesses, cognitive status, functional status, presence of geriatric syndromes, and level of caregiver support. Choosing a preventative medical intervention that will improve morbidity and mortality outcomes needs to consider both the estimated life expectancy and the time to benefit (Lee & Kim, 2018). In the case of centenarians whose life expectancy is somewhat limited, interventions that have a time to benefit of multiple years may simply take too long to be efficacious. An example, of such an intervention would be the initiation of statin therapy (that has a time to benefit of 2–5 years) in a centenarian. Shared decision-making discussions between patients, families, and health care professionals must include values and preferences of patient/family units.

With limited life expectancy and a lack of guidance from evidence-based medicine, health professionals, patients and caregivers may consider "deprescribing" (stopping) medications. Situations may arise (i.e., the need for hospice or a palliative care approach) where discussions to discontinue medications are part of the standard of clinical care. For patients with a history of myocardial infarction or angiography defined coronary artery disease, the deprescribing (withdrawal) of aspirin, beta-blockers, and statins should only be done through a careful shared decision-making process. Medication therapy should be continued for medications that provide relief for clinical symptoms, such as shortness of breath, orthopnea, and chest pain.

Although resting heart rate is generally unaffected, aging is associated with the loss of sinoatrial nodal cells and conduction abnormalities. As a result, centenarians are at increased risk of symptomatic bradycardia with the use of beta-blockers and the calcium channel blockers verapamil and diltiazem. Clinicians also need to be aware that acetylcholinesterase inhibitors (donepezil, rivastigmine, and galantamine) are a commonly prescribed non-heart medication that can cause bradycardia as a side effect.

Loop diuretics (furosemide and bumetanide) often provide relief for shortness of breath symptoms in congestive heart failure. By increasing urine production, loop diuretics can increase urinary incontinence symptoms. With a decrease in total body water, careful consideration should be used regarding diuretic therapy for patients with poor oral intake or those with volume loss due to diarrhea or vomiting. Frail older adults may also have an age-related decrease in the thirst response and many older adults use medications that can decrease appetite. Chronic kidney disease is common, and therefore, further caution should be used in the initiation of nephrotoxic medications and imaging contrast materials in centenarians. Blood monitoring of creatinine levels may be needed.

Efforts to avoid risk should not lead to the blanket withholding of procedural care. For example, a case series of intravenous thrombolysis for the treatment of acute ischemic stroke in four centenarians lead to two patients becoming functionally independent and there were no serious hemorrhagic adverse events (Baena Álvarez et al., 2021). Complications following coronary artery bypass surgery and percutaneous coronary intervention are higher in patients over the age of 80 years, but large-scale studies of outcomes among centenarians remain unknown. Transcatheter aortic valve replacement remains an option for frail older adults who are excessively high-risk candidates for aortic valve replacement.

4.8 Blood Pressure Evaluation and Management

Elevated blood pressure is associated with an increased risk of heart disease, congestive heart failure, stroke, and kidney disease. Clinically, these age-related decreases in vessel wall elasticity manifest in "normal" aging with a rise in systolic blood pressure and a widening of the pulse pressure (systolic minus diastolic pressure). A widening pulse pressure has been noted to be a risk factor for cardiovascular disease in middle aged and older adults that is independent of systolic hypertension (Franklin & Wong, 2016). A smaller pulse pressure with advanced aging is associated with a "slower rate of aging phenotype" (Newman et al., 2011). Both the systolic pressure and the pulse pressure tend to incline upward until 80 years of age. Among people over the age of 80 years, this trend appears to decline. (Cheng et al., 2012; Wang et al., 2019).

Variability in blood pressure seems to exist with regards to the specific birth cohort of the older adults. Newer cohorts of centenarians seem to have lower longitudinal blood pressures (Wang et al., 2019). In multiple study cohorts, systolic and diastolic blood pressures decline in the oldest-old (Richmond et al., 2011; Polonia et al., 2014; Zyczkowska et al., 2004). Of those centenarians with hypertension, most had an increased widening of the pulse pressure. However, these findings are not uniform across all centenarian cohorts. Blood pressures were higher among 1002 Chinese centenarians, with an average systolic and diastolic blood pressures of 151.32 mmHg ±22.67 and 75.10 mmHg ±11.90 respectively (Liu et al., 2021).

Current guidelines, such as the Joint National Committee (JNC) VIII have a strong recommendation (grade A) to initiate pharmacological treatment for blood pressures greater than or equal to 150/90 mm Hg in persons 60 years of age and older (James et al., 2014). The exact cutoffs for treatment may vary among published guidelines making studies of centenarians that report hypertension as a categorical variable more difficult to interpret. Because of the relative paucity of centenarians enrolled in hypertension-related clinical trials, guidelines for the treatment of hypertension in centenarians do not exist. But do the same rules apply to centenarians? Caution should be used before attempts to aggressively lower blood pressure beyond current, albeit debatable, hypertension guidelines. General geriatric prescribing principles should be followed. Medications should be started at the lowest possible dose and gently titrated upward. Potential drug-drug and drug-disease interactions should be taken into account. Patients should be assessed for medication side-effects.

Treatment goals should not be overly aggressive. Studies have noted that slightly elevated pressures are positively correlated with improved physical and mental performance. With advanced arterial stiffness, higher pressures potentially bring greater perfusion of blood to the organs, especially the heart and brain (Szewieczek et al., 2015). In a prospective study of Polish centenarians, elevated blood pressures tended to correlate with higher scores on functional assessments, such as the Katz Activities of Daily Living and Barthel Index (Szewieczek et al., 2015). These same functional measures were predictors of survival, as lower blood pressure in the oldest old may be associated with frailty, predisposing these individuals to falls and other geriatric syndromes (Szewieczek et al., 2015). While higher systolic blood pressure was associated with poorer cognitive function in 70-year-olds, the inverse was true among 90-year-olds and centenarians (Richmond et al., 2011; Kabayama et al., 2020).

4.9 Hyperlipidemia Management

Hyperlipidemia is an important risk factor for the development of atherosclerotic cardiovascular disease (ASCVD) and subsequently a determinant for premature death (Ducharme & Radhamma, 2008). Lipid lowering interventions directly correlate with decreased adverse cardiovascular events. Many lipid-lowering therapeutic trials do not take into account the very elderly, especially centenarians, and current guidelines recommend providers take a more individualized approach for those beyond 75 years of age. One study that looked at patients with significant coronary artery disease found that medication management in participants >80 years of age was associated with decreased mortality by 50% in post-hospitalized patients (Allen Maycock et al., 2002). Nonetheless, there are suggestions that by age 75 years, increased lipids in patients without atherosclerotic disease or diabetes may present as less of a risk factor for developing cardiovascular disease (Galioto et al., 2008).

Aging is associated with a decline in high-density lipoprotein (HDL) levels. However, among Ashkenazi Jewish centenarians, HDL levels are often comparable to younger adults (Milman et al., 2014). Offspring of these centenarians had even higher HDL levels inferring that the centenarians may have had even higher HDL levels when they were younger. Similarly, a cohort analysis of 400,000 persons noted a lower total cholesterol/HDL ration in the offspring of nonagenarians compared to the general cohort population (Vaarhorst et al., 2011).

Studies involving centenarian populations have found that elevated lipids may not be a primary factor that hinders life span, but instead may have a protective role. A positive correlation may exist between elevated cholesterol levels in centenarians and the ability to perform basic activities of daily living (ADL). A study of female Chinese centenarians revealed that higher LDL, triglyceride (TG), and HDL levels were associated with a greater capability to perform ADLs. A lower incidence of inflammation associated with high cholesterol may be the driving component to explain the decrease in disability in centenarians. This vulnerability to disease and inflammation is believed to be due to lipoproteins' ability to regulate multiple inflammatory markers, including cytokines, tumor necrosis factor, C-reactive proteins, and interleukin-6 (Liang et al., 2017). Another explanation is that those persons with lower lipoprotein levels may be individuals who are also malnourished and frail, increasing their risk of morbidity and mortality (Liang et al., 2017).

A longitudinal study that followed roughly 100,000 older adults for over 15 years revealed that those persons who started the study with lower LDL levels were hospitalized considerably more often for infectious causes versus those with higher LDL values (Ravnskov et al., 2016). Nine cohort studies following approximately 140,000 people for 10 – 30 years found an inverse correlation between total cholesterol and cancer incidence (Ravnskov et al., 2016). LDL binds to and inactivates a multitude of microorganisms, therefore low levels of such lipids are less likely to impede certain diseased states (Ravnskov et al., 2016). This correlation does not appear to be uniform. Among Chinese centenarians, lower levels of LDL, total cholesterol, and triglyceride were associated with a higher health-related quality of life (Wang et al., 2020). In a study of 6333 older adults (including 1385 centenarians and 1350 nonagenarians) higher levels of total cholesterol, LDL-C and superoxide dismutase activity were associated with greater cognitive decline (Lv et al., 2019).

In addition to the modifiable lifestyle choices that help to lower cholesterol levels, genetic variations in cholesterol synthesis may be a source of exceptional longevity seen in some centenarians. The gene that encodes apolipoprotein E (ApoE), which is responsible for transport of lipids and protein metabolism, has multiple alleles that have an effect on lipid levels (Santos-Lozano et al., 2016). The ApoE4 allele is associated with an increased risk of dyslipidemia, Alzheimer's disease, and mortality in centenarians (Santos-Lozano et al., 2016). In contrast, the ApoE alleles, e2 and e3, may have a positive relationship when studying exceptional longevity (Santos-Lozano et al., 2016). Other specific genes (FOXO3A, CETP) are associated with lipoprotein particle size may have alleles that can affect longevity (Abondio et al., 2019; Revelas et al., 2019). Despite these intriguing findings, there are no recommendations for genotyping patients for APOE or for any other gene.

Given these findings, extrapolating the morbidity and mortality benefits of lipid lowering therapy to centenarian patients remains unclear. The prescription of statins among patients over 80 years of age has increased despite the limited efficacy demonstrated in clinical trials (Gulliford et al., 2017; Petersen et al., 2010). This trend is likely due to the continuation of patients that started medication therapy in their sixties and seventies. Efforts to utilize dietary management to lower cholesterol levels can impair oral intake in patients with extreme longevity who have multiple age-related physiological changes that affect appetite and oral intake. With strong indications, such as established atherosclerotic cardiovascular disease (ASCVD), statins may be an acceptable adjunct to prevention in centenarians. Nonetheless, deprescribing of statins seems to be an upward trend with increasing age, especially in centenarians (Gulliford et al., 2017).

4.10 Congestive Heart Failure Diagnosis and Management

Heart failure is a significant cause of morbidity and mortality in the elderly population. The prevalence of this major comorbid state ranges between 32% to 60% among centenarians (Schmidt et al., 2018). Coronary atherosclerosis and hypertension are two major risk factors that increase the risk of developing congestive heart failure.

Heart failure is broken down into two major categories. Some patients present with a weakened heart that has a decreased ejection fraction. Other patients have a preserved ejection fraction, but their heart is rigid and less able to expand (relax) during diastole. Making the diagnosis of congestive heart failure relies on identifying characteristic clinical symptoms and signs on history and physical exam. Symptoms, including shortness of breath, fatigue, or the inability to exercise may be more ambiguous in the oldest old due to the presence of multiple comorbid illnesses and advanced age-related physiological changes. Additional symptoms of confusion, anorexia, and altered bowel movements may be seen among frail older adults with heart failure. Echocardiograms and the measurement of serum B-type natriuretic peptide (BNP) are often helpful in making the diagnosis. Using BNP levels to detect heart failure becomes more problematic in centenarians, as factors such as age, gender, renal function, and hemoglobin may skew the laboratory value (Rasmussen et al., 2019).

Fluid and dietary restrictions will be difficult to implement. Cardiac rehabilitation programs may not be feasible. Standard heart failure management criteria may not be effective in centenarians. Medication utilization in research studies seems to differ depending on the centenarian cohort. For example, German centenarians were less likely to be treated with beta-blockers, renin angiotensin inhibitors, and loop diuretics than octogenarians and nonagenarians with congestive heart failure (Schmidt et al., 2018). In contrast, centenarians from Finland and Sweden showed greater prescriptions rates, specifically with diuretics (Schmidt et al., 2018). Aldosterone inhibitors and neprilysin inhibitors were less likely to be used out of concern over the high prevalence of kidney disease as a comorbidity in centenarians with heart failure (Schmidt et al., 2018).

4.11 Atrial Fibrillation and the Use of Oral Anticoagulants

The risk of a stroke from atrial fibrillation increases with aging. Atrial fibrillation is a common disorder with a readily available pharmacological intervention. The use of oral anticoagulant medications for non-valvular atrial fibrillation lowers the risk of stroke by two-thirds. The CHA_2DS_2-VASc score is widely used to assess the annual risk of stroke from atrial fibrillation. The CHA_2DS_2-VASc score assigns one point for patients ages 65–74 years and two points for patients 75 years of age and above. Patients with a high CHA_2DS_2-VASc score have an annual risk of stroke of 10–12%. The assessment tool of atrial fibrillation stroke risk has only a moderate predictive value. Observational studies suggest a greater absolute benefit from oral anticoagulants for patients 80 years of age and older compared to younger patients (Patti et al., 2017; Xian et al., 2017).

The evidence to support the decision to use oral anticoagulants remains unclear for many "real-world" patients with competing risks including multi-morbidity, dementia, frailty, and limited life expectancy. Centenarians were not used in the validation studies of this tool and specific guidance for the management of atrial fibrillation in centenarians is lacking. Kheirbek, et al., identified that U.S. veteran centenarians were less likely to receive antiplatelet and anticoagulant therapy than octogenarians and nonagenarians (Kheirbek et al., 2018). Decisions to initiate or discontinue anticoagulant should follow a shared decision-making process.

4.12 Complementary Medical Interventions

There are no nutritional supplements or infusion therapies that will increase the likelihood that a person will live to 100 years of age. Despite intriguing research looking at the impact of specific nutritional compounds that can impair the molecular aging process, there are no nutritional supplements that have been proven to increase longevity. Addressing obesity leads to improved cardiovascular outcomes, and strict caloric restriction may have anti-aging benefits in humans. However, for persons accustomed to western eating habits the adherence to caloric restricted diets for extended periods of time is not feasible. Medications that mimic the effects of calorie restriction are an area of intense research interest. Another area of interest focuses on senolytic drugs (dasatinib, quercetin, fisetin, navitoclax) that may dampen the damaging effects that senescent cells have on surrounding cells (Kirkland & Tchkonia, 2020). At this time, none of these medications have been studied sufficiently in clinical trials to be recommended to patients. Metformin is a commonly used medication for the treatment of type II diabetes. Research is currently ongoing to identify potential anti-aging effects of this medication.

4.13 Conclusion

Even with an increasing centenarian population, major evidence gaps will persist in the cardiac care of patients with extreme longevity. Health care professionals should use geriatric medication prescribing principles prior to starting or escalating the dose of any cardiac medications. A geriatric assessment will provide important information for physicians, patients, and caregivers to have insightful shared decision-making discussions regarding cardiac diagnostic and treatment interventions. There are no evidence-based interventions that have been proven to increase the likelihood of living to an extreme old age. Recommendations beyond a "healthy lifestyle" and the avoidance of risky behaviors is lacking. With an ever-increasing understanding of molecular cell biology, it is likely that nutritional, immunologic, and genetic interventions will be developed over the next 10–20 years.

Acknowledgments This material is the result of work that was supported with resources and the use of facilities at the West Palm Beach VA Medical Center and the Orlando VA Healthcare System.

Disclaimer The contents do not represent the views of the Department of Veterans Affairs or the United States Government.

Multiple Choice Questions

1. Which of the following is the most important risk factor for multimorbidity?
   A. Tobacco
   B. Aging
   C. Obesity
   D. Diabetes mellitus
   CORRECT ANSWER: B

2. Which of the following cardiac medications should be used with caution in centenarians with congestive heart failure and poor oral intake?
   A. Aspirin
   B. Loop diuretics
   C. Beta blockers
   D. Calcium channel blockers
   CORRECT ANSWER: B

3. Which of the following medications can induce bradycardia in centenarians?
   A. Phenylephrine
   B. Albuterol
   C. Donepezil
   D. Ciprofloxacin
   CORRECT ANSWER: C

References

Abondio, P., Sazzini, M., Garagnani, P., Boattini, A., Monti, D., Franceschi, C., et al. (2019). The genetic variability of APOE in different human populations and its implications for longevity. *Genes, 10*, 222. https://doi.org/10.3390/genes10030222

Academy of Medical Sciences. (2018). Multimorbidity: A priority for global research. April 2018. https://acmedsci.ac.uk/filedownmrd/82222577. Accessed 15 Jan 2023.

Ailshire, J. A., Beltran-Sanchez, H., & Crimmins, E. M. (2015). Becoming centenarians: disease and functioning trajectories of older U.S. adults as they survive to 100. *Journals of Gerontology. Series A, Biological Sciences and Medical Sciences, 70*(2), 193–201.

Allen Maycock, C. A., Muhlestein, J. B., Horne, B. D., Carlquist, J. F., Bair, T. L., Pearson, R. R., et al. (2002). Statin therapy is associated with reduced mortality across all age groups of individuals with significant coronary disease, including very elderly patients. *Journal of the American College of Cardiology, 40*(10), 1777–1785.

Andersen, S. L., Sebastiani, P., Dworkis, D. A., Feldman, L., & Perls, T. T. (2012). Health span approximates life span among many supercentenarians: Compression of morbidity at the approximate limit of life span. *Journals of Gerontology. Series A, Biological Sciences and Medical Sciences, 67*(4), 395–405.

Andersen-Ranberg, K., Fjederholt, K. T., Madzak, A., Nybo, M., & Jeune, B. (2013). Cardiovascular diseases are largely underreported in Danish centenarians. *Age and Ageing, 42(2)*, 249–253.

Baena Álvarez, B., García-Madrona, S., Sainz Amo, R., Rodríguez Jorge, F., Gómez Corral, J., Vera Lechuga, R., et al. (2021). Intravenous thrombolysis for acute ischemic stroke in centenarians. *European Geriatric Medicine, 12*(4), 893–897.

Bridges, C., Edwards, F., Peterson, E., Coombs, L., & Ferguson, B. (2003). Cardiac surgery in nonagenarians and centenarians. *Journal of the American College of Surgeons, 197*(3), 347–356.

Cheng, S., Xanthakis, V., Sullivan, L. M., & Ramachandran, S. (2012). Blood pressure tracking over the adult life course: Patterns and correlates in the Framingham heart study. *Hypertension, 60*(6), 1393–1399.

da Silva, A. P., Valente, A., Chaves, C., Matos, A., Gil, A., Santos, A. C., et al. (2018). Characterization of Portuguese centenarian eating habits, nutritional biomarkers, and cardiovascular risk: A case control study. *Oxidative Medicine and Cellular Longevity, 218*, 5296168. https://doi.org/10.1155/2018/5296168

Ducharme, N., & Radhamma, R. (2008). Hyperlipidemia in the elderly. *Clinics in Geriatric Medicine, 24*(3), 471–487.

Evert, J., Lawler, E., Bogan, H., & Perls, T. (2003). Morbidity profiles of centenarians: Survivors, delayers, and escapers. *Journals of Gerontology. Series A, Biological Sciences and Medical Sciences, 58*(3), 232–237.

Franco, P. D., Capanema, B. S. V., Pereira, F. S., Barcia, S. O., Gil, P. R., & Mazo, G. Z. (2022). Frailty and physical activity in centenarians: A systematic review. *ABCS Heath Sciences, 47*, e022307. https://doi.org/10.7322/abcshs.202.1018.1747

Franklin, S. S., & Wong, N. D. (2016). Pulse pressure how valuable as a diagnostic and therapeutic tool? *Journal of the American College of Cardiology, 67*(4), 404–406.

Galioto, A., Dominguez, L. J., Pineo, A., Ferlisi, A., Putignano, E., Belvedere, M., et al. (2008). Cardiovascular risk factors for centenarians. *Experimental Gerontology, 43*, 106–113.

Gulliford, M., Ravindrarajah, R., Hamada, S., Jackson, S., & Charlton, J. (2017). Inception and deprescribing of statins in people aged over 80 years: Cohort study. *Age and Ageing, 46*(6), 1001–1005.

Hirata, T., Aria, Y., Yuasa, S., Abe, Y., Takayma, M., Sasaki, T., et al. (2020). Associations of cardiovascular biomarkers and plasma albumin with exceptional survival to advanced ages. *Nature Communications, 11*, 3820. https://doi.org/10.1038/s41467-020-17636-0

Ismail, K., Nussbaum, L., Sebastiani, P., Andersen, S., Perls, T., Barzilai, N., et al. (2016). Compression of morbidity is observed across cohorts with exceptional longevity. *Journal of the American Geriatrics Society, 64*(8), 1583–1591.

James, P. A., Oparil, S., Carter, B. L., Cushman, W., Dennison-Himmelfarb, C., Handler, J., et al. (2014). Evidence-based guidelines for the management of high blood pressure in adults—Report from the panel members appointed to the Eighth Joint National Committee (JNC8). *JAMA, 311*(5), 507–520.

Jiang, X., Lewis, C. E., Allen, N. B., Sidney, S., & Yaffe, K. (2023). Premature cardiovascular disease and brain health in midlife: The CARDIA Study. *Neurology, 25*. https://doi.org/10.1212/WNL.0000000000206825. Epub ahead of print.

Kabayama, M., Kamide, K., Gondo, Y., Masui, Y., Nakagawa, T., Ogawa, M., et al. (2020). The association of blood pressure with physical frailty and cognitive function in community-dwelling septuagenarians, octogenarians, and nonagenarians: The SONIC study. *Hypertension Research, 32*(12), 1421–1429.

Kheirbek, R. E., Fokar, A., Moore, H. J., Shara, N., Doukky, R., & Fletcher, R. D. (2018). Association between lifetime risk of atrial fibrillation and mortality in the oldest old. *Clinical Cardiology, 41*(5), 634–639.

Kirkland, J. K., & Tchkonia, T. (2020). Senolytic drugs: From discovery to translation. *Journal of Internal Medicine, 288*, 518–536.

Lee, S. J., & Kim, C. M. (2018). Individualizing prevention in older adults. *Journal of the American Geriatrics Society, 66*(2), 229–234.

Lee, D. R., Kawas, C. H., Gibbs, L., & Corrada, M. M. (2016). Prevalence of frailty and factors associated with frailty in individuals aged 90 and older: The 90+ study. *Journal of the American Geriatrics Society, 64*(11), 2257–2262.

Liang, Y., Vetrano, D. L., & Qiu, C. (2017). Serum total cholesterol and risk of cardiovascular and non-cardiovascular mortality in old age: A population-based study. *BMC Geriatrics, 17*(1), 294. https://doi.org/10.1186/s12877-017-0685-z

Liu, M., Kou, F., Yang, S., Wang, S., He, Y., & Zhang, W. (2021). Ideal cardiovascular health in the oldest-old and centenarians and its association with disability and health-related quality of life. *Frontiers in Cardiovascular Medicine, 8*, 603877. https://doi.org/10.3389/fcvm.2021.603877

Lv, Y., Mao, C., Yin, Z., Li, F., Wu, X., & Shi, X. (2019). Healthy ageing and biomarkers cohort study (HABBCS): A cohort profile. *BMJ Open, 9*, e026513.

Milman, S., Atzmon, G., Crandall, J., & Barzilai, N. (2014). Phenotypes and genotypes of high density lipoprotein cholesterol in exceptional longevity. *Current Vascular Pharmacology, 12*(5), 690–697.

Newman, A. B., Glynn, N. W., Taylor, C. A., Sebastiani, P., Perls, T. T., Mayeux, R., et al. (2011). Health and function of participants in the long life family study: A comparison with other cohorts. *Aging, 3*(1), 63–76.

Nguyen, H., Manolova, G., Daskalopoulou, C., Vitoratou, S., Prince, M., & Prina, A. M. (2019). Prevalence of multimorbidity in community settings: A systematic review and meta-analysis of observational studies. *Journal of Comorbidity, 9*, 2235042X19870934. https://doi.org/10.1177/2235042X19870934

Patti, G., Lucerna, M., Pecen, L., Siller-Matula, J. M., Cavallari, I., Kirchhof, P., et al. (2017). Thromboembolic risk, bleeding outcomes and effect of different antithrombotic strategies in very elderly patients with atrial fibrillation: A sub-analysis from the PREFER in AF (PREvention of thromboembolic events–European registry in atrial fibrillation). *Journal of the American Heart Association, 6*, e005657.

Petersen, L. K., Christensen, K., & Kragstrup, J. (2010). Lipid-lowering treatment to the end? A review of observational studies and RCTs on cholesterol and mortality in 80+ year olds? *Age and Ageing, 39*, 674–680.

Polonia, J., Martins, L., Pinto, F., & Nazare, J. (2014). Prevalence, awareness, treatment and control of hypertension and salt intake in Portugal. *Journal of Hypertension, 32*(6), 1211–1221.

Rasmussen, S. H., Andersen-Ranberg, K., Sanchez Dahl, J., Nybo, M., Jeune, B., Christensen, K., et al. (2019). Diagnosing heart failure in centenarians. *Journal of Geriatric Cardiology, 16*, 1–11.

Ravnskov, U., Diamond, D. M., Hama, R., Hamazaki, T., Hammarskjöld, B., Hynes, N., et al. (2016). Lack of an association or an inverse association between low-density-lipoprotein cholesterol and mortality in the elderly: A systematic review. *BMJ Open, 6*(6), e010401. https://doi.org/10.1136/bmjopen-2015-010401

Revelas, M., Thalamuthu, A., Oldmeadow, C., Evans, T.-J., Armstrong, N. J., Riveros, C., et al. (2019). Exceptional longevity and polygenic risk for cardiovascular health. *Genes*, 10. https://doi.org/10.3390/genes10030227

Richmond, R., Law, J., & Kay-Lambkin, F. (2011). Higher blood pressure associated with higher cognition and functionality among centenarians in Australia. *American Journal of Hypertension, 24*(3), 299–303.

Santos-Lozano, A., Santamarina, A., Pareja-Galeano, H., Sanchis-Gomar, F., Fiuza-Luces, C., Cristi-Montero, C., et al. (2016). The genetics of exceptional longevity: Insights from centenarians. *Maturitas, 90*, 49–57.

Schmidt, I. M., Kreutz, R., Dräger, D., Zwillich, C., Hörter, S., Kuhlmey, A., et al. (2018). Lower prescription rates in centenarians with heart failure and heart failure and kidney disease combined: Findings from a longitudinal cohort study of very old patients. *Drugs & Aging, 35*, 907–916.

Szewieczek, J., Francuz, T., Dulawa, J., Legierska, K., Hornik, B., Włodarczyk, I., et al. (2015). Functional measures, inflammatory markers and endothelin-1 as predictors of 360-day survival in centenarians. *Age, 37*(5), 85. https://doi.org/10.1007/s11357-015-9822-9

The New England Centenarian Study. Why study Centenarians? An Overview. https://www.bumc.bu.edu/centenarian/overview/. Accessed 27 Nov 2022.

Vaarhorst, A. A., Beekman, M., Suchiman, E. H., van Heemst, D., Houwing-Duistermaat, J. J., Westendorp, R. G., et al. (2011). Lipid metabolism in long-lived families: The Leiden longevity study. *Age, 33*, 219–227.

Wang, R., Vetrano, D. L., Liang, Y., & Qiu, C. (2019). The age-related blood pressure trajectories from young-old adults to centenarians: A cohort study. *International Journal of Cardiology, 296*, 141–148.

Wang, S., Yang, S., Jia, W., Cao, W., Han, K., Liu, M., et al. (2020). Relationships of lipids profile with health-related quality of life in Chinese centenarians. *Journal of Nutrition, Health & Aging, 24*(4), 404–411.

Wastesson, J. W., Canudas-Romo, V., Lindahl-Jacobsen, R., & Johnell, K. (2016). Remaining life expectancy with and without polypharmacy: A register-based study of Swedes aged 65 years and older. *Journal of the American Medical Directors Association, 17*(1), 31–35. https://doi.org/10.1016/j.jamda.2015.07.015. Epub 2015 Sep 2. PMID: 26341036; PMCID: PMC4699614.

Xian, Y., O'Brien, E. C., Liang, L., Xu, H., Schwamm, L. H., Fonarow, G. C., et al. (2017). Association of preceding antithrombic treatment with acute ischemic stroke severity and in-hospital outcomes among patients with atrial fibrillation. *JAMA, 317*(10), 1057–1067.

Xu, J. Q. (2016). *Mortality among centenarians in the United States, 2000–2014. NCHS data brief* (Vol. 233). National Center for Health Statistics.

Zhou, X., & Zhang, D. (2021). Multimorbidity in the elderly: A systematic bibliometric analysis of research output. *International Journal of Environmental Research and Public Health, 19*(1), 353. https://doi.org/10.3390/ijerph19010533

Zyczkowska, J., Klich-Raczka, A., Mossakowska, M., Gasowski, J., Wieczorowska-Tobis, K., & Grodzicki, T. (2004). Blood pressure in centenarians in Poland. *Journal of Human Hypertension, 18*(10), 713–716.

Chapter 5
Do Centenarians Get Dementia?

Jory Crull, Katherine Barlis, Olga Brawman-Mintzer, Christopher Blasy, and Jacobo Mintzer

Key Take Away Points
1. Cognitive impairment is not a necessary outcome of old age.
2. Lifestyle changes can be key in preserving brain health.

5.1 Introduction

To be able to call oneself a centenarian was once a rare exception but thanks to advances in science, medicine, and living conditions, we are seeing a rapidly growing number of individuals who are seemingly beating the odds and reaching these extreme ages. Some estimate that by the year 2100, approximately 25 million people world-wide will reach the age of 100 years old (Beker et al., 2020). Research is currently underway to better understand what can be done to maintain physical health for as long as possible, but what about cognitive health? In this chapter, we will explore what separates your typical age-related cognitive changes from that of dementia, clinical presentation of dementia, and its biological underpinnings. Importantly, we will discuss if aging without dementia is possible, and what work is currently being done with centenarians to investigate this question.

J. Crull · K. Barlis
Medical University of South Carolina, Charleston, SC, USA

Ralph H. Johnson VA Health Care System, Charleston, SC, USA
e-mail: crullj@musc.edu; Katherine.Barlis@va.gov

O. Brawman-Mintzer (✉) · C. Blasy · J. Mintzer
Ralph H. Johnson VA Health Care System, Charleston, SC, USA
e-mail: olga.brawman-mintzer@va.gov; Christopher.Blasy@va.gov; Jacobo.Mintzer@va.gov

R. E. Kheirbek, M. D. Llorente (eds.), *Current Perspectives on Centenarians*, International Perspectives on Aging 36,
https://doi.org/10.1007/978-3-031-30915-1_5

5.2 Illustrative Vignette

Dr. L is a well-known researcher at a major university. While at a party, he interrupts his dancing to have a casual conversation with a friend. The conversation focuses on the future of his research. He describes a dilemma he is facing when attempting to decide which direction his cutting-edge research should take in the next 5–10 years. There is nothing remarkable about this conversation among researchers other than the fact that Dr. L is 97 years old. What are the factors that have allowed Dr. L to have such a cognitive healthy life?

5.3 Pure-Aging (Stefanacci, 2022) Vs Dementia

As a person ages, there are various physiological changes which can be expected. Physical changes might include the degeneration of vision and hearing, or development of conditions such as arthritis, and osteoporosis (Stefanacci, 2022). Healthy older persons may show some cognitive alterations in various neuropsychological domains with changes in working memory, which deals with short term information, executive functioning, and processing speed (Toepper, 2017). These types of age-related changes define what is known as "pure-aging" and will eventually occur in anyone who lives long enough (Stefanacci, 2022).

While aging is an unavoidable and natural part of life, it also becomes the strongest risk factor for the development of dementia (Centers for Disease Control, 2019). Dementia itself is not a particular disease but a general term used to describe the impaired ability to remember, think, and make common everyday decisions. While a cognitively healthy person will inevitably experience some age-related memory decline, the memory deficits a person with dementia will experience are much more severe and are not considered to be a part of normal aging. However, since the onset of dementia is gradual, it can be difficult to differentiate from typical, age-related memory impairment, and is oftentimes first noticed by family members when function becomes impaired in the affected individual (Huang, 2022).

5.4 Dementia & Alzheimer's Disease

5.4.1 Overview & Risk Factors

Although there are many conditions which can lead to dementia, the most common cause is Alzheimer's disease (AD) which accounts for 60–80% of cases (Alzheimers Dement, 2020). While increasing age is the largest risk factor for the development of AD, roughly 5–15% of cases are familial, and half are typically related to mutations of specific genes such as APOE (Huang, 2021). Individuals who express two copies of the APOE-ε4 allele, for instance, have a roughly 10–30 times greater chance of developing AD by age 75 compared to those without the allele. Furthermore, vascular risk factors including hypertension, diabetes, dyslipidemia, and smoking have been shown to increase an individual's risk for developing AD, with current evidence suggesting that aggressive treatment of these risk factors can help lower the risk of developing dementia later in life.

Accumulation of extraneuronal protein fragments known as beta-amyloid plaques and intraneuronal neurofibrillary tangles (NFTs) of the tau protein in the brain make up the two pathological hallmarks of AD (Alzheimers Dement, 2020). Although the complete mechanism is not fully understood, it is hypothesized that the buildup of these beta-amyloid plaques triggers a subsequent increase of NFTs ultimately leading to neuronal death and damage to brain tissue. Further, changes in vasculature, the blood–brain barrier, the glymphatic system (waste-clearing system in the central nervous system), and other clearance systems of the brain such as the peripheral immune system, are involved in the complex, and yet to be fully ascertained, biological processes leading to AD (Scheltens et al., 2021). It is suspected that this overall damage to brain tissue is what leads to the development of dementia symptoms in affected individuals. Additionally, how quickly an affected person might progress from unnoticeable cognitive changes to clear problems with memory will vary depending on the individual's age, genetic makeup, race, gender, lifestyle, and other factors.

5.5 Symptoms & Progression of Dementia Due to Alzheimer's Disease

While the progression of dementia due to AD will vary for each person, a set of core symptoms exists on what is commonly referred to as the AD continuum, which consists of three distinct phases (Alzheimers Dement, 2020). The first is the preclinical AD phase, defined by measurable biomarkers, such as abnormal levels of beta-amyloid detected on positron emission tomography (PET) scans. It is important to note, during this phase the affected individual will display these abnormal biomarkers before they have developed any clinical symptoms such as memory loss. Once an individual displays these biomarkers and begins to exhibit cognitive problems, they have progressed into the second phase and can be diagnosed by a trained clinician as having mild cognitive impairment (MCI) due to AD. Those with MCI will have greater difficulty with memory and thinking compared to the usual age-related memory decline that is common in older individuals, however their everyday functioning typically remains unaffected (Huang, 2022). In many cases, family members or close friends may begin noticing the person's cognitive decline during this phase (Alzheimers Dement, 2020).

Dementia due to AD is the final phase of the AD continuum and is characterized by cognitive decline severe enough to impair the individual's everyday functioning

(Alzheimers Dement, 2020). This phase is further broken down into three stages which consists of early (mild), intermediate (moderate), and late (severe) dementia. During the early stage, while most individuals will be able to function independently, some assistance from others will likely be necessary as recent memory, critical thinking, or judgement may be impaired (Huang, 2022; Alzheimers Dement, 2020). Additionally, a person in the various stages may develop neuropsychiatric symptoms, such as increased anxiety, depression, apathy, and agitation (Huang, 2022).

The intermediate stage is oftentimes the longest stage for the affected person and is typically accompanied by significant loss of independence (Alzheimers Dement, 2020). While recent memory is notably more impaired, it is not yet completely lost (Huang, 2022). The affected individual will become more dependent on caregivers to assist with basic needs such as preparing meals, grooming, and finding their way around a once familiar environment. Personality and behavioral changes may continue to worsen, with some individuals demonstrating greater irritability or even physical aggression. Others may withdraw, become less talkative, and overall disinterested in many things.

In the late stage of AD, individuals will be completely dependent on others to care for their daily needs and will eventually become unable to communicate effectively (Alzheimers Dement, 2020). Extensive damage to the brain ultimately leaves individuals bedridden and may lead to incontinence, or the inability to swallow. These individuals are at much higher risk of developing systemic infections due to bed sores and may succumb to aspiration pneumonia when improperly swallowed food travels into the trachea instead of the esophagus.

5.6 Additional Causes of Dementia & Diagnosis

While AD is the most common cause of dementia, there are also non-AD types of dementia most often linked to cerebrovascular disease, Lewy-body disease, frontotemporal lobar degeneration (e.g. Pick's disease), Parkinson's disease, and hippocampal sclerosis (Huang, 2022; Alzheimers Dement, 2020). Adding to this, multiple prior studies have demonstrated that the majority of individuals with dementia demonstrate pathological evidence of more than one type, which is commonly referred to as mixed dementia (James et al., 2016). Differentiating between the different types of dementia involves an evaluation of an individual's medical history, and a standard neuropsychological testing (Huang, 2021). Additional laboratory testing and brain imaging, such as amyloid and tau PET can be performed to further assist in diagnostic accuracy.

5.7 Do Centenarians Get Dementia?

5.7.1 Incidence of Dementia in Centenarians

With prevalence and incidence rates of all causes of dementia steadily increasing exponentially after the age of 65 (Qiu & Fratiglioni, 2018), this leads to a question and the focus of this chapter – do centenarians get dementia? Indeed, results from cross-sectional studies have estimated that approximately 50% of centenarians exhibit clear signs of dementia, and another 25% display at least some symptoms of cognitive impairment (Beker et al., 2020). However, additional attention should be directed towards the remaining 25% who are considered to be cognitively healthy as these individuals provide evidence for the theory that aging without dementia is achievable. Additionally, it has been shown that not only do some centenarians completely escape the development of dementia, but many others also delay expressing clinical symptoms of dementia until very late ages allowing them to lead longer, cognitively healthy lives (Perls, 2004).

5.8 Dementia Risk & Protective Factors in Centenarians

While age is the biggest risk factor for developing dementia, the existence of dementia-free centenarians supports the idea that dementia is not inevitable. Studying the characteristics of centenarians and the factors associated with healthy aging into older adulthood can elucidate potential interventions for dementia throughout the lifespan. Much attention in the literature has therefore been devoted to determining whether centenarians have unique, inherited genes that allow them to survive into old age or a lifestyle that promotes healthy aging.

5.9 Genetic Factors

Various studies of centenarians have indicated that there is a familial component to longevity. This is often investigated by looking at the health and lifespan of the families of centenarians to see whether they show similar longevity. For example, research has shown that siblings of centenarians are more likely to live longer than their age-matched peers. One study reported that mortality rates of siblings of centenarians were about half of those of age-matched peers, with female siblings showing greater than a two-fold likelihood of reaching age 90 and male siblings having more than a five-fold likelihood compared to their peers (Willcox et al., 2006a).

These familial advantages also extend to children of centenarians, who are more likely to live longer compared to children of parents with average life expectancies (Terry et al., 2004). Beyond living longer, there is also evidence to suggest that centenarian children show health benefits compared to their peers. In particular, children of centenarians demonstrate reduced cardiovascular risk factors and may be less likely to have heart disease, hypertension, and diabetes (Terry et al., 2003). Researchers have attempted to differentiate whether these patterns are due to shared environmental factors among families, such as diet, or inherited genes. Current research suggests it is likely a combination of genetic and environmental factors, as some studies have identified unique gene variants that may be associated with longevity (Willcox et al., 2006b; Sebastiani et al., 2019a).

The most widely studied genetic risk factor for dementia in centenarians is the APOE gene. Given the established effect of APOE on risk for AD in the general population, research has examined whether these findings hold true in centenarians. Some studies have indeed found that the APOE gene affects both an individual's likelihood of reaching older age and the prevalence of dementia in centenarians. For example, inheriting the APOE-ε4 allele has shown associations with reduced likelihood of reaching extreme longevity, defined as the age achieved by less than 1% of the population (Sebastiani et al., 2019b). The APOE-ε4 allele has also been associated with increased mortality after reaching extreme longevity. At the same time, APOE-ε2ε2 and ε2ε3 carriers have shown increased likelihood of reaching extreme longevity compared to carriers of ε3ε3 (Sebastiani et al., 2019b). These patterns support the notion of increased risk with inheriting the ε4 allele and a protective effect of the ε2 allele for centenarians, similar to patterns in the general population.

To better assess whether the APOE gene serves as a risk factor for dementia in centenarians, researchers have examined whether it is associated with cognitive performance at an older age. Although some studies have found associations between the APOE genotype and cognitive function in centenarians, other studies did not find these associations to be present in people over 100 (Ishioka et al., 2016; Davey et al., 2013; Beker et al., 2021). Research has also suggested that the effect of the APOE gene in cognition may be moderated by factors such as gender and education level (Ishioka et al., 2016; Xiang et al., 2021). Additionally, specific proteins on the APOE ε2 allele have been identified as protective in the cognitive status of centenarians, suggesting that ε2 allele could be a future avenue for targeted interventions to prevent cognitive decline (Sebastiani et al., 2019a). Therefore, more research is necessary to determine the role of the APOE gene in dementia risk of centenarians and how this knowledge can be applied to further our understanding of dementia in the general population.

5.10 Physical Health and Cardiovascular Risk Factors

Although some risk factors for dementia cannot be modified, such as age and inherited genes, there are various modifiable risk factors that play a role in the chances of an individual to develop symptoms of dementia. For example, cardiovascular risk factors such as hypertension and coronary artery disease have established connections to increased risk of dementia, including Alzheimer's and vascular pathologies

(Song et al., 2021). One prominent way to control cardiovascular risk is through diet, as nutritional intake has shown numerous effects on health and aging (Leitão et al., 2022). In particular, a Mediterranean diet that focuses on plant-based foods and monounsaturated fats instead of saturated fats has shown promise in preventing or reducing cognitive decline with aging (Panza et al., 2004).

Examining the diets of centenarians can help identify potential ways that nutrition can impact longevity. Diet has been identified as a factor that could contribute to the presence of a high number of centenarians in some places of the world compared to others. The regions of Okinawa, Japan and Sardinia, Italy are two examples of places that have a higher percentage of centenarians than average for the country, and their diets share common features that are thought to contribute to this longevity (Willcox et al., 2006b; Buettner & Skemp, 2016; Wang et al., 2022). These dietary components include high concentrations of fruits and vegetables, which provide antioxidants, as well as increased whole grains. Diets of these regions also involve reduced amounts of saturated fats and meat (Willcox et al., 2006b; Buettner & Skemp, 2016; Wang et al., 2022). The dietary patterns common in centenarian populations resemble those associated with lower risk for dementia, which supports the notion that nutrition can be a powerful way to promote healthy aging and avoid cognitive decline throughout the lifespan (Leitão et al., 2022).

Further support for the importance of diet comes from studies showing that malnutrition is associated with cognitive decline in centenarians (Hai et al., 2017; Feng et al., 2022). In contrast, higher levels of plant-based nutrients are associated with better cognitive function in centenarians without dementia (Tanprasertsuk et al., 2021). Additionally, frequent intake of protein and limiting alcohol consumption have been associated with increased ability to independently perform activities of daily living in centenarians (Ozaki et al., 2007). Together, these findings suggest that it is particularly important for older adults to have adequate nutritional intake and that nutrition can serve as a protective factor against dementia even into late ages.

Another way to reduce cardiovascular risk factors is via physical activity. Given that physical activity is known to have a protective effect in reducing cognitive decline and risk for dementia, it is logical that these benefits will also be present for centenarians. As expected, regular exercise has shown significant correlations with increased ability to independently perform activities of daily living in centenarians (Ozaki et al., 2007). Furthermore, ability to perform activities of daily living is associated with increased cognitive performance in centenarians (Beker et al., 2021). Nonetheless, physical activity tends to decline with age, in part due to medical conditions or physiological changes in muscle and strength, and physical activity levels have been shown to continue to decline as centenarians age (Hernández-Vicente et al., 2019). Therefore, it is important to identify unique ways to alleviate sedentary behavior in centenarians to promote an active lifestyle despite any physical challenges.

5.11 Cognitive and Social Factors

Another modifiable factor that can affect risk for dementia includes cognitive and intellectual activities. Higher levels of education have been shown to correlate with reduced risk of dementia (Fratiglioni & Hui-Xin, 2007). Increased occupational complexity and participation in intellectually stimulating activities across the lifespan may also reduce or delay cognitive decline. One hypothesis for the mechanism behind these associations is that intellectual activities contribute to a cognitive reserve or brain reserve, in which individuals can better cope with age-related brain changes and delay showing symptoms even in the presence of brain pathology (Fratiglioni & Hui-Xin, 2007).

These beneficial effects of education have also been found in centenarians. Studies have shown that higher levels of education, as well as higher estimates of intelligence known as premorbid IQ, have been associated with increased cognitive function in centenarian populations (Ishioka et al., 2016; Beker et al., 2021). Not only can early-life education be protective, but higher lifetime cognitive activity and current cognitive activity levels in centenarians were correlated with higher cognitive performance (Beker et al., 2021; Kliegel et al., 2004). These results in centenarians suggest that engaging in intellectual and mentally stimulating activities can serve as a protective buffer from dementia.

Additionally, social activity has been demonstrated to play a role in cognition and reducing risk for dementia (Sommerlad et al., 2019). Higher levels of social support are associated with increased life satisfaction, ability to perform activities of daily living, and cognitive function among centenarians (MacDonald, 2007; Wu et al., 2017; Jopp et al., 2016; Wang et al., 2015). Spouses, children, or close friends of centenarians can serve as impactful sources of social support. In one study of centenarians, having more close friends and higher levels of social contact were correlated with increased cognitive performance (Wang et al., 2015). Given that social support has been identified as a protective factor in reducing risk for dementia, research suggests that participation in social activities throughout older adulthood can be helpful for increasing longevity and promoting cognitive function in centenarians.

5.12 Current Limitations in Centenarian Research

While former studies have provided estimates as to the prevalence rates of dementia among centenarians (Beker et al., 2020), it is important to note that the accuracy of these estimates have been called into question. This is largely due to the many limitations surrounding centenarian research which often leads to wide variations in the reporting of dementia prevalence among centenarians (Brodaty et al., 2016; Calvert Jr. et al., 2006; Poon et al., 2012). For example, in a literature review performed by Calvert and colleagues, they discovered multiple inconsistencies in the methods used by prior centenarian studies (Calvert Jr. et al., 2006). It was therefore concluded that these inconsistencies make it impossible to reach a definitive conclusion regarding the extent to which aging without dementia is ultimately achievable. In the discussion that follows, we review the most common limitations in centenarian research and considerations for future research.

5.13 Sample Size

A particular challenge centenarian studies face is when investigators are tasked with acquiring an adequate sample size. Acquiring an adequate sample size is essential to accurately detect meaningful differences within a sample which can then be generalized to a larger population (Biau et al., 2008). However, since centenarians make up such a small percentage of the population and are typically quite frail and fragile due to their extreme age, it can be challenging to obtain a sufficient number of individuals (Calvert Jr. et al., 2006). Additionally, while a significant number of centenarians reside in nursing homes (Fries et al., 2000), caution should be exercised when considering these individuals to be cognitively impaired. Their inability to live independently may not be due to cognitive impairment, but a result of social or physical circumstances that may limit their ability to live independently. Considering all these individuals to be cognitively impaired may result in an overestimation of the prevalence of cognitive impairment in this population (Calvert Jr. et al., 2006).

5.14 Convenience Sampling & Selection Bias

Difficulties surrounding the recruitment and enrollment of centenarians can further lead to selection bias due to investigators selecting subjects based off convenience (Calvert Jr. et al., 2006). Selection bias is especially detrimental when attempting to make distinctions between racial groups or special populations such as centenarians living in rural areas, and those in developing nations (Calvert Jr. et al., 2006). Multiple prior studies have shown that individuals who fit into one or more of these groups are at significantly higher risk of developing dementia due to risk factors such as limited access to healthcare, variations in health conditions, and lower institutional support (Alzheimers Dement, 2020; Van Patten & Tremont, 2020; Rosenthal & Fox, 2000). For perspective, the Alzheimer's Association reports that the likelihood of having dementia is approximately double for black/African Americans, and roughly one and a half times more likely for Hispanics/Latinos compared to dementia risk in caucasians (Alzheimers Dement, 2020). Despite this increased risk, these groups continue to be underrepresented in centenarian research further limiting accurate estimates of dementia prevalence among centenarians (Calvert Jr. et al., 2006).

5.15 Cognitive & Functional Assessments

Early research evaluating levels of cognitive impairment in centenarians utilized assessment methods generally used in clinical geriatric practice to diagnose dementia, including the DSM III-R and DSM-IV (Samuelsson et al., 1997; Ravaglia et al., 1999). However, it was discovered that these methods may not give reliable results when evaluating centenarians due to an extensive interview process, which proved to be very demanding for this group of individuals (Arosio et al., 2017). More recent research has instead focused on employing the Mini-Mental State Examination (MMSE) to evaluate cognitive impairment in centenarians.

The MMSE was specifically developed by a group of researchers who wished to address the difficulty of completing lengthy cognitive batteries with elderly patients, and particularly those suffering from dementia (Folstein et al., 1975). While the batteries available at the time required over 30 min to administer and score, the MMSE was able to be administered in only 5–10 min by concentrating solely on the cognitive aspects of mental functions such as orientation to time and place, attention and memory, concentration, language, and praxis (Arosio et al., 2017). To this day, the MMSE remains one of the most widely used instruments for assessing cognitive functioning.

However, while centenarian research most commonly utilizes the MMSE, it has been brought into question whether it is appropriate for evaluating cognitive impairment in these individuals (Arosio et al., 2017; Slavin et al., 2013). For example, a survey performed by Arioso et al. on the cognitive status of centenarians noted that since many centenarians experience visual, auditory, and tactile deficits, this can result in an inability to complete the final portion of the MMSE which includes reading text and copying a drawing (Arosio et al., 2017). This inability to complete the MMSE can lead to inaccurate reporting of dementia prevalence in centenarians.

Notably, in a review of 23 centenarian studies by Poon et al., it was found that a range of 27%–75% prevalence of dementia was being reported (Poon et al., 2012). Poon et al. asserted that this was likely due in part to a utilization of cognitive assessments which are not validated for use with centenarians potentially leading to haphazard results. Future research which aims to validate and standardize cognitive assessments for use with centenarians is essential for the most accurate estimates of dementia prevalence among this demographic.

5.16 Conclusion & Recommendations for the Future

Although dementia prevalence continues to rise around the world, many centenarians have shown that aging without developing dementia is achievable. There is still much we can learn from this incredible group of individuals. Studying the characteristics of centenarians and the factors associated with healthy aging into older adulthood can elucidate potential interventions for dementia throughout the lifespan. However, due to the limitations described earlier, it is difficult to reach a definitive conclusion regarding to what extent aging without dementia is ultimately achievable. To answer these questions, greater efforts must be made to address the current limitations in the literature. Albeit imperfect, one way to overcome the current limitation, to reveal protective mechanisms from AD pathology and cognitive impairment due to AD pathology, is to study family members of centenarians who are also predisposed to longer cognitive health spans. In doing so, this could ultimately result in a greater number of individuals that live longer and cognitively healthier lives.

Acknowledgements Acknowledgement to Arianne Fritts, MS for editing support.

End of Chapter Questions

1. What is the most common cause of dementia?
   (a) Lewy-body disease
   (b) Alzheimer's disease
   (c) Pick's disease
   (d) Cardiovascular disease
2. How can dementia be diagnosed clinically?
   (a) Taking a medical history & performing a neurological examination
   (b) Neuroimaging methods (ie. PET scan)
   (c) Neuropsychologic testing
   (d) All the above
3. What is the strongest risk factor for the development of dementia?
   (a) Diabetes
   (b) Family history
   (c) Age
   (d) Smoking

Answers: b, d, c

References

2020 Alzheimer's disease facts and figures. Alzheimer's Dement., 16: 391–460.
Arosio, B., et al. (2017). Cognitive status in the oldest old and centenarians: a condition crucial for quality of life methodologically difficult to assess. *Mechanisms of Ageing and Development*, 185–194.
Beker, N., et al. (2020). Longitudinal maintenance of cognitive health in centenarians in the 100-plus study. *JAMA Network Open*, e200094.

Beker, N., et al. (2021). Association of Cognitive Function Trajectories in centenarians with post-mortem neuropathology, physical health, and other risk factors for cognitive decline. *JAMA Network Open, 4*(1), e2031654.

Biau, D. J., Kerneis, S., & Porcher, R. (2008). Statistics in brief: The importance of sample size in the planning and interpretation of medical research. *Clinical Orthopaedics and Related Research, 466*(9), 2282–2288.

Brodaty, H., et al. (2016). ICC-dementia (international centenarian consortium – dementia): An international consortium to determine the prevalence and incidence of dementia in centenarians across diverse ethnoracial and sociocultural groups. *BMC Neurology, 16*, 52.

Buettner, D., & Skemp, S. (2016). Blue zones: Lessons from the World's longest lived. *American Journal of Lifestyle Medicine, 10*(5), 318–321.

Calvert, J. F., Jr., et al. (2006). Dementia-free survival among centenarians: An evidence-based review. *The Journals of Gerontology: Series A., 61*, 951–956.

Centers for Disease Control. (2019). What is Dementia? Available from: https://www.cdc.gov/aging/dementia/index.html

Davey, A., et al. (2013). Profiles of cognitive functioning in a population-based sample of centenarians using factor mixture analysis. *Experimental Aging Research, 39*(2), 125–144.

Feng, L., et al. (2022). Malnutrition is positively associated with cognitive decline in centenarians and oldest-old adults: A cross-sectional study. *eClinicalMedicine*, 47.

Folstein, M. F., Folstein, S. E., & Mchugh, P. R. (1975). "Mini-mental state" a practical method for grading the cognitive state of patients for the clinician*. *Journal of Psychiatric Research*, Pergamon Press, 189–198.

Fratiglioni, L., & Hui-Xin, W. (2007). Brain reserve hypothesis in dementia. *Journal of Alzheimer's Disease, 12*(1), 11–22.

Fries, B. E., et al. (2000). Accelerated dysfunction among the very oldest-old in nursing homes. *The Journals of Gerontology. Series A, Biological Sciences and Medical Sciences, 55*(6), M336–M341.

Hai, S., et al. (2017). Association between nutrition status and cognitive impairment among Chinese nonagenarians and centenarians. *International Journal of Gerontology, 11*(4), 215–219.

Hernández-Vicente, A., et al. (2019). Physical activity and sedentary behavior at the end of the human lifespan. *Journal of Aging and Physical Activity, 27*(4), 899–905.

Huang, J. (2021). Alzheimer disease – Neurologic disorders. Available from: https://www.merckmanuals.com/professional/neurologic-disorders/delirium-and-dementia/alzheimer-disease#

Huang, J. *Dementia – Neurologic Disorders*. 2021 [cited 2022 December 01]. Available from: https://www.merckmanuals.com/professional/neurologic-disorders/delirium-and-dementia/dementia

Ishioka, Y. L., et al. (2016). Effects of the APOE ε4 allele and education on cognitive function in Japanese centenarians. *Age, 38*(5–6), 495–503.

James, B. D., et al. (2016). TDP-43 stage, mixed pathologies, and clinical Alzheimer's-type dementia. *Brain, 139*(11), 2983–2993.

Jopp, D. S., et al. (2016). Physical, cognitive, social and mental health in near-centenarians and centenarians living in New York City: Findings from the Fordham centenarian study. *BMC Geriatrics, 16*(1), 1.

Kliegel, M., Zimprich, D., & Rott, C. (2004). Life-long intellectual activities mediate the predictive effect of early education on cognitive impairment in centenarians: A retrospective study. *Aging & Mental Health, 8*(5), 430–437.

Leitão, C., et al. (2022). The effect of nutrition on aging – A systematic review focusing on aging-related biomarkers. *Nutrients, 14*(3), 554.

MacDonald, M. (2007). Social support for centenarians' health, psychological well-being, and longevity. *Annual Review of Gerontology and Geriatrics, 27*(1), 107–127.

Ozaki, A., et al. (2007). The Japanese centenarian study: Autonomy was associated with health practices as well as physical status. *Journal of the American Geriatrics Society, 55*(1), 95–101.

Panza, F., et al. (2004). Mediterranean diet and cognitive decline. *Public Health Nutrition, 7*(7), 959–963.

Perls, T. (2004). Dementia-free centenarians. *Experimental Gerontology, 39*(11–12), 1587–1593.
Poon, L. W., et al. (2012). Understanding dementia prevalence among centenarians. *The Journals of Gerontology: Series A., 67A*, 358–365.
Qiu, C., & Fratiglioni, L. (2018). Aging without dementia is achievable: Current evidence from epidemiological research. *Journal of Alzheimer's Disease., 62*, 933–942.
Ravaglia, G., et al. (1999). Prevalence and severity of dementia among northern Italian centenarians. *Neurology, 53*(2), 416–418.
Rosenthal, T. C., & Fox, C. (2000). Access to health care for the rural elderly. *JAMA, 284*(16), 2034–2036.
Samuelsson, S. M., et al. (1997). The Swedish centenarian study: A multidisciplinary study of five consecutive cohorts at the age of 100. *International Journal of Aging and Human Development*, Baywood Publishing Inc., 223–253.
Scheltens, P., et al. (2021). Alzheimer's disease. *Lancet, 397*(10284), 1577–1590.
Sebastiani, P., et al. (2019a). A serum protein signature of APOE genotypes in centenarians. *Aging Cell, 18*(6), e13023.
Sebastiani, P., et al. (2019b). APOE alleles and extreme human longevity. *The Journals of Gerontology: Series A, 74*(1), 44–51.
Slavin, M. J., Brodaty, H., & Sachdev, P. S. (2013). Challenges of diagnosing dementia in the oldest old population. *The Journals of Gerontology. Series A, Biological Sciences and Medical Sciences, 68*(9), 1103–1111.
Sommerlad, A., et al. (2019). Association of social contact with dementia and cognition: 28-year follow-up of the Whitehall II cohort study. *PLoS Medicine, 16*(8), e1002862.
Song, R., et al. (2021). Association of cardiovascular risk burden with risk of dementia and brain pathologies: A population-based cohort study. *Alzheimer's & Dementia, 17*(12), 1914–1922.
Stefanacci, R. G. (2022). Overview of aging – Older People's health issues. Merck Manuals Consumer Version; Available from: https://www.merckmanuals.com/home/older-people%E2%80%99s-health-issues/the-aging-body/overview-of-aging
Tanprasertsuk, J., et al. (2021). Carotenoid-rich brain nutrient pattern is positively correlated with higher cognition and lower depression in the oldest old with no dementia. *Frontiers in Nutrition, 8*, 704691.
Terry, D. F., et al. (2003). Cardiovascular advantages among the offspring of centenarians. *The Journals of Gerontology. Series A, Biological Sciences and Medical Sciences, 58*(5), M425–M431.
Terry, D. F., et al. (2004). Lower all-cause, cardiovascular, and cancer mortality in centenarians' offspring. *Journal of the American Geriatrics Society, 52*(12), 2074–2076.
Toepper, M. (2017). Dissociating Normal aging from Alzheimer's disease: A view from cognitive neuroscience. *Journal of Alzheimer's Disease, 57*(2), 331–352.
Van Patten, R., & Tremont, G. (2020). Public knowledge of late-life cognitive decline and dementia in an international sample. *Dementia (London), 19*(6), 1758–1776.
Wang, B., He, P., & Dong, B. (2015). Associations between social networks, social contacts, and cognitive function among Chinese nonagenarians/centenarians. *Archives of Gerontology and Geriatrics, 60*(3), 522–527.
Wang, C., et al. (2022). Sardinian dietary analysis for longevity: A review of the literature. *Journal of Ethnic Foods, 9*(1), 33.
Willcox, B. J., et al. (2006a). Siblings of Okinawan centenarians share lifelong mortality advantages. *The Journals of Gerontology: Series A, 61*(4), 345–354.
Willcox, D. C., et al. (2006b). Genetic determinants of exceptional human longevity: Insights from the Okinawa centenarian study. *Age, 28*(4), 313–332.
Wu, T., et al. (2017). Factors associated with activities of daily life disability among centenarians in rural Chongqing, China: A cross-sectional study. *International Journal of Environmental Research and Public Health, 14*(11), 1364.
Xiang, Q., et al. (2021). Studying the interplay between apolipoprotein E and education on cognitive decline in centenarians using Bayesian Beta regression. *Frontiers in Genetics, 11*, 606831.

Chapter 6
Nutrition in Centenarians

Galya Bigman and Alice S. Ryan

Key Take Away Points

1. Traditional dietary patterns are associated with longevity and reduced risk of prevalent chronic diseases, in particular cardiovascular diseases.
2. While variations exist, traditional diets have certain common features among centenarians including: high consumption of seasonal foods, preferences for root vegetables and legumes, use of vegetable oils, and limited intake of whole fat dairy and other animal products as well as avoiding any intake of processed foods.
3. Caloric restriction is associated with slowing the aging process in many animal species and it might affect aging among human, though more studies are needed in this area.

G. Bigman
Veterans Affairs Maryland Health Care System, GRECC, Baltimore, MD, USA
e-mail: bigman.galya@gmail.com

A. S. Ryan (✉)
University of Maryland School of Medicine and Department of Veterans Affairs RR&D SRCS, Baltimore, MD, USA
e-mail: aryan@som.umaryland.edu

R. E. Kheirbek, M. D. Llorente (eds.), *Current Perspectives on Centenarians*, International Perspectives on Aging 36,
https://doi.org/10.1007/978-3-031-30915-1_6

6.1 Dietary Patterns and Longevity

6.1.1 Introduction

A dietary pattern is defined as the quantities, proportions, variety, or combination of different foods, drinks, and nutrients in diets and the frequency with which they are habitually consumed (United States Department of Agriculture, 2014). The components of a dietary pattern interact and have cumulative effects on health and longevity (Cespedes & Hu, 2015; Guasch-Ferré & Willett, 2021). Traditional diets such as Mediterranean, Okinawan, and Nordic diets describe an eating pattern that prevails in a certain geographical area and/or cultural heritage (Willcox et al., 2014). A diverse diet provides adequate nutritional quality, so there will be no widespread nutrient deficiency among a population, increasing their likelihood of survival.

Besides special food components with high nutritional values, traditional dietary patterns incorporate sustainable lifestyle behaviors passed from generation to generation over the years. It combines knowledge, abilities and practices of local cuisine, enriching not only food colors and aromas but also preserving nutritional values (Lorenzo et al., 2022). These eating behaviors emphasize the necessity of the connection of food with its natural environment and its seasonality as well as the importance of preparing and eating family-based meals and/or with other members of the community (Dominguez et al., 2021, 2022).

Since the mid-twentieth century, it has been observed that traditional diets are commonly seen in countries that have the lowest rates of chronic disease and the highest concentration of centenarians. These include Japan, the Mediterranean Basin (e.g., Italy, Greece), Europe (e.g., France, Spain), and the Nordic countries (Dominguez et al., 2022; Vasto et al., 2014). Within these places, there are even regions dubbed '*Blue Zones*' where people live the longest and are the healthiest: Okinawa, Japan; Sardinia, Italy; Nicoya, Costa Rica; Ikaria, Greece, and Loma Linda, California (Buettner, 2008; Buettner & Skemp, 2016).

This led to the development of studies that have intensively examined the components of traditional diets that promote health and longevity to benefit other populations (Dominguez et al., 2022; Guasch-Ferré & Willett, 2021; Teixeira et al., 2017; Yeung et al., 2021). Some studies provide scientific explanations for the long life expectancy and, most importantly, the long health span of centenarians despite having limited access to healthcare in some cases (Dominguez et al., 2022; Yeung et al., 2021). In particular, the Mediterranean dietary pattern has been extensively researched, where ample studies have proven that it reduces the risks for morbidity and mortality from chronic diseases (Guasch-Ferré & Willett, 2021), and therefore its principles have been incorporated into various dietary guidelines including those for Americans.

With mounting evidence for the beneficial nutrient components found in traditional diets, more modern dietary patterns have been developed. The purpose of these modified diets was to treat and or prevent a specific chronic health problem prevalent in Western regions, such as heart disease, diabetes, cancer, and dementia.

The popular modified dietary patterns include the Dietary Approaches to Stop Hypertension (DASH) (Filippou et al., 2020); the Portfolio diet designed to lower cholesterol levels (Chiavaroli et al., 2018), and the Mediterranean-DASH Diet Intervention for Neurodegenerative Delay (MIND) (van den Brink et al., 2019). Nutrition studies will construct a diet quality index (DQI) based on adherence to a specific dietary pattern, such as the Mediterranean diet score, in order to examine its relationship with aging and age-related diseases. (Jacobs Jr & Orlich, 2014). Another approach to examining the impact of dietary patterns on health is the posterior approach in which dietary patterns are derived from statistical modeling, such as factor analysis, using data from food records or food frequency questionnaires (FFQ) often resulting in two distinct patterns: Prudent/Traditional vs. Western (Jacobs Jr & Orlich, 2014).

In the following sections we will introduce and describe in detail traditional dietary patterns common among centenarians in different regions including the Mediterranean, Okinawan, and Nordic diets as well as the Southern European Atlantic Diet (SEAD). Also, we will discuss the scientific evidence on the relationships between traditional diets and chronic diseases and their potential effects on longevity.

6.1.2 Traditional Dietary Patterns

6.1.2.1 Japan and the Okinawan dietary patterns

Japan is well known for its long life expectancy. In 9/2022 Japan reached 72 centenarians per 100,000 population compared to the USA with 28 centenarians per 100,000 population (Japantimes, 2022). The traditional dietary cultures of Japan are collectively known as "*Washoku*" and were recognized on the United Nations Educational, Scientific and Cultural Organization (UNESCO) list of "Intangible Cultural Heritage." The guiding principles of *Washoku* are "a staple food —rice— which is complemented by a variety of side dishes, soup, and pickles" (Gabriel et al., 2018; Yoshiike et al., 2007). *Washoku* is characterized by high consumption of fish and soybean products and low consumption of animal fat and meat. It relies on the effective use of *umami* taste to enhance palatability. *Umami* translates to "pleasant savory taste" and is described as brothy or meaty. Most of the calories come from carbohydrates in rice, which make up 60–65% of total calories, while fats make up 20–25% and proteins make up 5–10% (Dominguez et al., 2022). Small portions of food, in particular seasonal items, are consumed at each meal, while having regular dietary habits with three meals a day. One eats until you are about 80% full (Dominguez et al., 2022; Pignolo, 2019; Willcox et al., 2009).

To preserve and promote their traditional dishes, in 2005, Japan released pictorial dietary guidelines. The pictorial guidelines describe four layers allocated in the inverted cone: the highest consisted of dishes containing grains (i.e., rice, noodles); the next layer comprised plant-based dishes (i.e., vegetables and soups); the third layer was composed of fish, meat, eggs, and soy-bean dishes; the fourth layer included fruit and dairy products (Yoshiike et al., 2007).

Within Japan, however, the longest-lived Japanese inhabit the southernmost islands, known as the Ryukyu Islands (or Okinawa prefecture) (Willcox et al., 2009, 2014). The traditional diet followed in Okinawa by its long-lived population is highly dense in nutrients and low in calories. This diet is different from the traditional Japanese diet, with up to 85% of calories coming from carbohydrates (plant-based foods), mainly in the form of root vegetables (orange and purple sweet potatoes), a high intake of phytochemicals from green and yellow vegetables (e.g., bitter melon, cabbage, carrots, Chinese okra, pumpkin, and green papaya), and whole grains (millet, wheat, rice, and noodles). Soybean-based foods are the main source of quality protein (e.g. tofu, miso, natto, and edamame).

The diet also is high in marine-sourced carotenoids, such as seaweed, algae, and kelp that are low in caloric density with a low omega-6/omega-3 ratio. The Okinawan diet is also low in saturated fats derived from a limited consumption of eggs, lean meats, and dairy products. Medicinal plants, garnishes, and spices (e.g., turmeric, mugwort, moringa, Okinawan peppers, and fennel seeds), tea and alcohol (*'Awamori'*, a rice-based distilled liquor) are moderately consumed among centenarians as well (Table 6.1) (Dominguez et al., 2022; Willcox et al., 2009, 2014).

6.1.2.2 The Mediterranean dietary pattern

According to UNESCO, the Mediterranean diet was recognized as an "Intangible Cultural Heritage of France, Italy, Greece, Spain and Morocco" in 2010 (UNESCO, 2013), thereby preserving the local biodiversity characteristics of Mediterranean countries and promoting a dietary pattern beneficial to human health (Ndlovu et al., 2019). Since the traditional cuisines differ slightly among Greece, Italy and other countries around the Mediterranean Sea there are different versions of the traditional Mediterranean diet. The consequence was to develop a Mediterranean diet pyramid emphasizing the amount and intake of certain foods from the diets of Crete, Greece and southern Italy (Table 6.1) (Bach-Faig et al., 2011; Monteagudo et al., 2015). During the mid-twentieth century, populations from these regions had the lowest incidence of cardiovascular diseases with life expectancies among the oldest in the world. Some of the regions still have a high concentration of centenarians. In Sardinia Italy for instance, the rate is 33.6 for every 100,000 inhabitants with exceptional male longevity (Wang et al., 2022). Also, on the small Greek island of Ikaria, there is a high rate of centenarians, where every third person lives to be over 90 years old and in reasonable health.

Traditionally, the Mediterranean diet consists largely of plant-derived foods and high intakes of fat derived from extra virgin (cold-pressed) olive oil (the chief source of dietary fat, for cooking and seasoning), tree nuts, and fatty fish. The diet provides about 40% of calories from fat, mostly monounsaturated and polyunsaturated fats, 40% from carbohydrates, preferably whole grain, and 20% of calories from protein. Specifically, the diet emphases daily consumption of colorful varied and seasonal

Table 6.1 Differences between servings in the Okinawan diet, Mediterranean diet, Nordic diet, and the Southern European Atlantic Diet (SEAD)

Components		Okinawan Diet[a]	Mediterranean Diet[b]	Nordic Diet[c]	SEAD[d]
Main Zone		Okinawa, Japan	Sardinia, Sicilian, Southern Italy. Ikaria, Greece, Crete	Denmark, Finland, Iceland, Norway, and Sweden.	Northern Portugal and Galicia, Spain
Vegetables		≥6 servings/day. Root and green-yellow vegetables e.g., sweet potato, bitter melon daikon radish, cabbage, carrots, okra, pumpkin, green papaya	≥2 servings/main meal (or ≥ 6 servings/day). Colorful varied and seasonal vegetables & leafy green vegetables. At least one of the serving should be raw. At most ≤3 servings/week of potatoes.	Vegetables/Root vegetables, >3 servings/day (or ≥ 500 per day) Potatoes, >2.5 servings/day	≥2 servings/day Brassicas, ≥3 servings/week Potatoes, ≥1 servings/day
Fresh fruits		1 servings/day. Tropical fruit	1–2 servings/main meal (or 3–6 servings/day)	Fruits (berries), >3 servings/day	≥3 servings/day
Carbohydrate	% Carbohydrates[e]	60–85%	40%	50%	40–60%
	Legumes	Soy, ≥2 servings/day	≥2 servings/week	No recommendation	2–3 servings/week of pulses.
	Grains/Cereal/Bread	Rice, 2–3 servings/day. Whole-grain, 6–7 servings/day Preferred low-glycemic index (millet, wheat, rice, noodles)	1–2 servings/main meal (or 3–6 servings/day). Unprocessed grains. Preferably whole grain (bread, pasta, rice, couscous).	Bread, 4–6 slices/day. Cereals, 1.5 servings/day (muesli, oat bran, barley flakes). Wholegrain pasta enriched with β-Glucans, 3 servings/week	6–8 servings/day

(continued)

Table 6.1 (continued)

Components		Okinawan Diet[a]	Mediterranean Diet[b]	Nordic Diet[c]	SEAD[d]
Protein	% Protein[e]	9–15%	20%	25%	15–20%
	Fish and/or Sea food	Fish, 2–3 servings/week. Oily fish with high Omega 3 fatty acids.	Fish and/or shellfish, ≥2 servings/week.	Fish, 3–5 servings/week Fatty freshwater or saltwater fish.	Fish and Seafood, 3–4 servings/week
	Meat/Poultry/ Pork	Restricted (Beef, poultry). Mostly ear lean pork.	Red meat, <2 servings/week (lean cuts) White (Poultry) meat, 2 servings/week Processed meat. < 1 serving/ week	Meat, ≤5 servings/week Poultry, ≤3 servings/week	Lean meat, 3–4 servings/week Pork/Poultry/ Game/Veal
	Dairy products	Limited consumption	2 servings/day. Low fat yoghurt, cheese and other fermented dairy products.	1–2 servings/week E.g., low-fat milk and fermented milk	3–4 servings/ day
	Eggs	Limited consumption	2–4 servings/week.	Egg, as long as the intake of cholesterol not exceeded the recommendation	3–4 servings/ week
Fat	% Fat[e]	6–28%	40%	25%	25–35%
	Vegetable oil	Frequent use of canola oil	Olive oil, 1 serving/main meal	Frequent use of canola oil	3–4 servings/ day of olive oil
	Nuts	Low	1–2 servings/day. Nuts and/or seeds	0.5 servings/day Mainly almonds (or 15 g/day)	4–6 servings/ week. Chestnuts, walnuts, almonds & hazelnuts
	% Saturated fat[e]	<7%	<10%	<8%	5–10%

Alcohol	Moderate. 'Awamori', a rice-based distilled liquor	Women 1 drink/day. Men 1–2 drinks/day. Wine/fermented beverages (beer) with meals.	Subjects' habitual amount e.g., low-alcohol beer in moderation.	Wine, ≥1 servings/day
Herbs, spices, or staple	Turmeric, mugwort, seaweed, kelp, bamboo shoots	Spices, herbs, garlic and onions for flavors and palatability to dishes and contribute to the reduction of salt addition.	Parsley, dill, mustard, horseradish, chive. bullion, mustard, vinaigrette, cooking wine, spices, soy sauce, oat-based non-dairy creamer, potato starch and yeast. Table salt with reduced sodium content	Olive oil is used as a dressing and in cooking.
Sweets	No added sugars/refined sweets	<2 servings/week.	Only during the weekends	A few times per month
Water/hot drink/beverages	Green tea, ≥3 servings/day	1.5–2.0 liter of water/day.	Tap water, tea/herb tea, filtered/ instant coffee. Fruits/berries/ vegetables juice.	6–8 servings/ day

[a] Willcox et al. (2009)
[b] Bach-Faig et al. (2011), Lorenzo et al., (2022), Monteagudo et al. (2015)
[c] Adamsson et al. (2012), Lorenzo et al. (2022)
[d] Calvo-Malvar et al. (2016), Lorenzo et al. (2022)
[e] % From the total kcal

vegetables including leafy green vegetables and fresh fruits, as well as unprocessed grains, mostly whole grains (bread, pasta, rice, couscous). Dairy products that are preferred are in the form of low fat yoghurt, cheese and other fermented dairy products. Several times per week, various types of pulses/legumes and nuts and seeds are consumed. Fish, red and processed meats are consumed in small portions. Low intakes of eggs serve as sources of high-grade proteins and occasional consumption of sweets, cakes, and dairy desserts in small amounts are seen. Herbs and spices for flavoring; drinking plenty of water as the main beverage; and consumption of wine in moderation (for women ≤1drink/day and 1– 2 drinks/day for men) always with meals (Table 6.1) (Davis et al., 2015; Dominguez et al., 2022; Martínez-González et al., 2017; Trichopoulou et al., 2014; Vasto et al., 2014).

6.1.2.3 The Nordic dietary pattern

As part of the Nordic dietary pattern (also known as the New Nordic Diet and Baltic Sea Diet), local foods are typically consumed in line with the Nordic dietary guidelines (Massara et al., 2022) that encourage the consumption of whole foods, sourced locally and in season. The diet was developed in Copenhagen as a model of a healthy and sustainable diet integrating gastronomic traditions and foods consumed in five Nordic countries: Denmark, Finland, Iceland, Norway, and Sweden (Meltzer et al., 2019). The dietary pattern recommends increasing the intake of vegetables (especially root vegetables like beets, turnips and carrots), pulses, fruits and berries (bilberries, lingonberries and strawberries), fish and seafood (especially fatty fish like salmon, tuna, sardines and mackerel to get omega-3 fatty acids), and nuts and seeds (Table 6.1).

Dietary guidelines recommend replacing refined cereals with wholegrain ones enriched with β-Glucans, such as rye, wheat, and oats. Similarly, butter is replaced with vegetable oils, particularly canola, rapeseed and olive oils, and high-fat dairy is switched with low-fat and fermented dairy products. The diet limits saturated fat and red meat and encourages the consumption of lean meats such as poultry and game. Additionally, it limits sugar-sweetened beverages, foods with added sugar, salt, and alcohol e.g., low-alcohol beer is consumed in moderation (Adamsson et al., 2012; Meltzer et al., 2019).

6.1.2.4 The Southern European Atlantic Diet (SEAD)

The Southern Europe Atlantic Diet (SEAD) is the traditional diet consumed in the Northwestern region of the Iberian Peninsula: Galicia (Spain) and northern Portugal. The diet is based on fresh, local, and seasonal ingredients. In this diet, there is a high intake of fish, seafood, cereals, potatoes, legumes, fruits, dairy products and vegetables. Meat, preferably lean meat, is consumed moderately as well as eggs and wine. The SEAD is considered more than a diet. It is a lifestyle where simple cooking techniques, respect for traditions, and the pleasure of eating together are constants (Cambeses-Franco et al., 2021; Lorenzo et al., 2022) (Table 6.1).

6.1.3 Dietary Patterns and Chronic Diseases

A large body of medical literature among various populations from across contrasting countries and cultures including those outside the Mediterranean region showed strong evidence for the benefits of the Mediterranean diet on several health outcomes. In particular, reduced risks for cardiovascular diseases and the associated risk factors of hypertension, obesity metabolic syndrome, and dyslipidemia are consistently found. Decreased cancer incidence and mortality, reduced risks for age-related cognitive dysfunction and lower incidence of neurodegenerative disorders are also seen (Becerra-Tomás et al., 2020; Guasch-Ferré & Willett, 2021; Rosato et al., 2019; Wu & Sun, 2017). For example, two meta-analysis studies of long-term cohorts and randomized trials strongly indicated a reduction of up to 38% in the risk of several cardiovascular outcomes among those who were in the highest versus the lowest category of Mediterranean diet adherence (Becerra-Tomás et al., 2020; Guasch-Ferré & Willett, 2021; Rosato et al., 2019). Another meta-analysis of longitudinal studies showed that higher adherence to the Mediterranean diet was associated with less cognitive decline (Wu & Sun, 2017).

In the Mediterranean diet, plant foods are consumed in high amounts (fruits, vegetables, bread and other cereals, potatoes, beans, nuts, and seeds), which provide vitamins, phytochemicals, antioxidants (e.g. vitamins C, E, and A), flavonoids, potassium, folate, minerals, and fibers. Moderate intakes of wine provide ethanol and polyphenols. A high intake of oleic acid abundant in olive oil and omega-3 fatty acids abundant in fish have plentiful nutrients and bioactive compounds and are thought to contribute to reducing the risk of age-related chronic diseases through anti-inflammatory, antithrombotic, antioxidative and anti-oncogenic pathways and favorable metabolic effects (Clinton et al., 2020).

Similar to the Mediterranean diet, the Okinawa diet showed associations with impressive health benefits, including lower risk for obesity, diabetes, and numerous age-associated diseases including cardiovascular diseases and certain cancers (Dominguez et al., 2022; Galbete et al., 2018; Massara et al., 2022; Willcox et al., 2009, 2014). Obesity prevalence is less than 4% in Japan, much less than the prevalence in Europe (15%) and in the USA (36%), where obesity largely contributes to the high prevalence of non-communicable diseases. Due to a large number of scarce intakes of saturated fats and large quantities of antioxidant and anti-inflammatory compounds in the Okinawa diet and the low omega-6/omega-3 ratio, the incidence of prostate, colon, and breast cancers is about 50% lower than in the rest of Japan. Moreover, people from Okinawa have a further reduced risk of cardiovascular and cerebrovascular disease than Japanese people living in metropolitan areas (Dominguez et al., 2022).

As for the Nordic diet, a recent study found that although people with higher adherence to such a diet showed a reduction in their risk of major cardiovascular disease outcomes and diabetes, the reduction was relatively small. The authors found similar reductions or greater reductions in the secondary outcomes of LDL-cholesterol, apolipoprotein B, insulin, body weight, body mass index, systolic blood pressure and other intermediate cardiometabolic risk factors (Massara et al., 2022). In the EPIC-Potsdam cohort study, participants were German, middle-aged, generally health, and followed for a mean of 10.6 years. Dietary scores to assess adherence to the Mediterranean diet and the Nordic diet were examined (separately). The incidence of major chronic diseases was then calculated and the health outcomes of the two diets compared. The authors concluded that the Nordic diet had a possible beneficial effect on myocardial infarction in the overall population and on stroke in men, while the Mediterranean diet conferred a lower risk of diabetes in the overall population and of myocardial infarction in women (Galbete et al., 2018).

Only a few studies have examined the link between the SEAD diet and a reduced risk of chronic diseases and mortality (Calvo-Malvar et al., 2016; Guallar-Castillón et al., 2013). Its foundations are controversial since they diverge from the Mediterranean diet and other healthy dietary patterns. However, some bioactive compounds in SEAD have shown health benefits and protection against chronic diseases (Calvo-Malvar et al., 2016; Guallar-Castillón et al., 2013; Lorenzo et al., 2022). For example, the diet includes grapes and red wine which contain compounds with reported anticancer properties such as resveratrol and flavonoids. Additional bioactive compounds thought to confer beneficial health effects in this diet include: glucosinolates from brassica vegetables, omega-3 fatty acids consumed from fish and seafood, sterols found in nuts and olive oil, and carotenoids abundant in colored fruits and vegetables (Lorenzo et al., 2022).

6.1.4 Dietary Patterns and Longevity

In most cases, traditional diets, including other healthy dietary patterns such as DASH, have been associated with reduced risk of chronic diseases and all-cause mortality, in particular cardiovascular mortality, thus increasing longevity. Several nutritional studies across countries and cultures among older people have replicated these results. In these studies, older people who followed the Mediterranean diet demonstrated a significant reduction in the risk of death. A meta-analysis of 29 prospective studies found a reduction of 10% in all-cause mortality for every 2-point increase in the Mediterranean diet score. This reduction was even higher in those who lived in the Mediterranean region compared with non-Mediterranean areas (Soltani et al., 2019). These findings suggest that adherence to a traditional Mediterranean diet is linked with enhanced longevity and may even help to slow the aging process (Guasch-Ferré & Willett, 2021).

The Okinawan diet like the Mediterranean diet is rich in fruits and vegetables and low in meat and processed foods. This diet is rich in antioxidants and anti-inflammatory compounds that may protect against the damage caused by free radicals, which can contribute to aging and the development of chronic diseases. Furthermore, the moderate caloric restriction practiced by some older Okinawans may further contribute to their longevity (Willcox et al., 2009, 2014). Among a seniors-ENRICA-1 cohort, which included 3165 individuals in Spain, it was shown that higher adherence to the SEAD was associated with lower all-cause mortality. The protective association between SEAD and all-cause death was of a similar magnitude to that found for the Mediterranean diet (Carballo-Casla et al., 2021).

6.1.5 Conclusion

There is considerable heterogeneity among the dietary patterns that have been reviewed, each of which reflects a cultural pattern related to a certain region and population. Nevertheless, they are all traditional diets from unique regions with high rates of centenarians and relatively healthy people. Each diet consists of different types of foods depending on its region, for example, types of fish, fruits and berries, root vegetables, different grains, and the amount of alcohol consumed (Lankinen et al., 2019). Therefore, it is unlikely that there is one particular dietary pattern that promotes exceptional health and longevity (Hausman et al., 2011a).

However, despite such variation, there are some similarities among those diets that might explain their advantages for health and longevity. Firstly, traditional diets are based mostly on plant-derived products and unprocessed foods. They emphasize the abundant use of vegetables especially root vegetables and legumes, and the preferred intake of whole-grain products. Olive oil is an invaluable source of unsaturated fat in the Mediterranean diet, and other healthy fats such as those in canola oil, are used in other diets. Another commonality is that all of these traditional diets restrict the use of saturated fat (whole dairy) and red and processed meat. However, animal protein intake has considerable variation. It is relatively low in some diets e.g., Okinawan and higher in others e.g., SEAD and the Nordic diet.

The traditional diet is accompanied by a cluster of activities, such as unique cooking techniques that preserve nutrients and bioactive compounds better than other culinary methods, such as frying (Lorenzo et al., 2022). Additional abilities and practices include using fresh plants and herbs from the garden or the forest if applicable. Also, one of the main eating habits of longest-living people is to finish eating before they are full. Lastly, traditional diets emphasize low intake (or even avoidance) of red meat, saturated fat and full-fat dairy products, refined grains, sweets, processed/ultra-processed foods, salt, and sugar-sweetened beverages, which are usually common in Western diets. As can be seen, the Western diet, which frequently consists of high quantities of saturated fat, processed foods, refined grains, high sugar and corn-syrup content, is often associated with harmful health outcomes including cardiovascular diseases, some cancers, diabetes, Alzheimer's disease, and several other chronic diseases as well as with elevated mortality rates (Jardim et al., 2021).

6.2 Energy Balance and Body Composition in Centenarians

6.2.1 Resting Metabolic Rate

Resting metabolic rate (RMR) typically accounts for the largest portion of energy needs and is defined as the energy required by the body in a resting condition. RMR comprises approximately 60–80% of daily energy expenditure and is largely dependent on body mass, age, sex, and genetics (Livingston & Kohlstadt, 2005). Moreover, RMR is related to fat-free mass (FFM). If RMR is not directly measured by indirect calorimetry, there are various predictive equations for estimating RMR that include age, weight, height, or lean body mass. Methods to best measure RMR in adults are reviewed elsewhere (Compher et al., 2006).

In general, RMR declines markedly with advancing age in sedentary populations (van Pelt et al., 2001). A review of the literature concluded that a reduction in RMR occurs with aging which cannot be explained by changes in body composition and the loss of fat-free mass, including atrophy or decreases in mass of high metabolic rate organs (St-Onge & Gallagher, 2010). These authors describe that the loss of FFM cannot fully explain the 5–25% decrease in RMR in healthy elderly. Further, there is indirect evidence that the metabolic rate of individual organs is lower in older compared with younger individuals.

There are limited studies examining RMR in advanced age. Only one study was identified after a thorough literature search that utilized indirect calorimetry to measure resting metabolism in centenarians. In a study comparing middle-aged ($n = 26$, <65 years), older ($n = 27$, 66–94 years), and very old ($n = 28$, ≥95 years), RMR was measured by a portable indirect calorimeter. The middle-aged and very old women had a similar RMR (1404 ± 216 vs. 1324 ± 222 kcal/d) which was higher than that of older women (1065 ± 303 kcal/d) (Rizzo et al., 2005). Although in the entire sample, RMR was associated with FFM, in the very old, only waist-to-hip ratio was associated with RMR suggesting body fat distribution is a contributing factor in the oldest age group. Furthermore, it is possible that genetics or lifestyle plays a role in protecting the decline in RMR in centenarians generally observed with aging.

Resting metabolic rate was higher in men than women Portuguese centenarians by bioimpedance analysis (1350 ± 189 vs. 1123 ± 174 kcal, respectively) and estimated using the Harris Benedict eq. (1019 ± 172 vs. 935 ± 103 kcal/d, respectively) (Pereira da Silva et al., 2016). Both methods are in agreement by Bland Altman analysis suggesting that RMR can be estimated if needed. Moreover, the authors suggest that these actual values for metabolism in the centenarians do not appear low and estimate that the overall mean metabolic age based on standard values for muscle mass and metabolic rate was well below chronologic age by about 15 years. Furthermore, RMR was strongly correlated with FFM ($r = 0.993$) demonstrating the influence of muscle mass on basal metabolism. Another study in approximately 250 Portuguese centenarians (100.3 ± 2 yrs), basal metabolism was lower in centenarians (1177 ± 202 kcal) compared to controls (mean age 67.5 ± 3 yrs) with low cardiovascular risk (1356 ± 171 kcal) or high cardiovascular risk profile (1561 ± 268 kcal) (da Silva et al., 2018).

6.2.2 Adiposity and Leanness

The most accurate method to assess body composition in adults over the age of 100 is not clear. In a cross-sectional study in women centenarians in Brazil (Duarte et al., 2019), two inexpensive and simple methods (skinfolds and bioimpedance) were utilized to determine fat and lean mass and compared against the criterion method of deuterium oxide, considered a gold standard. There were 24 women in the study, of whom 25% were bedridden and ~ 37% had normal cognition. The average number of medications and comorbidities was approximately 5 and 3.7, respectively. In this small sample, the average body mass index (BMI) was less than 22 kg/m^2. With either skinfolds or bioelectrical impedance analysis (BIA), the determination of fat mass was in better agreement with that obtained by deuterium oxide than the determination of lean mass. Depending on the equation employed for skinfold methods, lean mass calculated with the Durnin and Womersley equation had the highest agreement with deuterium oxide. Given that 25% of the sample required testing on the bed, these common methods were feasible. Yet, this study would suggest that different methods are needed to evaluate fat and lean mass in women centenarians. In an even smaller sample of 14 centenarians in Italy (Paolisso et al., 1996), lean mass by anthropometry and BIA were highly correlated. A systematic review of literature up to May 2022 evaluated the use of BIA to determine body composition and hydration status in centenarians (Mandala et al., 2023). Only four of over 2000 studies were eligible for review indicating the lack of research in this area. BIA overestimates lean mass and underestimates fat mass compared to deuterium oxide dilution analysis in women centenarians (Duarte et al., 2019). In contrast, two other studies report that BIA agrees with anthropometric measures of fat mass in centenarians (Pereira da Silva et al., 2016) (da Silva et al., 2018).

Body composition changes with aging are generally described to reflect an increase in percent body fat and decrease in lean mass, and specific increases in abdominal fat mass. However, studies of body composition in centenarians are somewhat limited. A study conducted in Northern Italy, examined anthropometrics in 41 centenarian healthy free-living residents and compared their values to elderly groups and reference values (Ravaglia et al., 1997). Men were significantly taller and heavier than women centenarians without differences in BMI. Further, there were no differences in Waist-Hip Ratio (WHR) among centenarians but men over 90 years had central adiposity whereas women had peripheral adiposity by skinfold measurements. The centenarians had lower muscle and fat mass than nonagenarians.

Finally, anthropometric values were much lower than corresponding reference values in US and European surveys; however, the age-groups for reference values ranged from 65–74 or 85+ for certain American and European elderly subjects which at the time of this cross-sectional study illustrated the lack of normative values for adults over the age of 90 years and centenarians. In 252 Portuguese centenarians, the majority were of normal weight by BMI; yet, 25% were underweight and ~ 13% were overweight who tended to be women and men, respectively (Pereira da Silva et al., 2016). The authors further examined the prevalence of obesity by BIABias and reported it as 6% in the overall sample, although it was higher using anthropometric skinfold eqs. (43–77%). Using skinfold thickness at various sites and equations to predict body fat and density, Rizzo et al. (2005) found an average percent body fat of 25% in "long-lived" (>95 years old) participants which was significantly higher than adult subjects aged <65 years. The very old also had significantly lower BMI, fat mass, and FFM than middle-aged and older women. In approximately 1000 China Hainan centenarians, from the China Hainan Centenarian Cohort Study (CHCCS) (Yang et al., 2021), the average BMI was 18.1, and 57% were underweight, 39% was normal weight, 2.8% were overweight, and < 1% were obese (defined as BMI > =28 kg/m^2). Furthermore, the majority (88%) had a normal waist circumference and less than 12% were classified as obese by waist circumference (waist circumference (WC) > =90 cm in men and WC > =85 cm in women). In the China Hainan Centenarian Cohort Study, centenarian women had significantly reduced weight, height, waist circumference than females aged 80–99 years (Fu et al., 2021).

In centenarians from the state of Georgia, U.S. of whom almost 85% were women, 79% were white, and more than half lived in the community. The majority (~44%) were of normal weight range (Hausman et al., 2011b). In addition, over 30% had a BMI of ≤20 kg/m^2 and were classified as underweight, whereas almost 25% were classified as overweight/obese (BMI ≥25 kg/m^2). Moreover, triceps skinfold and mid-arm circumference of centenarians in the lowest BMI classification were on average below the 5th percentile for females compared to the National Health and Nutrition Examination Survey (NHANES) data. The median BMI for men and women was approximately 23 and 22 kg/m^2 respectively in centenarians from Warsaw Poland and fell within the normal range for most centenarians (Kollajtis-Dolowy et al., 2007). Likewise, in centenarians living in Okinawa, Japan, the average BMI was approximately 20 kg/m^2 in both men and women, was not different in male centenarians than male elderly but was significantly lower in women centenarians than elderly women (Chan et al., 1997).

6.2.3 Sarcopenia

Sarcopenia, originally described as a general loss of muscle mass that occurs with aging (Evans & Campbell, 1993), has undergone considerable study to determine clinical cutpoints. Lean mass measured by dual-energy x-ray absorptiometry is employed and compared to a young reference population (Baumgartner et al., 1998). Equations that utilize body size or body fat, strength and function (Cawthon et al., 2014; Cruz-Jentoft et al., 2010a; Fielding et al., 2011; Morley et al., 2011) were developed to define sarcopenia. Sarcopenia increases the risk for subsequent injury and disability (Baumgartner et al., 1998; Cruz-Jentoft et al., 2010b; Delmonico et al., 2007) and predicts hospitalization and death (Bianchi et al., 2015).

In the limited studies that specifically tested sarcopenia in centenarians, sarcopenia as defined using FFM was highly prevalent, seen in almost 68% in a large (~250) sample of men and women Portuguese centenarians (da Silva et al., 2018; Pereira da Silva et al., 2016). The importance of skeletal muscle mass for longevity was investigated in the Project of Longevity and Aging in Dujiangyan in China (Wang et al., 2019). Appendicular skeletal muscle mass (ASM) was estimated in 738 adults over the age of 90, using equations validated in the Chinese population that included body weight, height, sex, and age. Interestingly, arm span was used a surrogate for height due to vertebral compression and kyphosis in some of the participants. Survival status was examined over a 4-year follow-up period. The 4-year mortality was ~52%. Moreover, low muscle mass index (SMI) was associated with a higher risk of death in women but not men.

6.3 Caloric Restriction Without Malnutrition

6.3.1 Introduction

Nutritional and lifestyle interventions have long been thought to improve longevity. Caloric restriction (CR) has been investigated to determine whether it can delay the onset and progression of aging-related metabolic disease. Caloric restriction is defined as habitual restriction in calorie intake without a reduction in essential nutrients. In several non-human primate species, CR has shown to result in an extension of lifespan (Anderson & Weindruch, 2012). A review by Heilbronn and Ravussin (2003) report that CR extends lifespan by 50–300% in numerous animal species including yeast, flies, and rodents. With the study of preclinical models, physiological mechanisms by which CR extends lifespan have been identified and include reductions in metabolic activity, oxidative stress, autophagy, and inflammation (Speakman & Mitchell, 2011).

Additional mechanisms responsible for the effects of caloric restriction on longevity and disease in animal models include changes in nutrient responsive signaling genes, reduced insulin resistance, and reduction in adiposity. A review of processes involved in longevity regulation in short-lived species demonstrates that longevity is associated with a reduction in the activity of growth pathways and a switch to metabolic patterns associated with fasting (Longo & Anderson, 2022).

6.3.2 Caloric Restriction Diet for Longevity and Impact on Metabolism

The Biosphere experiment was an initial investigation in 1991, in which eight adults (4 women, 4 men) were sealed inside a self-contained ecological space (Biosphere 2) for 2 years to test caloric restriction and aging (Walford et al., 1995). The experiment reduced food production and energy consumption by the crewmembers over time from expected (2500 kcal per person per day to 1750–2100 kcal/day). The diet was rich in nutrients of vegetables, fruits, nuts, grains, and legumes, with small amounts of dairy, eggs, and meat with added vitamin and mineral supplements including vitamin B_{12}, folic acid, vitamin D, Vitamin E and ascorbic acid (Walford et al., 1999). The nature of the diet was meant to mimic diets of rodents shown to enhance health, lower disease incidence, and retard aging. Results of the experiment demonstrated loss of body weight in both men (19%) and women (13%), large reductions in systolic and diastolic blood pressures (22–25%), favorable changes in metabolic parameters including reductions in glucose, insulin and cholesterol levels. At this time, it is unknown whether the 2 years in the Biosphere led to longevity in this small sample.

The National Institute on Aging supported a 2-year trial of healthy adults randomized to 25% calorie restriction (n = 143) or maintenance of current diet (n = 75). Adults in the Comprehensive Assessment of Long-term Effects of Reducing Intake of Energy Phase 2 (CALERIE) study were between the ages of 18 and 51 years (mean age ~ 37 years) and nonobese (BMI 21.9–28.0 kg/m^2). The CR group had an 11.9% decrease in body weight, waist circumference and FFM compared to the control group with men losing more FFM than women (Das et al., 2017). The CALERIE study demonstrated that caloric restriction in humans induces a loss of total body weight (Most et al., 2018) and greater insulin sensitivity (Ravussin et al., 2015). Moreover, CR was associated with reduced risk factors for cardiovascular disease (Kraus et al., 2019) and improved biomarkers of liver health (Dorling et al., 2021). Furthermore, CR which did not have an exercise component, did not alter aerobic capacity or muscular strength when expressed per body weight in the CALERIE 2 study (Racette et al., 2017). As treadmill time and work rate increased at the 2-year mark, the authors contend that long-term, modest CR does not adversely affect cardiorespiratory function in healthy adults (Racette et al., 2017). Moreover, there was (1) little effect of CR on most appetite parameters except increased hunger and thirst ratings of which the magnitude had little clinical significance and

(2) consistent adherence to the CR until week 20 after which it declined suggesting that long-term compliance is challenging (Dorling et al., 2020). These results suggest that strategies may need to be developed for long-term adherence to CR if it is to impact longevity. Belsky et al., (2017) compared chronological age and biological age determined with the Klemera–Doubal Method (KDM) in adults in the CALERIE study. The biomarkers included serum albumin, alkaline phosphatase, C-reactive protein, total cholesterol, creatinine, glycated hemoglobin, systolic blood pressure, urea nitrogen, uric acid, and white blood cell count. Results indicate that CALERIE participants randomized to the trial's caloric restriction arm experienced slower biological aging as compared to participants randomized to ad libitum group which was not accounted for by the amount of weight loss. Further, the pace of biological aging among CALERIE participants randomized to the caloric-restriction arm was slower for participants who achieved more caloric restriction indicating that the greater amounts of caloric restriction are important in slowing the aging process. Using blood DNA methylation patterns and the CALERIE trial for validation, Belsky et al. later developed a composite termed the Pace-of-Aging which confirmed the delayed pace of aging in the CALERIE study (Belsky et al., 2020). The reader is referred to several published reviews of findings from the CALERIE studies for more complete details and results of the trials.

One review describes how CR may modify primary and secondary aging (Flanagan et al., 2020). Another study reviewed the changes in anthropometrics, energy metabolism, cardiometabolic health, inflammation and immune function, physical fitness, health behaviors, and mental health in response to weight loss (1-year) and weight loss maintenance (2-year) (Kebbe et al., 2021). One study has examined timing of eating in centenarians in Abruzzo, Italy and demonstrated that an early dinner and CR lapse of approximately 17 h was an important contributor to the longevity of that group of centenarians (Angelino et al., 2022). More work in the area of CR as well as meal timing may provide additional insights into the biological mechanisms for the extension of a healthy lifespan and lead to geroprotective therapies and strategies in humans.

6.4 Chapter Conclusion

In summary, centenarians from various regions across the world differ in their diets, body measures, and other healthy habits from the general population. Although these differences do exist, it appears that nutrition in conjunction with related activities plays an imperative role in their exceptional long lives. However, more studies in specific areas of nutrition research are needed to understand the magnitude of such an impact. Included are centenarians'body composition and resting metabolic rate, as well as whether they affect longevity independently. In addition, although studies on animals have shown that CR can increase lifespan and improve health by reducing the risk of age-related diseases, its impact on human health and longevity is still not fully understood.

Multiple Choice Questions

1. All of the following are commonly found food items in traditional diets except:
   A. Root vegetables
   B. Processed meats
   C. Whole grains
   D. Legumes
   CORRECT ANSWER: B

2. Which of the following is the definition of sarcopenia?
   A. Loss of appetite
   B. Loss of movement
   C. Loss of muscle mass
   D. Loss of weight
   CORRECT ANSWER: C

3. Which of the following dietary patterns contribute to slowing of the aging process?
   A. Caloric restriction
   B. Heavy alcohol consumption
   C. Consuming an animal-based diet
   D. Eating every 3–4 hours
   CORRECT ANSWER: A

References

Adamsson, V., Reumark, A., Cederholm, T., Vessby, B., Risérus, U., & Johansson, G. (2012). What is a healthy Nordic diet? Foods and nutrients in the NORDIET study. *Food & Nutrition Research, 56*. https://doi.org/10.3402/fnr.v56i0.18189

Anderson, R. M., & Weindruch, R. (2012). The caloric restriction paradigm: Implications for healthy human aging. *American Journal of Human Biology, 24*(2), 101–106. https://doi.org/10.1002/ajhb.22243

Angelino, D., Pietrangeli, F., & Serafini, M. (2022). Early dinner time and caloric restriction lapse contribute to the Longevity of Nonagenarians and Centenarians of the Italian Abruzzo Region: A Cross-Sectional Study. *Frontiers in Nutrition, 9*, 863106. https://doi.org/10.3389/fnut.2022.863106

Bach-Faig, A., Berry, E., Lairon, D., Reguant, J., Trichopoulou, A., Dernini, S., et al. (2011). Mediterranean diet pyramid today. Science and cultural updates. *Public Health Nutrition, 14*(12A), 2274–2284. https://doi.org/10.1017/S1368980011002515

Baumgartner, R. N., Koehler, K. M., Gallagher, D., Romero, L., Heymsfield, S. B., Ross, R. R., et al. (1998). Epidemiology of sarcopenia among the elderly in New Mexico. *American Journal of Epidemiology, 147*(8), 755–763. Retrieved from http://www.ncbi.nlm.nih.gov/pubmed/9554417

Becerra-Tomás, N., Blanco Mejía, S., Viguiliouk, E., Khan, T., Kendall, C. W. C., Kahleova, H., Rahelić, D., Sievenpiper, J. L., & Salas-Salvadó, J. (2020). Mediterranean diet, cardiovascular disease and mortality in diabetes: A systematic review and meta-analysis of prospective cohort studies and randomized clinical trials. *Critical Reviews in Food Science and Nutrition, 60*(7), 1207–1227. https://doi.org/10.1080/10408398.2019.1565281

Belsky, D. W., Huffman, K. M., Pieper, C. F., Shalev, I., & Kraus, W. E. (2017). Change in the rate of biological aging in response to caloric restriction: CALERIE biobank analysis. *The Journals of Gerontology. Series A, Biological Sciences and Medical Sciences, 73*(1), 4–10. https://doi.org/10.1093/gerona/glx096

Belsky, D. W., Caspi, A., Arseneault, L., Baccarelli, A., Corcoran, D. L., Gao, X., et al. (2020). Quantification of the pace of biological aging in humans through a blood test, the DunedinPoAm DNA methylation algorithm. *eLife, 9*. https://doi.org/10.7554/eLife.54870

Bianchi, L., Ferrucci, L., Cherubini, A., Maggio, M., Bandinelli, S., Savino, E., et al. (2015). The predictive value of the EWGSOP definition of sarcopenia: Results from the InCHIANTI Study. *The Journals of Gerontology. Series A, Biological Sciences and Medical Sciences*. https://doi.org/10.1093/gerona/glv129

Buettner, D. (2008). *The Blue Zone: Lessons for living longer from the people who've lived the longest*. National Geographic Society.

Buettner, D., & Skemp, S. (2016). Blue Zones: Lessons from the World's longest lived. *American Journal of Lifestyle Medicine, 10*(5), 318–321. https://doi.org/10.1177/1559827616637066

Calvo-Malvar, M. M., Leis, R., Benítez-Estévez, A. J., Sánchez-Castro, J., & Gude, F. (2016). A randomised, family-focused dietary intervention to evaluate the Atlantic diet: The GALIAT study protocol. *BMC Public Health, 16*(1), 820. https://doi.org/10.1186/s12889-016-3441-y

Cambeses-Franco, C., González-García, S., Feijoo, G., & Moreira, M. T. (2021). Encompassing health and nutrition with the adherence to the environmentally sustainable New Nordic Diet in Southern Europe. *Journal of Cleaner Production, 327*, 129470. https://doi.org/10.1016/j.jclepro.2021.129470

Carballo-Casla, A., Ortolá, R., García-Esquinas, E., Oliveira, A., Sotos-Prieto, M., Lopes, C., Lopez-Garcia, E., & Rodríguez-Artalejo, F. (2021). The Southern European Atlantic Diet and all-cause mortality in older adults. *BMC Medicine, 19*(1), 36. https://doi.org/10.1186/s12916-021-01911-y

Cawthon, P. M., Peters, K. W., Shardell, M. D., McLean, R. R., Dam, T. T., Kenny, A. M., et al. (2014). Cutpoints for low appendicular lean mass that identify older adults with clinically significant weakness. *The Journals of Gerontology. Series A, Biological Sciences and Medical Sciences, 69*(5), 567–575. https://doi.org/10.1093/gerona/glu023

Cespedes, E. M., & Hu, F. B. (2015). Dietary patterns: From nutritional epidemiologic analysis to national guidelines. *The American Journal of Clinical Nutrition, 101*(5), 899–900. https://doi.org/10.3945/ajcn.115.110213

Chan, Y. C., Suzuki, M., & Yamamoto, S. (1997). Dietary, anthropometric, hematological and biochemical assessment of the nutritional status of centenarians and elderly people in Okinawa, Japan. *Journal of the American College of Nutrition, 16*(3), 229–235. https://doi.org/10.1080/07315724.1997.10718679

Chiavaroli, L., Nishi, S. K., Khan, T. A., Braunstein, C. R., Glenn, A. J., Mejia, S. B., Rahelić, D., Kahleová, H., Salas-Salvadó, J., Jenkins, D. J. A., Kendall, C. W. C., & Sievenpiper, J. L. (2018). Portfolio dietary pattern and cardiovascular disease: A systematic review and meta-analysis of controlled trials. *Progress in Cardiovascular Diseases, 61*(1), 43–53. https://doi.org/10.1016/j.pcad.2018.05.004

Clinton, S. K., Giovannucci, E. L., & Hursting, S. D. (2020). The World Cancer Research Fund/American Institute for Cancer Research third expert report on diet, nutrition, physical activity, and cancer: Impact and future directions. *The Journal of Nutrition, 150*(4), 663–671. https://doi.org/10.1093/jn/nxz268

Compher, C., Frankenfield, D., Keim, N., Roth-Yousey, L., & Evidence Analysis Working, G. (2006). Best practice methods to apply to measurement of resting metabolic rate in adults: A systematic review. *Journal of the American Dietetic Association, 106*(6), 881–903. https://doi.org/10.1016/j.jada.2006.02.009

Cruz-Jentoft, A. J., Baeyens, J. P., Bauer, J. M., Boirie, Y., Cederholm, T., Landi, F., et al. (2010a). Sarcopenia: European consensus on definition and diagnosis: Report of the European Working Group on Sarcopenia in Older People. *Age and Ageing, 39*(4), 412–423. https://doi.org/10.1093/ageing/afq034

Cruz-Jentoft, A. J., Landi, F., Topinkova, E., & Michel, J. P. (2010b). Understanding sarcopenia as a geriatric syndrome. *Current Opinion in Clinical Nutrition and Metabolic Care, 13*(1), 1–7. https://doi.org/10.1097/MCO.0b013e328333c1c1

da Silva, A. P., Valente, A., Chaves, C., Matos, A., Gil, A., Santos, A. C., et al. (2018). Characterization of Portuguese Centenarian Eating Habits, Nutritional Biomarkers, and Cardiovascular Risk: A Case Control Study. *Oxidative Medicine and Cellular Longevity, 2018*, 5296168. https://doi.org/10.1155/2018/5296168

Das, S. K., Roberts, S. B., Bhapkar, M. V., Villareal, D. T., Fontana, L., Martin, C. K., et al. (2017). Body-composition changes in the Comprehensive Assessment of Long-term Effects of Reducing Intake of Energy (CALERIE)-2 study: A 2-y randomized controlled trial of calorie restriction in nonobese humans. *The American Journal of Clinical Nutrition, 105*(4), 913–927. https://doi.org/10.3945/ajcn.116.137232

Davis, C., Bryan, J., Hodgson, J., & Murphy, K. (2015). Definition of the Mediterranean Diet; a Literature Review. *Nutrients, 7*(11), 9139–9153. https://doi.org/10.3390/nu7115459

Delmonico, M. J., Harris, T. B., Lee, J. S., Visser, M., Nevitt, M., Kritchevsky, S. B., et al. (2007). Alternative definitions of sarcopenia, lower extremity performance, and functional impairment with aging in older men and women. *Journal of the American Geriatrics Society, 55*(5), 769–774. https://doi.org/10.1111/j.1532-5415.2007.01140.x

Dominguez, L. J., Di Bella, G., Veronese, N., & Barbagallo, M. (2021). Impact of Mediterranean Diet on Chronic Non-Communicable Diseases and Longevity. *Nutrients, 13*(6), 2028. https://doi.org/10.3390/nu13062028

Dominguez, L. J., Veronese, N., Baiamonte, E., Guarrera, M., Parisi, A., Ruffolo, C., Tagliaferri, F., & Barbagallo, M. (2022). Healthy aging and dietary patterns. *Nutrients, 14*(4), 889. https://doi.org/10.3390/nu14040889

Dorling, J. L., Das, S. K., Racette, S. B., Apolzan, J. W., Zhang, D., Pieper, C. F., et al. (2020). Changes in body weight, adherence, and appetite during 2 years of calorie restriction: The CALERIE 2 randomized clinical trial. *European Journal of Clinical Nutrition, 74*(8), 1210–1220. https://doi.org/10.1038/s41430-020-0593-8

Dorling, J. L., Ravussin, E., Redman, L. M., Bhapkar, M., Huffman, K. M., Racette, S. B., et al. (2021). Effect of 2 years of calorie restriction on liver biomarkers: Results from the CALERIE phase 2 randomized controlled trial. *European Journal of Nutrition, 60*(3), 1633–1643. https://doi.org/10.1007/s00394-020-02361-7

Duarte, M. G., Duarte, P. O., Pelichek, A., Ferriolli, E., Moriguti, J. C., Pfrimer, K., & Lima, N. K. (2019). Comparison of body composition analysis methods among centenary women: Seeking simpler methods. *SAGE Open Med, 7*, 2050312119865126. https://doi.org/10.1177/2050312119865126

Evans, W. J., & Campbell, W. W. (1993). Sarcopenia and age-related changes in body composition and functional capacity. *The Journal of Nutrition, 123*(2 Suppl), 465–468. Retrieved from http://www.ncbi.nlm.nih.gov/pubmed/8429405

Fielding, R. A., Vellas, B., Evans, W. J., Bhasin, S., Morley, J. E., Newman, A. B., et al. (2011). Sarcopenia: An undiagnosed condition in older adults. Current consensus definition: Prevalence, etiology, and consequences. International working group on sarcopenia. *Journal of the American Medical Directors Association, 12*(4), 249–256. https://doi.org/10.1016/j.jamda.2011.01.003

Filippou, C. D., Tsioufis, C. P., Thomopoulos, C. G., Mihas, C. C., Dimitriadis, K. S., Sotiropoulou, L. I., Chrysochoou, C. A., Nihoyannopoulos, P. I., & Tousoulis, D. M. (2020). Dietary Approaches to Stop Hypertension (DASH) Diet and blood pressure reduction in adults with and without Hypertension: A systematic review and meta-analysis of randomized controlled trials. *Advances in Nutrition (Bethesda, Md.), 11*(5), 1150–1160. https://doi.org/10.1093/advances/nmaa041

Flanagan, E. W., Most, J., Mey, J. T., & Redman, L. M. (2020). Calorie restriction and aging in humans. *Annual Review of Nutrition, 40*, 105–133. https://doi.org/10.1146/annurev-nutr-122319-034601

Fu, S., Ping, P., Li, Y., Li, B., Zhao, Y., Yao, Y., & Zhang, P. (2021). Centenarian longevity had inverse relationships with nutritional status and abdominal obesity and positive relationships with sex hormones and bone turnover in the oldest females. *Journal of Translational Medicine, 19*(1), 436. https://doi.org/10.1186/s12967-021-03115-7

Gabriel, A. S., Ninomiya, K., & Uneyama, H. (2018). The Role of the Japanese Traditional Diet in Healthy and Sustainable Dietary Patterns around the World. *Nutrients, 10*(2), 173. https://doi.org/10.3390/nu10020173

Galbete, C., Kröger, J., Jannasch, F., Iqbal, K., Schwingshackl, L., Schwedhelm, C., Weikert, C., Boeing, H., & Schulze, M. B. (2018). Nordic diet, Mediterranean diet, and the risk of chronic diseases: The EPIC-Potsdam study. *BMC Medicine, 16*(1), 99. https://doi.org/10.1186/s12916-018-1082-y

Guallar-Castillón, P., Oliveira, A., Lopes, C., López-García, E., & Rodríguez-Artalejo, F. (2013). The Southern European Atlantic Diet is associated with lower concentrations of markers of coronary risk. *Atherosclerosis, 226*(2), 502–509. https://doi.org/10.1016/j.atherosclerosis.2012.11.035

Guasch-Ferré, M., & Willett, W. C. (2021). The Mediterranean diet and health: A comprehensive overview. *Journal of Internal Medicine, 290*(3), 549–566. https://doi.org/10.1111/joim.13333

Hausman, D. B., Fischer, J. G., & Johnson, M. A. (2011a). Nutrition in centenarians. *Maturitas, 68*(3), 203–209. https://doi.org/10.1016/j.maturitas.2011.01.003

Hausman, D. B., Johnson, M. A., Davey, A., & Poon, L. W. (2011b). Body mass index is associated with dietary patterns and health conditions in Georgia centenarians. *Journal of Aging Research, 2011*, 138015. https://doi.org/10.4061/2011/138015

Heilbronn, L. K., & Ravussin, E. (2003). Calorie restriction and aging: Review of the literature and implications for studies in humans. *The American Journal of Clinical Nutrition, 78*(3), 361–369. https://doi.org/10.1093/ajcn/78.3.361

Jacobs, D. R., Jr., & Orlich, M. J. (2014). Diet pattern and longevity: Do simple rules suffice? A commentary. *The American Journal of Clinical Nutrition, 100 Suppl 1(1)*, 313S–319S. https://doi.org/10.3945/ajcn.113.071340

Japantimes. (2022). https://www.japantimes.co.jp/news/2022/09/16/national/japan-record-centenarians/

Jardim, M. Z., Costa, B. V. L., Pessoa, M. C., & Duarte, C. K. (2021). Ultra-processed foods increase noncommunicable chronic disease risk. *Nutrition Research (New York, N.Y.), 95*, 19–34. https://doi.org/10.1016/j.nutres.2021.08.006

Kebbe, M., Sparks, J. R., Flanagan, E. W., & Redman, L. M. (2021). Beyond weight loss: Current perspectives on the impact of calorie restriction on healthspan and lifespan. *Expert Review of Endocrinology and Metabolism, 16*(3), 95–108. https://doi.org/10.1080/17446651.2021.1922077

Kollajtis-Dolowy, A., Pietruszka, B., Kaluza, J., Pawliniska-Chmara, R., Broczek, K., & Mossakowska, M. (2007). The nutritional habits among centenarians living in Warsaw. *Roczniki Państwowego Zakładu Higieny, 58*(1), 279–286. Retrieved from https://www.ncbi.nlm.nih.gov/pubmed/17711123

Kraus, W. E., Bhapkar, M., Huffman, K. M., Pieper, C. F., Krupa Das, S., Redman, L. M., et al. (2019). 2 years of calorie restriction and cardiometabolic risk (CALERIE): Exploratory outcomes of a multicentre, phase 2, randomised controlled trial. *The Lancet Diabetes and Endocrinology, 7*(9), 673–683. https://doi.org/10.1016/S2213-8587(19)30151-2

Lankinen, M., Uusitupa, M., & Schwab, U. (2019). Nordic Diet and Inflammation-A review of observational and intervention studies. *Nutrients, 11*(6), 1369. https://doi.org/10.3390/nu11061369

Livingston, E. H., & Kohlstadt, I. (2005). Simplified resting metabolic rate-predicting formulas for normal-sized and obese individuals. *Obesity Research, 13*(7), 1255–1262. https://doi.org/10.1038/oby.2005.149

Longo, V. D., & Anderson, R. M. (2022). Nutrition, longevity and disease: From molecular mechanisms to interventions. *Cell, 185*(9), 1455–1470. https://doi.org/10.1016/j.cell.2022.04.002

Lorenzo, P. M., Izquierdo, A. G., Rodriguez-Carnero, G., Fernández-Pombo, A., Iglesias, A., Carreira, M. C., Tejera, C., Bellido, D., Martinez-Olmos, M. A., Leis, R., Casanueva, F. F., & Crujeiras, A. B. (2022). Epigenetic effects of healthy foods and lifestyle habits from the Southern European Atlantic Diet Pattern: A narrative review. *Advances in Nutrition (Bethesda, Md.), 13*(5), 1725–1747. https://doi.org/10.1093/advances/nmac038

Mandala, C., Veronese, N., Dominguez, L. J., Candore, G., Accardi, G., Smith, L., et al. (2023). Use of bioelectrical impedance analysis in centenarians: A systematic review. *Aging Clinical and Experimental Research, 35*(1), 1–7. https://doi.org/10.1007/s40520-022-02282-x

Martínez-González, M. Á., Hershey, M. S., Zazpe, I., & Trichopoulou, A. (2017). Transferability of the Mediterranean Diet to Non-Mediterranean Countries. What is and what is not the Mediterranean Diet. *Nutrients, 9*(11), 1226. https://doi.org/10.3390/nu9111226

Massara, P., Zurbau, A., Glenn, A. J., Chiavaroli, L., Khan, T. A., Viguiliouk, E., Mejia, S. B., Comelli, E. M., Chen, V., Schwab, U., Risérus, U., Uusitupa, M., Aas, A. M., Hermansen, K., Thorsdottir, I., Rahelić, D., Kahleová, H., Salas-Salvadó, J., Kendall, C. W. C., & Sievenpiper, J. L. (2022). Nordic dietary patterns and cardiometabolic outcomes: A systematic review and meta-analysis of prospective cohort studies and randomised controlled trials. *Diabetologia, 65*(12), 2011–2031. https://doi.org/10.1007/s00125-022-05760-z

Meltzer, H. M., Brantsæter, A. L., Trolle, E., Eneroth, H., Fogelholm, M., Ydersbond, T. A., & Birgisdottir, B. E. (2019). Environmental sustainability perspectives of the Nordic Diet. *Nutrients, 11*(9), 2248. https://doi.org/10.3390/nu11092248

Monteagudo, C., Mariscal-Arcas, M., Rivas, A., Lorenzo-Tovar, M. L., Tur, J. A., & Olea-Serrano, F. (2015). Proposal of a Mediterranean Diet serving score. *PLoS One, 10*(6), e0128594. https://doi.org/10.1371/journal.pone.0128594

Morley, J. E., Abbatecola, A. M., Argiles, J. M., Baracos, V., Bauer, J., Bhasin, S., et al. (2011). Sarcopenia with limited mobility: An international consensus. *Journal of the American Medical Directors Association, 12*(6), 403–409. https://doi.org/10.1016/j.jamda.2011.04.014

Most, J., Gilmore, L. A., Smith, S. R., Han, H., Ravussin, E., & Redman, L. M. (2018). Significant improvement in cardiometabolic health in healthy nonobese individuals during caloric restriction-induced weight loss and weight loss maintenance. *American Journal of Physiology. Endocrinology and Metabolism, 314*(4), E396–E405. https://doi.org/10.1152/ajpendo.00261.2017

Ndlovu, T., van Jaarsveld, F., & Caleb, O. J. (2019). French and Mediterranean-style diets: Contradictions, misconceptions and scientific facts-A review. *Food Research International (Ottawa, Ont.), 116*, 840–858. https://doi.org/10.1016/j.foodres.2018.09.020

Paolisso, G., Gambardella, A., Ammendola, S., D'Amore, A., Balbi, V., Varricchio, M., & D'Onofrio, F. (1996). Glucose tolerance and insulin action in healthy centenarians. *The American Journal of Physiology, 270*(5 Pt 1), E890–E894. https://doi.org/10.1152/ajpendo.1996.270.5.E890

Pereira da Silva, A., Matos, A., Valente, A., Gil, A., Alonso, I., Ribeiro, R., et al. (2016). Body composition assessment and nutritional status evaluation in men and women Portuguese Centenarians. *The Journal of Nutrition, Health & Aging, 20*(3), 256–266. https://doi.org/10.1007/s12603-015-0566-0

Pignolo, R. J. (2019). Exceptional Human Longevity. *Mayo Clinic Proceedings, 94*(1), 110–124. https://doi.org/10.1016/j.mayocp.2018.10.005

Racette, S. B., Rochon, J., Uhrich, M. L., Villareal, D. T., Das, S. K., Fontana, L., et al. (2017). Effects of two years of calorie restriction on aerobic capacity and muscle strength. *Medicine and Science in Sports and Exercise, 49*(11), 2240–2249. https://doi.org/10.1249/MSS.0000000000001353

Ravaglia, G., Morini, P., Forti, P., Maioli, F., Boschi, F., Bernardi, M., & Gasbarrini, G. (1997). Anthropometric characteristics of healthy Italian nonagenarians and centenarians. *The British Journal of Nutrition, 77*(1), 9–17. https://doi.org/10.1017/s0007114500002841

Ravussin, E., Redman, L. M., Rochon, J., Das, S. K., Fontana, L., Kraus, W. E., et al. (2015). A 2-year randomized controlled trial of human caloric restriction: Feasibility and effects on predictors of health Span and longevity. *The Journals of Gerontology. Series A, Biological Sciences and Medical Sciences, 70*(9), 1097–1104. https://doi.org/10.1093/gerona/glv057

Rizzo, M. R., Mari, D., Barbieri, M., Ragno, E., Grella, R., Provenzano, R., et al. (2005). Resting metabolic rate and respiratory quotient in human longevity. *The Journal of Clinical Endocrinology and Metabolism, 90*(1), 409–413. https://doi.org/10.1210/jc.2004-0390

Rosato, V., Temple, N. J., La Vecchia, C., Castellan, G., Tavani, A., & Guercio, V. (2019). Mediterranean diet and cardiovascular disease: A systematic review and meta-analysis of observational studies. *European Journal of Nutrition, 58*(1), 173–191. https://doi.org/10.1007/s00394-017-1582-0

Soltani, S., Jayedi, A., Shab-Bidar, S., Becerra-Tomás, N., & Salas-Salvadó, J. (2019). Adherence to the Mediterranean Diet in Relation to All-Cause Mortality: A Systematic Review and Dose-Response Meta-Analysis of Prospective Cohort Studies. *Advances in Nutrition (Bethesda, Md.), 10*(6), 1029–1039. https://doi.org/10.1093/advances/nmz041

Speakman, J. R., & Mitchell, S. E. (2011). Caloric restriction. *Molecular Aspects of Medicine, 32*(3), 159–221. https://doi.org/10.1016/j.mam.2011.07.001

St-Onge, M. P., & Gallagher, D. (2010). Body composition changes with aging: The cause or the result of alterations in metabolic rate and macronutrient oxidation? *Nutrition, 26*(2), 152–155. https://doi.org/10.1016/j.nut.2009.07.004

Teixeira, L., Araújo, L., Jopp, D., & Ribeiro, O. (2017). Centenarians in Europe. *Maturitas, 104*, 90–95. https://doi.org/10.1016/j.maturitas.2017.08.005

Trichopoulou, A., Martínez-González, M. A., Tong, T. Y., Forouhi, N. G., Khandelwal, S., Prabhakaran, D., Mozaffarian, D., & de Lorgeril, M. (2014). Definitions and potential health benefits of the Mediterranean diet: Views from experts around the world. *BMC Medicine, 12*, 112. https://doi.org/10.1186/1741-7015-12-112

UNESCO. (2013). *Representative list of the Intangible Cultural Heritage of Humanity Representative list of the intangible cultural heritage of humanity*. Paris, France.

US Department of Agriculture. (2014). Center for Nutrition Policy and Promotion, Nutrition Evidence Library, Dietary Patterns Technical Expert Collaborative. A Series of Systematic Reviews on the Relationship Between Dietary Patterns and Health Outcomes. https://nesr.usda.gov/sites/default/files/2019-06/DietaryPatternsReport-FullFinal2.pdf. Published 2014. Accessed January 23, 2022.

van den Brink, A. C., Brouwer-Brolsma, E. M., Berendsen, A. A. M., & van de Rest, O. (2019). The Mediterranean, Dietary Approaches to Stop Hypertension (DASH), and Mediterranean-DASH Intervention for Neurodegenerative Delay (MIND) Diets Are Associated with Less Cognitive Decline and a Lower Risk of Alzheimer's Disease-A Review. *Advances in Nutrition (Bethesda, Md.), 10*(6), 1040–1065. https://doi.org/10.1093/advances/nmz054

van Pelt, R. E., Dinneno, F. A., Seals, D. R., & Jones, P. P. (2001). Age-related decline in RMR in physically active men: Relation to exercise volume and energy intake. *American Journal of Physiology. Endocrinology and Metabolism, 281*(3), E633–E639. https://doi.org/10.1152/ajpendo.2001.281.3.E633

Vasto, S., Buscemi, S., Barera, A., Di Carlo, M., Accardi, G., & Caruso, C. (2014). Mediterranean diet and healthy ageing: A Sicilian perspective. *Gerontology, 60*(6), 508–518. https://doi.org/10.1159/000363060

Walford, R. L., Weber, L., & Panov, S. (1995). Caloric restriction and aging as viewed from Biosphere 2. *Receptor, 5*(1), 29–33. Retrieved from https://www.ncbi.nlm.nih.gov/pubmed/7613481

Walford, R. L., Mock, D., MacCallum, T., & Laseter, J. L. (1999). Physiologic changes in humans subjected to severe, selective calorie restriction for two years in biosphere 2: Health, aging, and toxicological perspectives. *Toxicological Sciences, 52*(2 Suppl), 61–65. Retrieved from https://www.ncbi.nlm.nih.gov/pubmed/10630592

Wang, H., Hai, S., Liu, Y., Liu, Y., & Dong, B. (2019). Skeletal muscle mass as a mortality predictor among nonagenarians and centenarians: A prospective cohort study. *Scientific Reports, 9*(1), 2420. https://doi.org/10.1038/s41598-019-38893-0

Wang, C., Murgia, M. A., Baptista, J., et al. (2022). Sardinian dietary analysis for longevity: A review of the literature. *Journal of Ethnicity Food, 9*, 33. https://doi.org/10.1186/s42779-022-00152-5

Willcox, D. C., Willcox, B. J., Todoriki, H., & Suzuki, M. (2009). The Okinawan diet: Health implications of a low-calorie, nutrient-dense, antioxidant-rich dietary pattern low in glycemic load. *Journal of the American College of Nutrition, 28*(Suppl), 500S–516S. https://doi.org/10.1080/07315724.2009.10718117

Willcox, D. C., Scapagnini, G., & Willcox, B. J. (2014). Healthy aging diets other than the Mediterranean: A focus on the Okinawan diet. *Mechanisms of Ageing and Development, 136-137*, 148–162. https://doi.org/10.1016/j.mad.2014.01.002

Wu, L., & Sun, D. (2017). Adherence to Mediterranean diet and risk of developing cognitive disorders: An updated systematic review and meta-analysis of prospective cohort studies. *Scientific Reports, 7*, 41317. https://doi.org/10.1038/srep41317

Yang, S., Wang, S., Tai, P., Jia, W., Han, K., Liu, M., & He, Y. (2021). Central and peripheral adiposity had different effect on disability in centenarians. *Front Endocrinol (Lausanne), 12*, 635205. https://doi.org/10.3389/fendo.2021.635205

Yeung, S. S. Y., Kwan, M., & Woo, J. (2021). Healthy diet for healthy aging. *Nutrients, 13*(12), 4310. https://doi.org/10.3390/nu13124310

Yoshiike, N., Hayashi, F., Takemi, Y., Mizoguchi, K., & Seino, F. (2007). A new food guide in Japan: The Japanese food guide spinning top. *Nutrition Reviews, 65*(4), 149–154. https://doi.org/10.1111/j.1753-4887.2007.tb00294.x

Chapter 7
Physical Activity in Centenarians

Alice S. Ryan and Margarita S. Treuth

Key Take Away Points
1. Physical activity has a positive impact on longevity in adults.
2. Centenarians often present with slower gait speed, poor balance, and reduced strength.
3. Centenarians can benefit from cardiorespiratory and muscle strengthening exercises.

7.1 The Role of Physical Activity in Promoting Longevity

7.1.1 Introduction

Modification of one's lifestyle through healthy behaviors can impact the aging process. Critical to this 'lifestyle' component is physical activity, which is defined as any bodily movement produced by the contraction of skeletal muscles that results in an increase in caloric requirements over resting energy expenditure. It has been well established that regular physical activity reduces the risk of many diseases including cardiovascular disease (hypertension, dyslipidemia), cancer, and diabetes. Exercise is a type of physical activity consisting of planned, structured, and repetitive bodily

A. S. Ryan (✉)
University of Maryland School of Medicine and Department of Veterans Affairs RR&D SRCS, Baltimore, MD, USA
e-mail: aryan@som.umaryland.edu

M. S. Treuth
Salisbury University, School of Health Sciences, Salisbury, MD, USA
e-mail: mstreuth@salisbury.edu

R. E. Kheirbek, M. D. Llorente (eds.), *Current Perspectives on Centenarians*, International Perspectives on Aging 36,
https://doi.org/10.1007/978-3-031-30915-1_7

movement done to improve and/or maintain one or more components of physical fitness. The American College of Sports Medicine has a position stand which contains specific recommendations for healthy adults for the quantity and quality of exercise to develop and maintain cardiorespiratory, musculoskeletal and neuromotor fitness (Garber et al., 2011). Recommendations for adults include accumulating at least 150 min of moderate to vigorous intensity physical activity or 75 min of vigorous intensity physical activity per week (Services, 2018). Reducing physical inactivity or reducing sedentary time is also recommended as well as advocating that some physical activity is better than none. Despite these recommendations, the oldest adults (>65 years) have the lowest rates of adherence to physical activity guidelines of aerobic activity from the National Health and Nutrition Examination Surveys from 2007 to 2016 compared to all other age groups (Du et al., 2019). Moreover, increases in time spent in sedentary behavior were observed in the older age groups. Meeting guidelines for physical activity plays a vital role in healthy aging and evaluating physical activity, exercise, and fitness in centenarians may provide a better understanding of the role of physical activity in promoting longevity.

Illustative Vignette

Dr. Smith is a lively centenarian who always made physical activity and fitness a priority in her life. From a young age, she walked miles to school, played basketball, and loved to dance. She was a concert violinist and played the piano. She continually stayed active, whether through taking walks in the park, stationary cycling during her lunch breaks, playing with her eight children, or even just doing household chores.

As she aged, she continued to make exercise a part of her daily routine. She started to use her smart phone to track her walking mileage every day. On her daily walks, she is cognizant of her surroundings because of her fear of falling. She was aware that she needed to keep her muscles strong and her bones solid.

But it was not only her physical health that benefited from her active lifestyle. Regular exercise has been shown to boost mood, reduce stress and anxiety, and improve overall cognitive function. Dr. Smith always felt sharp and mentally alert, which helped her to continue to stay engaged and active in her work and her community.

Dr. Smith's commitment to physical activity and fitness paid off in her later years. Despite being 100 years old, she is still able to walk unassisted, climb stairs, and even do some light strengthening exercises using handheld weights. Her good health allows her to enjoy her golden years to the fullest, as she is able to travel, spend time with her family and friends, and continue to do other things she loved, like playing the piano.

Her love for physical activity and fitness and positive attitude in life plays a major role in her longevity. Studies have shown that regular physical activity can help to reduce the risk of chronic diseases, such as heart disease, diabetes, and cancer, which are common causes of death.

Dr. Smith's story is a testament to the importance of physical activity and fitness in maintaining both quality of life and longevity.

7.1.2 Physical Activity Patterns and Longevity

How much and what type of physical activity is needed to enhance longevity? Examining physical activity patterns in centenarians may help answer this challenging question. However, initial investigations of how physical activity patterns may influence health span came from prospective cohort studies in various populations. Quantification of physical activity levels is estimated by questionnaires or directly via activity tracking.

An early study which prospectively followed Harvard College alumni in the early 1960's through 1988 or to the age of 90, examined adoption or maintenance of physical activity and its influence on mortality rates (Paffenbarger et al., 1994). Men who increased their physical activity (via walking, stair climbing, sports, or recreational activities) had a relative risk of death of 0.72 compared to 1.0 for less active men. This early study in the US demonstrated that adopting an active lifestyle influenced longevity.

A cohort study (Wen et al., 2011) involving 416,175 Taiwanese individuals, examined weekly exercise, specifically the leisure-time physical activity calculated as a product of intensity (metabolic equivalent) and duration (hours) of exercise. Survey responses were then categorized into inactive, or low, medium, high, or very high activity. Compared to the inactive group, those in the low activity group (92 min/week or 15 min/day) had a 3 year longer life expectancy (Wen et al., 2011). An early paper which reported on data from the National Health and Nutrition Survey and the National Health Interview Study concluded that somewhat-active and active non-Hispanic white men had a life expectancy that was 1.2 years longer at age 80 years than for the inactive men (Janssen et al., 2013). Also utilizing data from the National Health and Nutrition Survey, Del Pozo Cruz et al. (2021) later examined light-intensity physical activity and life expectancy in 6636 participants after a mean follow-up of 11 years. In this study, light-intensity physical activity was measured using an objective criterion, accelerometry, and the life expectancy (years of life gained) was estimated on surviving up to 85 years of age. Findings indicated that years of life gained at age 45 and 65 years were 2.51 and 1.52 years, respectively for those categorized in the light leisure time physical activity group suggesting that even a low level of physical activity is beneficial to life expectancy even if this benefit is less in the elderly.

Physical inactivity worldwide is a major public health issue. One study (Lee et al., 2012) aimed to estimate gain in life expectancy at the population level if inactive persons became active. Using life-table analysis to estimate these gains in the population, Lee et al. reported that elimination of physical inactivity would increase the life expectancy of the world's population by 0.68 (range 0.41–0.95) years. A review by Venturelli et al. (2012) describes the physical capacity of centenarians and evaluates how exercise impacts their health and longevity. There is likely a wide interindividual physical activity variability in centenarians.

The cellular mechanism to explain the longevity has been hypothesized to be related to reduced oxidative damage (Andersen et al., 1998). In a study of 41 centenarians from Funen, Denmark, antioxidative enzymes in erythrocytes were compared to elderly people (Andersen et al., 1998). The centenarians between 100–105 years of age had lower superoxide dismutase levels and a higher glutathione reductase activity than the younger group. Moreover, centenarians with better IADL levels had the highest glutathione activity. Thus, the centenarians had reduced oxidative damage which might play a role in their longevity.

In summary, these studies indicate that some physical activity is better than none, and that even low levels of physical activity have beneficial effects on life expectancy. Although these reports did not focus on centenarians, even some low level of physical activity has a positive impact.

7.2 Physical Activity and Its Role in Improving Quality of Life

7.2.1 Physical Activity Levels in Centenarians

Studies that quantify the actual physical activity levels in terms of the quantity and mode of activity in centenarians are sparse, yet there is evidence that some centenarians have an active lifestyle. In terms of modes of physical activity in centenarians, walking is considered a low-level activity and a means of ambulation and is likely the most common type of physical activity in this population.

In a small sample of 18 Spanish centenarians (age 100–103 years), Hernandez-Vicente et al. (2019) measured physical activity using an Actigraph accelerometer to quantify activity counts per minute and steps/day. Interestingly, these centenarians averaged 17.6 ± 7.1 counts per min and 455 ± 237 steps per day. This was significantly lower than nonagenarians (age 90–98 years), with their data suggesting that the "decline in physical activity continues to worsen until the end of the human lifespan". This study also reported that the most active time of the day was in the morning, showing a peak of activity between 10 am and noon. Although this study was unique to quantify the steps/day, the sample was predominately women who were institutionalized. In a follow-up study (Hernandez-Vicente et al., 2022), the authors determined cut-point-free metrics for physical activity that were positively associated with functional independence and cognitive and physical capacities which could be utilized in larger, and diversified populations of centenarians.

It is also necessary to consider the role of inactivity on quality of life, as reducing sedentary behavior is a targeted goal to achieve a healthy lifestyle. In 878 Chinese centenarians (19.7% men, 80.3% women) aged 100–117 years, most of the centenarians were not physically active as determined by interview (Li et al., 2014). In addition, 23% of the study centenarians considered taking a walk their favorite activity and 33% preferred to rest, and 18.6% preferred to chat. Moreover, 64% were able to take care of themselves. Thus, data by questionnaires indicate that almost a quarter of centenarians enjoy walking but more prefer a sedentary day.

In summary, there is limited direct evidence of physical activity levels using accelerometry in centenarians. However, both levels of activity and inactivity have an impact on healthy aging.

7.3 Components of Physical Activity in Centenarians

7.3.1 Muscular Strength

Resistance exercise is one component that is recommended in the PA guidelines for Americans (Services, 2018) and the 2020 World Health Organization guidelines (Bull et al., 2020). It is recommended that adults do muscle-strengthening activities of moderate or greater intensity that involve all major muscle groups on two or more days a week. It is well established that there is a decrease in muscle mass and strength with aging. Muscular strength, necessary for activities of daily living (ADL's), can be easily measured as grip strength using a hand-grip dynamometer.

In a 44-year prospective study of men from the Honolulu Heart Program/ Honolulu-Asia Aging Study, there were 47 centenarians (≥100 years) and 545 nonagenarians (90–99 years) of whom grip strength was measured in midlife (Rantanen et al., 2012). The centenarians were more likely to be in the highest third of grip strength in midlife (OR = 2.52) and participated in physical activity outside work (OR = 1.13 per daily hour). Similar but weaker associations were observed in the nonagenarians. Interestingly, having a long-lived mother (≥80 years compared to 60 years) also indicated resilience to aging. These findings suggest that both muscular strength and physical activity are important predictors of exceptional longevity.

In a prospective cohort study of 81 nonagenarians and centenarians, handgrip strength was assessed to examine the association between this variable and cancer diagnosis (Saez de Asteasu et al., 2022). All participants had multiple comorbidities. The mean handgrip strength observed in the entire sample of nonagenarians and centenarians was 17.65 ± 7.73 kg. Furthermore, those participants without a cancer diagnosis had a higher handgrip strength than peers with cancer (Saez de Asteasu et al., 2022). However, the handgrip strength reported here is relatively low compared to younger adults demonstrating a marked decline in strength in individuals over 90+ years of age.

In the Georgia centenarian study (Poon et al., 2007), the community dwellers had 50% higher grip strength than the skilled nursing facility residents. Specifically, the community dwellers average of the right and left grip strength was 8.96 kg compared to the skilled nursing facility residents who demonstrated a grip strength of 3.89 kg. Leg extension strength was similar between the two groups. It was noted that 30% of both groups were moderately impaired and 25% of each group had a complaint of weakness. The authors suggest that the care and assistance provided in the skilled nursing facility enables the participant to 'match' the decreased strength that was measured (Poon et al., 2007).

A recent publication by Matsumoto et al. sought to provide reference values for physical performance measures including hand grip strength for Japanese oldest old in the Septuagenarians, Octogenarians, and Nonagenarians Investigation with Centenarians (SONIC) study (Matsumoto et al., 2022). Sex-specific reference values are 24.1 ± 5.4 kg and 14.4 ± 4.0 kg in hand grip strength for men and women, respectively. Moreover, hand grip strength was lower in individuals who were in their nineties, than those in the 80's cohort and 70's cohort. The decline in grip strength with age was similar across each 10-year age cohort for both sexes. Twenty percent of the 90-year-olds were unable to perform the sit-and-stand test which was used to examine physical performance. This rate was considerably higher than the other age cohorts indicating a rapid decline in lower limb function form age 80 to age 90. The authors conclude with reference values for hand grip strength in Japanese oldest old and caution that the technique utilized to measure hand grip strength (standing vs. sitting) must be considered if other researchers use these reference values.

In a case study of a 99 year-old patient with knee osteoarthritis, it was hypothesized that strength training would result in muscle hypertrophy. The participant underwent 24 sessions of unilateral free-weight resistance training (knee extensor) to examine changes in muscle mass (Scarpelli et al., 2021). The training resulted in a 12% increase in muscle cross-sectional area and 8% increase in muscle thickness of the vastus lateralis by ultrasound. Although the timed up and go (TUG) test which assess functional performance scores did not significantly change, the resistance training may have prevented a decline in functionality performance.

It is evident that there is a continual decline in strength with aging as evidenced by these few studies. The inability to complete certain activities, e.g. sit-to-stand, in centenarians is common; however, the case study discussed shows promise that improving strength in centenarians can be attained with muscular training.

7.3.2 Cardiorespiratory Fitness

Physical fitness has generally been described as a set of attributes or characteristics individuals have or achieve that relate to their ability to perform physical activity and activities of daily living. Maximal oxygen consumption (VO_2max) is highest in aerobic athletes, such as cyclists, runners, rowers and swimmers. Measurement of VO_2max is generally considered the gold standard for assessing aerobic capacity and best accomplished specific to training mode. VO_2max declines with age even in highly trained adults. There are very limited studies utilizing graded maximal exercise tests to test cardiorespiratory fitness in centenarians. Exercise capacity on a cycle ergometer and lung function measured by spirometry was compared between eight female centenarians (98–102 years old) and eight young females (18–22 years) (Venturelli et al., 2013). At rest, pulmonary ventilation (breathing frequency tidal volume), gas exchange (oxygen uptake, carbon dioxide production), and metabolism (respiratory exchange ratio) were not different between groups. Results from the graded maximal cycle test indicated that peak work rate and VO_2 were significantly reduced in the centenarians. VO_2 peak ranged between 6.1–9.3 ml/kg/min and averaged 7.5 ml/kg/min in this sample of centenarians. The older participants had a significantly elevated breathing frequency and a tendency for a reduced tidal volume. The authors found a reduced oxygen cost of work as illustrated by the slope of the VO_2/work rate in the centenarians which they hypothesized plays a vital role in maintaining physical function and longevity in the centenarians.

In a novel case study, an elite centenarian cyclist from France who cycled between the ages of 15 and 25 years returned to cycling at age 101 and was followed for 2 years (Billat et al., 2017). During the 2-year period, he trained 5000 km/year with the majority of mileage completed at a "light" intensity by RPE (rating of perceived exertion) with the remaining 20% at a "hard" intensity. Not only did maximal oxygen consumption (VO_2max) increase 13%, but peak power output increased almost 40%. Also remarkable was his initial high VO_2max of 31.9 ml/kg/min, a value comparable to a sedentary male half his age. This case is a unique example of an improvement in aerobic capacity and performance at a very old age.

Similar to what has been observed with the decline in strength, maximal oxygen uptake decreases with advancing age. However, the case study does support that an improvement in cardiorespiratory fitness can be attained with aerobic training.

7.3.3 *Neuromotor Fitness*

7.3.3.1 Frailty

According to the American College of Sports Medicine, neuromotor exercise training is a component of the position stand (Services, 2018). Neuromotor exercise training refers to motor skills that involve balance, gait, coordination, agility, and proprioceptive training. In centenarians, balance and gait are necessary for adequate ambulation. Some studies have assessed these parameters and incorporated them into answering questions about frailty, activities of daily living (ADL), and other indicators of healthy aging.

In the 5-COOP studies (Herr et al., 2018), investigators assessed frailty in a sample of over 1200 centenarians from five countries including Japan, France, Switzerland, Denmark, and Sweden. Two of the five indicators of frailty were slow walking speed and low physical activity, of which these were reported in 77.6% and 72.5% of the participants (Herr et al., 2018). Only weakness, as a frailty indicator, was reported more frequently (84.2%). The group summarized their findings to highlight that reaching 100 years of age is rarely observed without frailty. A study of 1043 Chinese centenarians of whom the majority were females in the China Longitudinal Healthy Longevity Survey also reported a lack of exercise associated with frailty (Zhang & Xu, 2022).

the FTSST was 18.63 ± 10.93 s, and 34% of these frail adults needed assistance with this test. In addition, the TUG took 20.22 ± 15.71 sec, with 27% of the adults needing assistance.

7.3.3.3 Balance

Older adults are recommended to perform multicomponent physical activity that includes balance training in addition to aerobic and muscle-strengthening activities. The Short Physical Performance Battery (SPPB) measures balance, gait, strength, and endurance on a scale of 0–12 with higher scores indicating higher lower limb function (Guralnik et al., 1994).

The Japanese SONIC study evaluated SPPB and found that tandem balance was higher in men than women and declined from age 70's to 90's cohort (Matsumoto et al., 2022). In another study of adults aged 90 or older in Dujiangyan China, Hao et al. (Hao et al., 2015) examined the association between falls and physical activity. The marker of physical activity was evaluated by former and current exercisers and farm work. This study reported that current habitual farm work and exercise had a significant odds ratio for falls, after adjusting for many variables (e.g. age, gender, body mass index, education, lifestyle, vision, temperament). The results indicated that current exercise was associated with a lower risk of falls, and former exercise played a more important role in prevalence of falls in women than current habitual farm work (Hao et al., 2015).

Poor balance can increase the risk for falls. The risk of falling and fall-related problems increases with age. As many falls can be prevented, it would be prudent to further investigate balance in centenarians given the limited information in this area.

7.4 Chapter Conclusion

Physical activity has a positive effect on health, and may be one highly important lifestyle factor influencing a centenarian's longevity. Studies that assessed the components of physical fitness have demonstrated a wide variability in muscular strength, cardiorespiratory fitness, and neuromotor fitness among centenarians. There is relatively little research on the improvements that can be attained with structured physical activity interventions in centenarians, although a few case studies point to highly active centenarians. It may also be of importance to investigate the lifestyle patterns of centenarians to help elucidate the best modality of activity that not only improves overall wellness, but that is safe and enjoyable for centenarians.

Multiple Choice Questions

1. Physical activity includes all of the following components except:
   A. Cardiorespiratory Fitness
   B. Neuromotor Fitness
   C. Nutrition
   D. Muscular Strength
   CORRECT ANSWER: C

2. Neuromotor exercise training refers to all of the following except?
   A. Coordination
   B. Proprioceptive Training
   C. Agility
   D. VO_2max
   CORRECT ANSWER: D

3. Which of the following measures would NOT be included in a test for balance?
   A. Ability to stand with the eyes closed
   B. Shoulder flexibility
   C. Gait
   D. Tandem walking
   CORRECT ANSWER: B

References

Andersen, H. R., Jeune, B., Nybo, H., Nielsen, J. B., Andersen-Ranberg, K., & Grandjean, P. (1998). Low activity of superoxide dismutase and high activity of glutathione reductase in erythrocytes from centenarians. *Age and Ageing, 27*(5), 643–648. https://doi.org/10.1093/ageing/27.5.643

Billat, V., Dhonneur, G., Mille-Hamard, L., Le Moyec, L., Momken, I., Launay, T., et al. (2017). Case studies in physiology: Maximal oxygen consumption and performance in a centenarian cyclist. *Journal of Applied Physiology (Bethesda, MD: 1985), 122*(3), 430–434. https://doi.org/10.1152/japplphysiol.00569.2016

Bull, F. C., Al-Ansari, S. S., Biddle, S., Borodulin, K., Buman, M. P., Cardon, G., et al. (2020). World Health Organization 2020 guidelines on physical activity and sedentary behaviour. *British Journal of Sports Medicine, 54*(24), 1451–1462. https://doi.org/10.1136/bjsports-2020-102955

Chan, Y. C., Suzuki, M., & Yamamoto, S. (1997). Dietary, anthropometric, hematological and biochemical assessment of the nutritional status of centenarians and elderly people in Okinawa, Japan. *Journal of the American College of Nutrition, 16*(3), 229–235. https://doi.org/10.1080/07315724.1997.10718679

Del Pozo Cruz, B., Biddle, S. J. H., Gardiner, P. A., & Ding, D. (2021). Light-intensity physical activity and life expectancy: National Health and nutrition survey. *American Journal of Preventive Medicine, 61*(3), 428–433. https://doi.org/10.1016/j.amepre.2021.02.012

Du, Y., Liu, B., Sun, Y., Snetselaar, L. G., Wallace, R. B., & Bao, W. (2019). Trends in adherence to the physical activity guidelines for Americans for aerobic activity and time spent on sedentary behavior among US Adults, 2007 to 2016. *JAMA Network Open, 2*(7), e197597. https://doi.org/10.1001/jamanetworkopen.2019.7597

Garber, C. E., Blissmer, B., Deschenes, M. R., Franklin, B. A., Lamonte, M. J., Lee, I. M., et al. (2011). American College of Sports Medicine position stand. Quantity and quality of exercise for developing and maintaining cardiorespiratory, musculoskeletal, and neuromotor fitness in apparently healthy adults: Guidance for prescribing exercise. *Medicine and Science in Sports and Exercise, 43*(7), 1334–1359. https://doi.org/10.1249/MSS.0b013e318213fefb

Guralnik, J. M., Simonsick, E. M., Ferrucci, L., Glynn, R. J., Berkman, L. F., Blazer, D. G., et al. (1994). A short physical performance battery assessing lower extremity function: Association with self-reported disability and prediction of mortality and nursing home admission. *Journal of Gerontology, 49*(2), M85–M94. Retrieved from PM:8126356.

Hao, Q., Yang, M., Luo, L., Hai, S., Ding, X., & Dong, B. (2015). The association of falls and various physical activities in Chinese nonagenarians/centenarians. *Archives of Gerontology and Geriatrics, 61*(1), 21–26. https://doi.org/10.1016/j.archger.2015.04.008

Hernandez-Vicente, A., Santos-Lozano, A., Mayolas-Pi, C., Rodriguez-Romo, G., Pareja-Galeano, H., Bustamante, N., et al. (2019). Physical activity and sedentary behavior at the end of the human lifespan. *Journal of Aging and Physical Activity, 27*(4), 899–905. https://doi.org/10.1123/japa.2018-0122

Hernandez-Vicente, A., Marin-Puyalto, J., Pueyo, E., Vicente-Rodriguez, G., & Garatachea, N. (2022). Physical activity in centenarians beyond cut-point-based accelerometer metrics. *International Journal of Environmental Research and Public Health, 19*(18). https://doi.org/10.3390/ijerph191811384

Herr, M., Jeune, B., Fors, S., Andersen-Ranberg, K., Ankri, J., Arai, Y., et al. (2018). Frailty and associated factors among centenarians in the 5-COOP countries. *Gerontology, 64*(6), 521–531. https://doi.org/10.1159/000489955

Janssen, I., Carson, V., Lee, I. M., Katzmarzyk, P. T., & Blair, S. N. (2013). Years of life gained due to leisure-time physical activity in the U.S. *American Journal of Preventive Medicine, 44*(1), 23–29. https://doi.org/10.1016/j.amepre.2012.09.056

Katz, S., Ford, A. B., Moskowitz, R. W., Jackson, B. A., & Jaffe, M. W. (1963). Studies of illness in the aged. The Index of Adl: A standardized measure of biological and psychosocial function. *JAMA, 185*, 914–919. https://doi.org/10.1001/jama.1963.03060120024016

Kim, H., Lee, T., Lee, S., Kim, K., Lee, S., Kam, S., et al. (2012). Factors associated with ADL and IADL dependency among Korean centenarians: Reaching the 100-year-old life transition. *International Journal of Aging & Human Development, 74*(3), 243–264. https://doi.org/10.2190/AG.74.3.e

Lawton, M. P., & Brody, E. M. (1969). Assessment of older people: Self-maintaining and instrumental activities of daily living. *Gerontologist, 9*(3), 179–186. Retrieved from https://www.ncbi.nlm.nih.gov/pubmed/5349366

Lee, I. M., Shiroma, E. J., Lobelo, F., Puska, P., Blair, S. N., Katzmarzyk, P. T., & Lancet Physical Activity Series Working, G. (2012). Effect of physical inactivity on major non-communicable diseases worldwide: An analysis of burden of disease and life expectancy. *Lancet, 380*(9838), 219–229. https://doi.org/10.1016/S0140-6736(12)61031-9

Li, Y., Bai, Y., Tao, Q. L., Zeng, H., Han, L. L., Luo, M. Y., et al. (2014). Lifestyle of Chinese centenarians and their key beneficial factors in Chongqing, China. *Asia Pacific Journal of Clinical Nutrition, 23*(2), 309–314. https://doi.org/10.6133/apjcn.2014.23.2.05

Martin, P., MacDonald, M., Margrett, J., Siegler, I., Poon, L. W., Jazwinski, S. M., et al. (2013). Correlates of functional capacity among centenarians. *Journal of Applied Gerontology, 32*(3), 324–346. https://doi.org/10.1177/0733464811420563

Matsumoto, K., Gondo, Y., Masui, Y., Yasumoto, S., Yoshida, Y., Ikebe, K., et al. (2022). Physical performance reference values for Japanese oldest old: A SONIC study. *BMC Geriatrics, 22*(1), 748. https://doi.org/10.1186/s12877-022-03299-7

Nozaki, H., Nohara, Y., Ashitomi, I., Zukeran, R., Inafuku, T., Akisaka, M., & Suzuki, M. (1998). [Serum albumin level and activities of daily living in centenarians]. *Nihon Ronen Igakkai Zasshi, 35*(10), 741–747. https://doi.org/10.3143/geriatrics.35.741.

Ozaki, A., Uchiyama, M., Tagaya, H., Ohida, T., & Ogihara, R. (2007). The Japanese centenarian study: Autonomy was associated with health practices as well as physical status. *Journal of the American Geriatrics Society, 55*(1), 95–101. https://doi.org/10.1111/j.1532-5415.2006.01019.x

Paffenbarger, R. S., Jr., Kampert, J. B., Lee, I. M., Hyde, R. T., Leung, R. W., & Wing, A. L. (1994). Changes in physical activity and other lifeway patterns influencing longevity. *Medicine and Science in Sports and Exercise, 26*(7), 857–865. Retrieved from https://www.ncbi.nlm.nih.gov/pubmed/7934759

Poon, L. W., Jazwinski, M., Green, R. C., Woodard, J. L., Martin, P., Rodgers, W. L., et al. (2007). Methodological considerations in studying centenarians: Lessons learned from the Georgia centenarian studies. *Annual Review of Gerontology & Geriatrics, 27*(1), 231–264. Retrieved from https://www.ncbi.nlm.nih.gov/pubmed/21852888

Rantanen, T., Masaki, K., He, Q., Ross, G. W., Willcox, B. J., & White, L. (2012). Midlife muscle strength and human longevity up to age 100 years: A 44-year prospective study among a decedent cohort. *Age (Dordrecht, Netherlands), 34*(3), 563–570. https://doi.org/10.1007/s11357-011-9256-y

Ravaglia, G., Forti, P., Maioli, F., Boschi, F., Cicognani, A., Bernardi, M., et al. (1997). Determinants of functional status in healthy Italian nonagenarians and centenarians: A comprehensive functional assessment by the instruments of geriatric practice. *Journal of the American Geriatrics Society, 45*(10), 1196–1202. https://doi.org/10.1111/j.1532-5415.1997.tb03769.x

Saez de Asteasu, M. L., Steffens, T., Ramirez-Velez, R., Cadore, E. L., Izquierdo, M., & Pietta-Dias, C. (2022). Low handgrip strength is associated with higher cancer prevalence in frail nonagenarians and centenarians. *Experimental Gerontology, 165*, 111862. https://doi.org/10.1016/j.exger.2022.111862

Scarpelli, M. C., Bergamasco, J. G. A., Arruda, E. A. B., Cook, S. B., & Libardi, C. A. (2021). Resistance training with partial blood flow restriction in a 99-year-old individual: A case report. *Front Sports Act Living, 3*, 671764. https://doi.org/10.3389/fspor.2021.671764

Services, U. S. D. o. H. a. H. (2018). *Physical activity guidelines for Americans*, 2nd edn.

Shimizu, K., Takeda, S., Noji, H., Hirose, N., Ebihara, Y., Arai, Y., et al. (2003). Dietary patterns and further survival in Japanese centenarians. *Journal of Nutritional Science and Vitaminology (Tokyo), 49*(2), 133–138. https://doi.org/10.3177/jnsv.49.133

Venturelli, M., Schena, F., & Richardson, R. S. (2012). The role of exercise capacity in the health and longevity of centenarians. *Maturitas, 73*(2), 115–120. https://doi.org/10.1016/j.maturitas.2012.07.009

Venturelli, M., Schena, F., Scarsini, R., Muti, E., & Richardson, R. S. (2013). Limitations to exercise in female centenarians: Evidence that muscular efficiency tempers the impact of failing lungs. *Age (Dordrecht, Netherlands), 35*(3), 861–870. https://doi.org/10.1007/s11357-011-9379-1

Wang, H., Hai, S., Liu, Y., Liu, Y., & Dong, B. (2019). Skeletal muscle mass as a mortality predictor among nonagenarians and centenarians: A prospective cohort study. *Scientific Reports, 9*(1), 2420. https://doi.org/10.1038/s41598-019-38893-0

Wen, C. P., Wai, J. P., Tsai, M. K., Yang, Y. C., Cheng, T. Y., Lee, M. C., et al. (2011). Minimum amount of physical activity for reduced mortality and extended life expectancy: A prospective cohort study. *Lancet, 378*(9798), 1244–1253. https://doi.org/10.1016/S0140-6736(11)60749-6

Winograd, C. H., Lemsky, C. M., Nevitt, M. C., Nordstrom, T. M., Stewart, A. L., Miller, C. J., & Bloch, D. A. (1994). Development of a physical performance and mobility examination. *Journal of the American Geriatrics Society, 42*(7), 743–749. https://doi.org/10.1111/j.1532-5415.1994.tb06535.x

Wu, Y., Wang, L., Cai, Z., Bao, L., Ai, P., & Ai, Z. (2017). Prevalence and risk factors of low health literacy: A community-based study in Shanghai, China. *International Journal of Environmental Research and Public Health, 14*(6). https://doi.org/10.3390/ijerph14060628

Yang, S., Wang, S., Tai, P., Jia, W., Han, K., Liu, M., & He, Y. (2021). Central and peripheral adiposity had different effect on disability in centenarians. *Front Endocrinol (Lausanne), 12*, 635205. https://doi.org/10.3389/fendo.2021.635205

Zeng, Y., Feng, Q., Hesketh, T., Christensen, K., & Vaupel, J. W. (2017). Survival, disabilities in activities of daily living, and physical and cognitive functioning among the oldest-old in China: A cohort study. *Lancet, 389*(10079), 1619–1629. https://doi.org/10.1016/S0140-6736(17)30548-2

Zhang, J., & Xu, L. (2022). Frailty and associated factors among Chinese centenarians. *The Journal of Nutrition, Health & Aging, 26*(8), 806–813. https://doi.org/10.1007/s12603-022-1831-7

Chapter 8
African American Centenarians

Rita Hargrave and Kanya Nesbeth

Key Take Away Points

1. African American centenarians have survived extensive socio-economic, educational, and healthcare disparities across their lifespan. These psychosocial challenges have produced devastating biological, psychological and social effects.
2. Despite this history, African American centenarians comprise 12% of all centenarians, similar to their ethnic/racial representation in the adult population of the United States. Family, friends, community, religious resources, and adaptive psychological strategies have contributed immensely to their survival.
3. Further research into African American centenarians' life trajectory and process of aging may help advocate for in advocating for increased community, state and federal support for this population's health and emotional well-being.

Illustrative Case Vignette Virginia McLaurin made headline news when she danced with President and Mrs. Obama at the age of 106 (by her report), as part of a Black History Month celebration in 2016 (National Archives, 2022; Ives, 2022). She was born at home into a sharecropper family in South Carolina. Ms. McLauin stated that her birth was recorded in a family Bible in 1909. However, official South Carolina records listed her birth year as 1916. She grew up in the Jim Crow South and left school in the eighthgrade to get married. She moved north as part of

R. Hargrave, M.D., F.A.P.A. (✉)
Consultant, University of California, Davis Alzheimer Disease Center-East Bay Division, Walnut Creek, CA, USA

PG-4 Resident, Howard University School of Medicine, Department of Pyschiatry, Washington, DC, USA
e-mail: ecarenet@yahoo.com

K. Nesbeth, M.D.
Washington, USA

R. E. Kheirbek, M. D. Llorente (eds.), *Current Perspectives on Centenarians*, International Perspectives on Aging 36,
https://doi.org/10.1007/978-3-031-30915-1_8

the Great Migration of millions of southern African-Americans and eventually settled in Washington, D.C. In her new home she worked as a seamstress, a domestic helper, laundry manager, and shipyard worker. In her "retirement", she volunteered 40 hours per week as a foster grandparent at a local school and as a voting advocate. She received many community service volunteer awards from several Washington, D.C. mayors, and the President's Volunteer Service Award in 2016. She passed away in 2022 at the age of 113. While Ms. McLaurin's acclaim may be unusual, her life experiences are illustrative of many other African American centenarians. Despite many racially based social obstacles (e.g. discrimination in education, employment, housing, and healthcare) which impacted her world, Ms. McLaurin pursued her long life with a sense of purpose, passion and community connectedness.

8.1 Introduction

African American centenarians represent a diverse cohort of individuals of mixed ethnic and cultural heritage. Beginning with the seventeenth-century international slave trade, millions of people participated in a forced relocation resulting in a diaspora from West and Central Africa to many parts of the world, including the Carribean, South America, Central America and the United States. Despite centuries of socio-economic, educational and health care disparities, African American centenarians comprise 12% of all centenarians in the United States, similar to their ethnic/racial representation in the adult population of the United States (2017 Profile of 2African Americans).

Prior ethno-geriatric research has focused on biological and psychosociological differences between African American compared to White older adults (Boen & Hummer, 2019). Few studies have described the unique adaptive and resilience strategies of the African American older adults and centenarians, and the nature of the networks and communities that have supported and sustained them (Boen & Hummer, 2019). Since most studies on cross-cultural health disparities are based on cross-sectional data, the currently available literature fails to explore the cumulative impact of lifetime inequities, racial/ethnic marginalization, implicit bias and the subsequent disparities of access to behavioral health, medical and wellness care. The COVID-19 pandemic produced a disproportionately large impact on the economic well-being, health and life-expectancy of African Americans. These burdens were devastating to African American older adults who were particularly vulnerable to the exposed health care and social service gaps in the United States. Future research approaches should focus on to improving our understanding of the life course African American centenarians, to take into account these cumulative effects. More nuanced, comprehensive research should focus on identifying strategies to improve social supports, health and wellness care, and political advocacy for African American centenarians and their caregivers. This chapter will explore the existing literature on the impact of biological and psychosocial forces and COVID-19 pandemic and the development of resilience strategies on the lives of African American centenarians.

8.2 Biological Aspects

8.2.1 Black-White Cross-over Mortality Paradox

For decades an ongoing debate has raged concerning the existence of a "crossover effect" in the mortality risk of the U.S. non-Hispanic Black and non-Hispanic White populations. The Black-White Mortality Crossover effect occurs when the higher age-specific mortality risk of one subpopulation (e.g., African Americans) converges with and then becomes lower than the age-specific mortality risk of another subpopulation (e.g., non-Hispanic whites) (Evert et al., 2003). The Black-White difference in mortality rates is widest in young adulthood, and then rates converge with increasing age until a crossover occurs at about age 85 years, after which African American older adults exhibit a lower mortality rate relative to older white adults (Lariscy, 2017; Roth et al., 2016). The proposed hypotheses for the Black-White paradox include the 1) select survivor cohort, 2) poor data quy, 3) cohort effects and 4) self-reported quality of health.

Select Survivor Cohort African Americans compared to Whites more frequently experience to adverse health outcomes due to multiple factors including health vulnerabilities, reduced access to medical care and social determinants of health. As a result, African Americans compared to Whites have a shorter life expectancy, and generally die at younger ages. Some investigators suggest that centenarians can be classified by three distinct morbidity profiles: Survivors, Delayers, and Escapers (Evert et al., 2003). Survivors profile, or those who have had a diagnosis of an age-associated illness prior to the age of 80. Delayers are individuals who delayed the onset of age-associated illness until at least the age of 80. Escapers were individuals who attained their 100th year of life without the diagnosis of common age-associated illnesses, is a select cohort of African Americans with enhanced survival rates relative to the same birth cohort of Whites (Evert et al., 2003). Compression of morbidity may be as a contributing factor for the development of select survivor cohorts. Ismail et al. (2016) reported that subgroup of Ashkenazi Jewish centenarians participating in the Longevity Genes Project (LGP) and the New England Centenarian Study (NECS) exhibited morbidity compression. Compression of morbidity may have delayed the onset of majorage-related diseases, compared to younger reference groups (Ismail, et al. 2016). These findings are consistent with previous research and may be generalizable to other cohorts. Future large scale comparative studies need to examine validity of the concepts of compression of morbidity and distinct morbidity profiles among of African American centenarians.

Poor Data Quality The Black-White mortality crossover paradox has been linked to inaccuracies in data collection due to unmatched or uncounted deaths and age misreporting on death certificates (Barnes & Bates, 2017). Age misreporting (i.e., overstatement of age) on death certificates may be more common among African Americans than Whites. Hill et al. noted that only 53% of death certificates report accurate ages, and that errors of 5 years or greater existed in 10% of the records (Hill et al., 1997). This reporting error could bias mortality rate estimates downward among the oldest adults (Barnes & Bates, 2017). Inaccurate death records may hinder accurate estimates of ethnic/racial differences in mortality data of African American compared to White older adults (Lariscy, 2017).

Cohort Effects Some investigators suggest that cohort effects drive the Black-White mortality crossover paradox. The relationship between cohort characteristics and mortality risk extends the heterogeneity argument, which proposes that disparate cohort processes affect the divergent life course and mortality risks of African American compared to and White populations (Masters, 2012). Cohort effects are also fundamental to the "life course theory." The Life Course Theory conceptualizes health as an integrated continuum that describes how the interaction of biological, behavioral, psychological, social, and environmental factors across an individual's life shape health trajectory outcomes. The principles of the Life Course Theory promote looking beyond the narrow lens of a single disease process in isolation from other factors. The Life Course Theory underscores how social, economic, and environmental factors are driving forces of persistent inequalities in healthcare among African Americans and other marginalized populations (U.S. Department of Health, Human Services 2010). The lived experiences of the current cohort of African American and White older adults have changed dramatically over the twentieth century. The Life Course Theory offers a unique perspective on how psychosocial force shape the morbidity and mortality risks of African American and White older adults (Ben-Shlomo & Kuh, 2002).

Self-Reported Quality of Health Previous research has identified a positive association between poor self-reported health and higher mortality risk particularly among Whites, younger populations, and individuals with greater education. But Roth et al. reported that African Americans, compared to Whites, have a lower association between poor self-reported health and mortality, even after adjusting for demographics and health history covariates (Roth et al., 2016). The authors proposed that this lower association between self-reported health and mortality among African Americans is due to other factors and mechanisms besides race/ethnicity. Roth et al. suggest that future research which provides a more comprehensive examination of behavioral, social, and cultural factors, as well as social determinants of health would improve and advance our understanding of the Black-White mortality crossover effect among older adults in the United States. (Roth et al., 2016).

8.3 Impact of the COVID-19 Pandemic

The COVID-19 pandemic resulted in devastating effects on older adults in African Americans and other marinalized ethnic/racial minorities. COVID-19 accounted for most of the overall reduction in 2020 life expectancy at birth, with extensive racial/

ethnic disparities in the mortality risk (Andrasfay & Goldman, 2022). In 2020, African American and Latino populations experienced reductions in life expectancy at birth which were more than twice as large as that of the White population. Further, despite the widespread distribution in 2021 of effective vaccines that could have mitigated the overall severity and mortality of COVID-19, vaccination rates have been lower among racial/ethnic minority groups. As a result, health and wellness disparities persisted in those communities (Andrasfay & Goldman, 2022). The U.S. population experienced a decline in life expectancy at birth in 2021 of 2.2 years from 2019, 0.6 years more than estimated for 2020. The corresponding reductions estimated for the Black and Latino populations were nearly twice that for Whites. (Andrasfay & Goldman, 2022).

The disproportionate impact of COVID-19 on older populations and African American, Latinos, and other racial/ethnic minority groups underscored their precarious position in terms of higher levels of potential exposure, elevated risk for poorer disease outcomes, and disproportionately high mortality rates (Chatters et al., 2020). COVID-19 revealed how racism and ageism continue to shape attitudes, medical practice, and policies concerning older adults and racial/ethnicminority groups and the resultant outcomes (Chatters et al., 2020; Khazan, 2020). Tragically, persons who are both older and members of racial and ethnic minority groups, particularly African American and Latino older adults, continue to suffer disproportionately from COVID-19 when compared to older White adults. The aftermath of COVID will likely affect the morbidity, mortality, and life course of future cohorts of African American centenarians. Future research should explore the long-term effects of COVID on morbidity, mortality, and quality of life for African American older adults in the U.S.

8.4 Sociological Aspects of Aging

Some authors suggest that the rate of improved individual health over time was equivalent across different regions of the U.S. (Northeast, Midwest, West, South). (Abeliansky et al., 2020). The authors attributed this steady trend of improved health among older Americans to improved access to health care and effective public health programs. Public health programs such as smoking cessation campaigns have led to greatly improved public education about the health-damaging impact of smoking and resulted in reduced rates of smoking (Abeliansky et al., 2020).

Ferraro and other investigators have suggested that the cumulative inequity should be incorporated into gerontological research to explore how the process of early and accumulated social inequities shape the physical and mental life course of older adults (Ferraro & Shippee, 2009). "Cumulative inequality (CI) theory specifies that social systems generate inequality, which manifests over the life course via demographic and developmental processes, and that personal trajectories are shaped by the accumulation of risk, available resources, perceived trajectories, and human agency…" and "may lead to premature mortality" (Ferraro & Shippee, 2009).

Cumulative inequity theory provides a useful perspective for examination of the lifetime trajectory of African American centenarians. The frailty index (FI) is a component of the cumulative inequity theory (Mitnitski et al., 2002). The FI measures older individual's health status and serves as a proxy measure of aging and vulnerability (Mitnitski et al., 2002). FI calculates the proportion of deficits present in an individual out of the total number of age-related health variables (Mitnitski et al., 2002). These deficits include diseases, signs, symptoms, laboratory abnormalities, cognitive impairments, and disabilities in activities of daily living (Mitnitski et al., 2002). Longitudinal data analysis indicates that FI for Whites improves at a rate of 1.3–1.5% per year of birth, consistent with estimated rates reported among European populations (Abeliansky et al., 2020). However the rate of age-associated improvement among African Americans is substantially lower (Abeliansky et al., 2020). The authors suggest that African American older adults experienced less benefit from the improving health status described for White older adults in the United States. This persistent health deficit among African American compared to White older adults may be due to both static and dynamic inequality. Due to static inequality, African American (compared to White) adults struggle to overcome persistent obstacles to accessing the most up-to-date diagnostic and treatment services (Abeliansky et al., 2020). The authors posit that dynamic inequality in terms of obstacles to healthcare access and education between Whites and African Americans have become larger over time (Abeliansky et al., 2020). Outreach and educational programs based on the cumulative inequity theory and the lived experience of African American older adults could facilitate the development and mobilization of resources (personal, group, and social) that promote human agency and shape health literacy, illness prevention, and behavioral health initiatives (Ferraro & Shippee, 2009). This longitudinal, more comprehensive ethnogeriatric perspective is particularly relevant for African American centenarians, many of whom have survived despite early and enduring inequalities, multiple medical and psychosocial risks and restricted opportunities. **A significant and longstanding body of research suggests that provider and institutional bias and discrimination contribute to racial health disparities, and resulting in ethnic/racial differences in diagnosis, prognosis, and treatment decisions** (Tong & Artiga, 2021). Racially based inequalities in healthcare and socio-economic status (SES) are also pervasive drivers of health inequalities (Phelan & Link, 2015). Recent studies suggest that other social forces such as inequities in power, prestige, freedom, and neighborhood context, exert tremendous impacts on wellness and healthcare of African Americans independent of SES (Phelan & Link, 2015). Numerous authors have noted that health care providers appear to exhibit implicit bias in terms of positive attitudes toward Whites and negative attitudes toward people of color (Hall et al., 2015). However there is little existing literature on the combined impact of ageism and implicit racial/ethnic bias on the health and well-being of African American centenarians. Future studies should utilize more comprehensive methods to examine the complex relationship between implicit bias, ethnicity, age, and healthcare outcomes. Interventions focused on reducing implicit bias among health care professionals are critical to reducing health disparities for African American centenarians.

8.5 Psychological Aspects of Aging

8.5.1 Black- White Mental Health Paradox

There is a paucity of research on psychiatric disorders and mental health among African American in general and especially among African American older adults (Taylor et al., 2019). Determining comparative rates of psychiatric disorders can be difficult since the definition of older adults varies depending on the research group from those over 50 years old to those over 60. Several researchers have explored the intersection of ethnicity and mental health in relation to the Black-White mental health epidemiological paradox. The Black White mental health paradox refers to the observation that African Americans, compared to non-Latino Whites have lower or similar rates of mental disorders (Barnes et.al., 2013). Yet, research has generally paid less attention to how such findings may vary across different socio-economic levels (Tobin et al., 2022). Though their study did not include data on centenarians or near centenarians, Taylor et al. reported that older compared to younger African Americans experienced lower rates of psychiatric disorders (Taylor et al., 2019). In addition, this mental health advantage found among African Americans when compared with Whites widened after adjusting for socioeconomic factors (Taylor et al., 2019; Erving et al., 2019). A highly understudied, but a consistent finding is that suicide rates among older African Americans (aged 65–74) are lower than suicide rates in any other racial group of American seniors (Curtin & Hedegaard, 2019). Future research directions should address current gaps in our knowledge regarding the correlates and risk factors for centenarians and near centenarians for specific disorders (e.g., PTSD, anxiety disorders), the impact of incarceration, homelessness, and other life experiences and trajectories on African American centenarians. In addition, examination of the coping strategies used by older African Americans (e.g. drawing upon family, friends, community and religious resources) will improve our understanding of these factors contributors to longevity of African American centanarians and may help to promote the development of similar strategies for other racial and ethnic groups (Taylor et al., 2019).

The prevalence and incidence of Alzheimer's disease among African Americans is higher compared to Whites (Rajan et al., 2019). Rajan et al. found that the rates were approximately twice as high among African Americans compared to European Americans. More recently, Power and colleagues found that the prevalence and incidence of dementia remained substantially higher among African-American compared with non-Hispanic White individuals in the US from 2000 to 2016 (Power et al., 2021). The frequency of dementia remains higher among African American centenarians compared to White centenarians (87.2% of African American versus 73.2% of white centenarian study participants) (Poon et al., 2012). The authors hypothesize that reasons for racial differences may include known disease risk factors (such as hypertension, diabetes mellitus, and stroke) and lower educational attainment, both of which occur with greater frequency among African Americans. However dementia in centenarians is not inevitable. 12.5% of African American centenarian study participants exhibited no dementia.

8.6 Religion and Spirituality

A 2020 review of comparative studies on religion and mental health and well-being among African American and Latino older adults suggests that religious involvement can be a protective factor against a wide range of mental health problems, including depression, substance use disorders, suicide, anxiety disorders, and depressive symptoms (Nguyen, 2020). The author described differences in the impact of the multiple dimensions of religiosity and mental health among African Americans, Latinos, and non-Latino Whites. The author discussed the limitations of the current literature and proposed future directions for research on religion and mental health in racial/ethnic minority populations of older adults. The authors underscored how an improved understanding of the mental health effects of religion on African American older adults could contribute to the developing and implementing of more culturally competent practices and interventions.

Religiosity is especially important for older blacks as a buffer against the negative consequences of discrimination and hopelessness. For many older adults, aging brings is an increased awareness of the finality of life and more frequent experiences of death, including the death of a spouse or other family members and friends of similar age (Mitchell et al., 2020). African American older adults may therefore turn to religion to a greater extent as a way of coping with and finding meaning in these major life events (Silverstein & Bengtson, 2018). Mitchell noted that a large percentage of the older African Americans in their study were born between 1912 and 1960, many of whom came of age during the Civil Rights Movement. During that unique historical period, the Black Church played a powerful role in the everyday lives of African Americans. Prominent ministers and congregational leaders provided messages of faith and resilience to combat discrimination, domestic terrorism and adversity. Future research should explore whether the powerful social influence of the Black church on current and future cohorts of African American centenarians.

8.7 Resilience Strategies

The health and well-being of African Americans is often described in terms of significant disparities, such as higher disease prevalence, greater comorbidities, poorer health outcomes, and earlier mortality. Little attention has been historically devoted to the narrative that for centuries African Americans have demonstrated the sustained ability to survive an evolving array of social, economic, and environmental adversarial forces. (Taylor et al., 2019). The individual and collective resilience of African Americans has often been overlooked. Generations of African Americans have employed adaptive psychological strategies such as control of beliefs, increased personal growth, and maintaining a sense of life purpose (Springfield et al., 2022). The **Pfund study reported that having a clear life purpose** may help buffer against the detrimental effects of depressive symptoms, cognitive decline and loneliness (Pfund et. al., 2022). The authors indicated that the buffering effects of a sense of purpose on subjective cognitive decline were stronger for African American compared to White older adults. **The authors suggest that f**uture research should examine how purpose-promoting programs support healthy cognitive aging, particularly among African American older adults. Future scientific exploration of resilience strategies should focus on how marginalized African American centenarians bounce back from chronic adversities, ranging from daily microaggressions to legally sanctioned, chronic oppression (Taylor et al., 2019).

Life course theory explores how individuals are affected by chronological age, social roles, and historical time, resulting in differences in developmental trajectories (Elder & Rockwell, 1979). The life course patterns of ethnic minorities are often influenced by cumulative intergenerational inequality or the transmission of inequality across multiple generations over time (Ferraro & Shippee, 2009). Oral historical narratives describing cumulative inequality among long-lived African American individuals have received inadequate attention in the gerontological literature. No published research has explored the life course experiences of a large representative sample of exceptionally long-lived African American men and women. However interviews with a small sample of African American older adults (Heinz et al., 2021) identified two themes. First, historical time and place influence perceptions of participants' family lineage, segregation, discrimination, racism, and societal changes. Second, participants employed a variety of resource buffers against inequality. The participants also discussed subthemes of support and cultural connectedness, religion and spirituality, and self-reliance. (Heinz et al., 2021). The authors suggested that research should utilize a person-centered psychosociological research strategy to uncover a broader range of adaptive strategies used by African American centenarians.

8.8 Conclusion

There needs to be more examination of the biological and psychosocial aspects and resilience strategies of African American centenarians. Future research on African American centenarians should include representative samples drawn from various geographic locations, socio-economic, and educational backgrounds to elucidate this unique group of individuals' medical, psychosocial and behavioral health needs. Future research with African American centenarians may be helpful in advocating for increased community, state, and federal support for this population.

Multiple Choice Questions

1. Which of the following groups of seniors (aged 65–74) have the lowest suicide rates?
   A. Non Hispanic Whites
   B. Non Hispanic Blacks
   C. Non Hispanic Asians
   D. Hispanics
   CORRECT ANSWER: B
2. When does the Black White Mortality Cross-Over Effect occur?
   A. In late life, after age 85
   B. In middle age
   C. In young adulthood
   D. In infancy
   CORRECT ANSWER: A
3. Which of the following are reported to contribute to resiliency among African American centenarians?
   A. Support and cultural connectedness
   B. Religion and spirituality
   C. Self-reliance
   D. All of the above
   CORRECT ANSWER: D

References

Abeliansky, A. L., Erel, D., & Strulik, H. (2020). Aging in the USA: Similarities and disparities across time and space. *Scientific Reports, 10*(1), 14309. https://doi.org/10.1038/s41598-020-71269-3

Andrasfay, T., & Goldman, N. (2022). Reductions in US life expectancy during the COVID-19 pandemic by race and ethnicity: Is 2021 a repetition of 2020? *medRxiv [Preprint]*. https://doi.org/10.1101/2021.10.17.21265117

Barnes, D. M., & Bates, L. M. (2017). Do racial patterns in psychological distress shed light on the black–white depression paradox? A systematic review. *Social Psychiatry and Psychiatric Epidemiology, 52*, 913–928. https://doi.org/10.1007/s00127-017-1394-9

Barnes, D. M., Keyes, K. M., & Bates, L. M. (2013). Racial differences in depression in the United States: How do subgroup analyses inform a paradox? *Social Psychiatry and Psychiatric Epidemiology, 48*(12), 1941–1949. https://doi.org/10.1007/s00127-013-0718-7

Ben-Shlomo, Y., & Kuh, D. (2002). A life course approach to chronic disease epidemiology: Conceptual models, empirical challenges and interdisciplinary perspectives. *International Journal of Epidemiology, 31*, 285–293. https://doi.org/10.1093/ije/31.2.285

Boen, C. E., & Hummer, R. A. (2019). Longer-but harder-lives? The Hispanic health paradox and the social determinants of racial, ethnic, and immigrant-native health disparities from midlife through late life. *Journal of Health and Social Behavior, 60*(4), 434–452. https://doi.org/10.1177/0022146519884538

CDC. Covid Data Tracker. https://covid.cdc.gov/covid-data-tracker/#datatracker-home

Chatters, L. M., Taylor, H. O., & Taylor, R. J. (2020). Older black Americans during COVID-19: Race and age double jeopardy. *Health Education & Behavior, 47*(6), 855–860. https://doi.org/10.1177/1090198120965513

Curtin SC, Hedegaard H. (2019). Suicide rates for females and males by race and ethnicity: United States, 1999 and 2017. Available at: Products - Health E Stats - Suicide Rates for females and males by race/ethnicity: United States: 1999 and 2014 (cdc.gov). Accessed 14 Jan 2023.

Elder, G. H., & Rockwell, R. C. (1979). The life-course and human development: An ecological perspective. *International Journal of Behavioral Development, 2*, 1–21. https://doi.org/10.1177/016502547900200101

Erving, C. L., Thomas, C. S., & Frazier, C. (2019). Is the black-white mental health paradox consistent across gender and psychiatric disorders? *American Journal of Epidemiology, 188*(2), 314–322. https://doi.org/10.1093/aje/kwy224

Evert J, Lawler E, Bogan H, Perls T. (2003) Morbidity profiles of centenarians: survivors, delayers, and escapers. *The Journals of Gerontology. Series A, Biological Sciences and Medical Sciences, 58*(3):232–237

Ferraro, K. F., & Shippee, T. P. (2009). Aging and cumulative inequality: How does inequality get under the skin? *The Gerontologist, 49*(3), 333–343. https://doi.org/10.1093/geront/gnp034

Hall, W. J., Chapman, M. V., Lee, K. M., Merino, Y. M., Thomas, T. W., Payne, B. K., Eng, E., Day, S. H., & Coyne-Beasley, T. (2015). Implicit racial/ethnic bias among health care professionals and its influence on health care outcomes: A systematic review. *American Journal of Public Health, 105*(12), e60–e76. https://doi.org/10.2105/AJPH.2015.302903

Heinz, M., Bishop, A. J., & Finchum, T. (2021). The lived experiences of African American centenarians: Narrative exploration from a life course theory perspective. *The Gerontologist, 61*(8), 1266–1276. https://doi.org/10.1093/geront/gnab052

Hill, M. E., Preston, S. H., Elo, I. T., & Rosenwaike, I. (1997). Age-linked institutions and age reporting among older African Americans. *Social Forces, 75*(3), 1007–1030. https://doi.org/10.2307/2580528

Ismail, K., Nussbaum, L., Sebastiani, P., Andersen, S., Perls, T., Barzilai, N., & Milman, S. (2016). Compression of morbidity is observed across cohorts with exceptional longevity. *Journal of the American Geriatrics Society, 64*(8), 1583–1591. https://doi.org/10.1111/jgs.14222

Ives M. (2022). Virginia McLaurin Dies; Sharecroppers' Daughter Who Danced with the Obamas. Available at: Virginia McLaurin Dies; Sharecroppers' Daughter Who Danced With the Obamas- The New York Times (nytimes.com). Accessed 14 Jan 2023.

Khazan O. (2020). A failure of empathy led to 200,000 deaths. It has deep roots. The Atlantic. https://www.theatlantic.com/politics/archive/2020/09/covid-death-toll-us-empathy-elderly/616379/

Lariscy, J. T. (2017). Black–White disparities in adult mortality: Implications of differential record linkage for understanding the mortality crossover. *Population Research and Policy Review, 36*, 137–156.

Masters, R. K. (2012). Uncrossing the U.S black-white mortality crossover: The role of cohort forces in life course mortality risk. *Demography, 49*(3), 773–796. https://doi.org/10.1007/s13524-012-0107-y

Mitchell, U. A., Gutierrez-Kapheim, M., Nguyen, A. W., & Al-Amin, N. (2020). Hopelessness among middle-aged and older blacks: The negative impact of discrimination and protecting power of social and religious resources. *Innov Aging, 4*(5), igaa044. https://doi.org/10.1093/geroni/igaa044

Mitnitski, A. B., Graham, J. E., Mogilner, A. J., & Rockwood, K. (2002). Frailty, fitness and late-life mortality in relation to chronological and biological age. *BMC Geriatrics, 2*, 1. https://doi.org/10.1186/1471-2318-2-1

National Archives. (2022). Rediscovering black history – DC's favorite centenarian: A tribute to Virginia McLaurin. Available at: https://rediscovering-black-history.blogs.archives.gov/2022/11/17. Accessed 14 Jan 2023.

Nguyen, A. W. (2020). Religion and Mental Health in Racial and Ethnic Minority Populations: A Review of the Literature. *Innov Aging, 4*(5), igaa035. https://doi.org/10.1093/geroni/igaa035

Pfund, G. N., Spears, I., Norton, S. A., Bogdan, R., Oltmanns, T. F., & Hill, P. L. (2022). Sense of purpose as a potential buffer between mental health and subjective cognitive decline. *International Psychogeriatrics, 16*, 1–11. https://doi.org/10.1017/S1041610222000680

Phelan, J. C., & Link, B. G. (2015). Is racism a fundamental cause of inequalities in health? *The Annual Review of Sociology, 41*, 311–330. https://doi.org/10.1146/annurev-soc-073014-112305

Poon, L. W., Woodard, J. L., Stephen Miller, L., Green, R., Gearing, M., Davey, A., Arnold, J., Martin, P., Siegler, I. C., Nahapetyan, L., Kim, Y. S., & Markesbery, W. (2012). Understanding dementia prevalence among centenarians. *J Gerontol A Biol Sci Med Sci, 67*(4), 358–365. https://doi.org/10.1093/gerona/glr250. Epub 2012 Mar 1. PMID: 22389466; PMCID: PMC3309877).

Power, M. C., Bennett, E. E., Turner, R. W., Dowling, N. M., Ciarleglio, A., Glymour, M. M., & Gianattasio, K. Z. (2021). Trends in Relative Incidence and Prevalence of Dementia Across Non-Hispanic Black and White Individuals in the United States, 2000–2016. *JAMA Neurol, 78*(3), 275–284. https://doi.org/10.1001/jamaneurol.2020.4471. PMID: 33252617; PMCID: PMC7953306).

Rajan, K. B., Weuve, J., Barnes, L. L., Wilson, R. S., & Evans, D. A. (2019). Prevalence and incidence of clinically diagnosed Alzheimer's disease dementia from 1994 to 2012 in a population study. *Alzheimers Dement, 15*(1), 1–7. https://doi.org/10.1016/j.jalz.2018.07.216. Epub 2018 Sep 7. PMID: 30195482; PMCID: PMC6531287.

Roth, D. L., Skarupski, K. A., Crews, D. C., Howard, V. J., & Locher, J. L. (2016). Distinct age and self-rated health crossover mortality effects for African Americans: Evidence from a national cohort study. *Social Science & Medicine, 156*, 12–20. https://doi.org/10.1016/j.socscimed.2016.03.019

Silverstein, M., & Bengtson, V. L. (2018). Return to religion? Predictors of religious change among baby-boomers in their transition to later life. *Journal of Population Ageing, 11*(1), 7–21. https://doi.org/10.1007/s12062-017-9216-0

Springfield, S., Qin, F., Hedlin, H., Eaton, C. B., Rosal, M. C., Taylor, H., Staudinger, U. M., & Stefanick, M. L. (2022). Modifiable Resources and Resilience in Racially and Ethnically Diverse Older Women: Implications for Health Outcomes and Interventions. *Int J Environ Res Public Health, 19*(12), 7089. https://doi.org/10.1007/s00127-013-0718-7. Epub 2013 Jun 4. PMID: 23732705; PMCID: PMC3834079.

Taylor, R. J., Chatters, L. M., & Taylor, H. O. (2019). Race and objective social isolation: Older African Americans, black Caribbeans, and non-Hispanic whites. *The Journals of Gerontology. Series B, Psychological Sciences and Social Sciences, 74*(8), 1429–1440. https://doi.org/10.1093/geronb/gby114

Tobin, C. T., Erving, C. L., Hargrove, T. W., & Satcher, L. A. (2022). Is the black-white mental health paradox consistent across age, gender, and psychiatric disorders? *Aging & Mental Health, 26*(1), 196–204. https://doi.org/10.1080/13607863.2020.1855627

Tong M, Artiga S. (2021). Use of race in clinical diagnosis and decision making: Overview and implications. https://www.kff.org/racial-equity-and-health-policy/issue-brief/use-of-race-in-clinical-diagnosis-and-decision-making-overview-and-implications/#:~:text=Racial%20stereotyping%20of%20disease%20an

Chapter 9
The Hispanic Paradox: Is There a Hispanic Mortality Advantage?

Danya P. Anouti, Alexander Z. Beard, Maritza Buenaver, and Maria D. Llorente

Key Take Away Points

1. US Hispanics have longer life expectancy than other US populations, including NHW despite a worse health outcomes profile including higher rates of central obesity, low levels of physical activity, lower educational level, lower socioeconomic status, and discrimination. This phenomenon is known as the Hispanic Paradox.
2. Factors, such as strong family and social supports, protective dietary habits, and optimism have all been proposed as reasons for the Hispanic Paradox.
3. Acculturation may decrease the longevity advantage.

9.1 Introduction

Hispanics are a diverse and complex group and are now the largest minority population in the United States. Like the rest of the country, this group is also aging. Despite experiencing hardships in arriving to the US, and multiple societal

D. P. Anouti · A. Z. Beard
Department of Psychiatry, George Washington University School of Medicine, Washington, DC, USA

M. Buenaver
Oklahoma City VA Health Care System, Oklahoma CIty, OK, USA

M. D. Llorente (✉)
Department of Veterans Affairs, Washington, DC, USA

Department of Psychiatry, Georgetown University School of Medicine, Washington, DC, USA
e-mail: Maria.Llorente@va.gov

R. E. Kheirbek, M. D. Llorente (eds.), *Current Perspectives on Centenarians*, International Perspectives on Aging 36,
https://doi.org/10.1007/978-3-031-30915-1_9

disadvantages that should compromise their health, US Latinos demonstrate a longevity advantage (the Hispanic Paradox) when compared to the majority population. This chapter will review the demographic, social determinants, physical and mental health of US Latinos, and compare these features to those of the majority US population, non-Hispanic Whites (NHW). Evidence demonstrating the Hispanic Paradox, as well as possible reasons for these findings are provided. Some of the unique contributors to resilience and successful aging among Latinos will be described.

9.2 Illustrative Vignette

CL is a vibrant 102-year-old never married Mexican woman who identifies as Catholic. She has a medical history of hypertension, chronic kidney disease (stage II), multiple yeast infections, bowel and bladder incontinence, and mild cognitive impairment. She grew up, spent most of her life in Mexico City, and then migrated to the United States (U.S.) in the 1980s to live with her only daughter and her daughter's family. She helped raise her two grandchildren. While one of eight children, she is the last surviving sibling. Her family describes her as "always happy," "life loving," and "vivacious". She enjoys eating *ceviche* and *helado* for dessert, dancing to mariachi music, taking long walks where she can enjoy nature, and attending church every Sunday. When her daughter died, she moved in with her granddaughter where she gets to spend time with her great grandchildren.

9.3 Is It Hispanic, Latino, Chicano, or Latinx?

The terms Hispanic, Latino, Chicano, and Latinx have all been used to describe diverse, multinational groups of people, each with their own unique history, culture, geography, and reasons for migration. What unites these groups is a common language, Spanish and some shared cultural aspects. It is important to understand these terms, and their origins, as well as preferences expressed by the people these terms are intended to represent. The word Hispanic originates from *Hispania*, a Latin language term for the region that would later become the nation of Spain (Merriam-Webster, 2022a, b, c, d). Of note, Hispania is also related to the Spanish language word for Spain, *España*. One definition used is "of, relating to, or being a person of Latin American descent and especially of Cuban, Mexican, or Puerto Rican origin living in the U.S."· It is notable that Hispanic is a term used primarily in the United States, as emphasized in this definition. Another listed definition is "of, or relating to, the people, speech, or culture of Spain". This term therefore excludes persons from countries without direct ties to Spain, such as Brazil, Haiti, Suriname, Guyana, and French Guiana and others who have ties to colonial powers other than Spain. The term "Hispanic" first gained popularity and use throughout the 1960s and 1970s as a part of the civil rights movement in the US (Blakemore, 2022.) At the time, there was recognition that the lack of data describing Hispanic/Latino populations made it difficult to guide appropriate legislation or government policies. In 1970, the US Census asked people if they were "persons of Spanish origin"; however, this led to confusion as not everyone can directly trace their roots directly to Spain. In 1980, the question changed to ask if people were "of Spanish/Hispanic origin or descent". This was accompanied by a public service advertising campaign by the federal government which led to popularization of the term.

There are potential concerns in using the term Hispanic. It is inexorably tied to the colonial past of Spain and its impact on the indigenous peoples of the Americas. This has led to the popularity of another term, Latino. Latino is defined as "a native or inhabitant of Latin America" and alternatively as "a person of Latin American origin living in the U.S." (Merriam-Webster, 2022a, b, c, d). While the term has existed possibly since the early 1800s, it started to gain popularity in the 1970s and ultimately was added to the US Census in 2000 in a question that asks if the person is "Spanish/Hispanic/Latino" (Cohn, 2010).

Chicano is a term for those specifically of Mexican heritage who were born in the United States (Merriam-Webster, 2022a, b, c, d). There is some debate on the origin of the term but the prevailing theory is that it originates from dropping the first syllable in *Mexicano*, and replacing the "x" with the "ch" sound: Xicano to Chicano (Zaragoza, 2017). This term similarly gained popularity in the 1960s and 1970s as a part of civil rights movements in the US (Estrada, 2015). Chicano is considered to be an acceptable term for Mexican American persons, but is not typically used to refer to other Latino subgroups.

The term "Latinx" is a new term which was initially suggested as an attempt to find a gender-neutral alternative to Latino or Latina (Merriam-Webster, 2022a, b, c, d). In the Spanish language, nouns and adjectives are assigned a masculine or feminine gender. A word ending with -o is considered masculine or gender neutral and the ending -a is considered feminine (Harris, 1991). While Latinx has been used in some academic contexts (Torres, 2018), it has received significant negative backlash among US Latinos, and as a result, has not only not significantly received widespread usage, but has been heavily criticized. This term is viewed by many Latinos as offensive, "x'ing" out the Latino culture and language, and replacing it with an English word (Lopez Torregrosa, 2021). First, the -x as a neutral letter may work in English, but it does not follow the structure of Spanish and there is no clear way to pronounce "Latinx" in Spanish. Second, polling data of Latino/Hispanic people in 2020 showed that only 3% use the term, and a similar questionnaire in 2021 showed usage had dropped to 2% (Bendixen & Amandi International, 2021; Noe-Bustamante et al., 2020). In the 2021 poll, 40% of participants indicated that the term "Latinx" bothers or offends them. Only 23% had heard of the term previously. As a result, in 2021, the League of United Latin American Citizens, the largest and oldest Hispanic civil rights organization in the US, dropped Latinx from all official communications (Gamboa, 2021). In the 2021 poll referenced above, participants were asked which terms come closest to describing their ethnic background with 68% choosing Hispanic and 21% choosing Latino/Latina. The 2020 data showed a similar result with 61% choosing Hispanic and 29% choosing Latino/Latina. While both terms are generally considered to be acceptable, Hispanic is preferred. Further, it would be a preferred gender-neutral term to refer to those individuals who identify as non-binary. Currently, the US Census uses "Hispanic or Latino" to ask about ethnicity (U.S. Department of Commerce, 2022). Recently, opinion editorials are starting to suggest referring to the person's country of origin rather than attempting to come up with a term to describe such a vast geographic and cultural space (Austin & Johnson, 2012; Bernstein, 2021). Unfortunately, there is very limited data, and in some cases no data at all, that drill down to the specific country of origin for much of the medical research conducted in US Hispanic populations. When the data is available, this chapter will describe it, but in general, the terms "Latino" and "Hispanic" are used throughout interchangeably.

9.4 Latino Seniors: Demographics, Social Determinants and Health

9.4.1 Demographics and Changing Future Trends

The US Hispanic population will grow to 112 million by 2050, accounting for 28% of the total population (Hummer & Hayward, 2015). In 2019, about one third of all Latinos living in the US were born outside the country (Funk & Lopez, 2022). Approximately half of Hispanics live in California, Florida, and Texas. In many large metropolitan areas, Hispanics often live in segregated and predominantly Hispanic neighborhoods. The areas with higher Latino segregation tend to be those where large Latino populations have traditionally lived and been established, such as Los Angeles, Chicago, or the northeast. Newer destinations for Latinos are less segregated, particularly in the southeast or Midwest, with the fastest growth rates in North and South Dakota. Segregation levels among Hispanics are modestly declining.

This population is also aging, with Hispanics 65 and older projected to increase five-fold between 2012 and 2050. By 2060, the number of Hispanics aged 65 and older in the US is projected to increase to 19.9 million and will comprise 21% of the older population (US Department of Health & Human Services, 2020). In 2017, there were nearly 7300 Hispanic centenarians in the US (1955 men and 5340 women). Prior to the COVID-19 pandemic, US Hispanics had the longest life expectancy at 81.8 years compared to 78.5 years for NHW and Asians, and 74.9 years for Blacks (Feldman & Bassett, 2021). As a result of the pandemic, life expectancy fell for all groups, but the greatest decline was seen among Hispanics, dropping to 78.8 years. A recent study confirmed these findings, based on official death counts, but this same impact on life expectancy was not seen in 21 peer countries. (Woolf et al. 2022). The main reason proposed for this disproportionate impact for US Hispanics was increased COVID-19 infection and mortality associated with risk factors that Hispanics are more likely to experience. These include crowded living conditions, frontline jobs with high exposure, dependence on public transportation, lower access to healthcare, and greater rates of comorbid medical conditions.

9.4.2 *Diversity Among Hispanics and Longevity*

Hispanics have a unique heritage with high levels of admixture of west African, European, and native American ancestry. They have varied histories and reasons for migrating to the US, as well. Persons born in Mexico, or of Mexican ancestry are the largest US subgroup, representing approximately 60% of US Latinos (Funk & Lopez, 2022). The next largest group are of Puerto Rican descent, accounting for 9.7% of US Latinos and are born US citizens. Cubans, Salvadorans, Dominicans, Guatemalans and Hondurans each have a million or more population residing in the US in 2019. While centenarian data is not currently available for all Hispanic countries, Table 9.1 demonstrates some of the variability in reaching 100 years in several. The peninsula of Nicoya, Costa Rica is included for an extreme age comparison. Nicoya is one of the "Blue Zones": geographic locations recognized for having clusters of centenarians (Buettner & Skemp, 2016). Nicoyan men have longevity advantages. A 60-year-old Nicoyan male has a seven-fold increased chance of becoming a centenarian compared to a Japanese male. This advantage disappears if the man leaves this area, and is associated with lower levels of biomarkers of cardiovascular risk, and therefore, cardiovascular mortality. Nicoyans are leaner, suffer fewer functional disabilities, and their DNA exhibits less telomere shortening. The Nicoya diet consists of complex carbohydrates with low glycemic index and high fiber content, and consists of beans, fruits and vegetables, with small amounts of meat. Between 2000 and 2014, the death rate for centenarians living in the US was highest for NHW, and lowest for Hispanic centenarians (Xu, 2016).

Table 9.1 Centenarians per 100,000 population by country

Hispanic country	Centenarians per 100,000 residents	% Female centenarians
Mexico	18.3	64
Argentina	15.5	67
Cuba	13.24	60.3
Puerto Rico	45	74
Nicoya, Costa Rica	**128**	**N/A**
Spain	3.4	79

INEGI (2020), Clarin (2020), Museo Virtual de Ecologia Humana (2018), Buchholz (2021), Rosero-Bixby et al. (2013), Gimeno-Miguel et al. (2019)

9.4.3 *Social Determinants*

As the largest minority group in the US, understanding the social determinants of health of US Hispanics is critically important. According to the Centers for Disease Control, social determinants of health (SDOH) are defined as "conditions in the places where people live, learn, work, and play that affect a wide range of health and quality-of-life risks and outcomes" (CDC, 2021). There are 5 general domains of SDOH: economic stability, education access and quality, neighborhood and built environment, social/community context, and health care access and quality. Addressing social determinants of health may reduce health disparities. Among Hispanics, although many groups do experience adversity, there are social determinants that, in some cases, may serve as protective, and having a better understanding may improve healthcare outcomes for others, including the majority population (Healthy People, 2030).

9.4.3.1 Economic Stability

While the number of Latinos in skilled and higher-paid jobs has increased, Latinos remain overrepresented in lower-wage occupations and underrepresented in higher-wage ones. Latinos are also generally paid less than non-Latino Whites working in the same types of jobs. As a result, the annual median income for Latinos is lower than for NHW (McKinsey and Co., 2021). In 2019, the poverty rate for older Latinos was higher than that among all older Americans (17% v. 8.9%) (US Department of Health and Human Services, 2020).

9.4.3.2 Education Access and Quality

Educational attainment among Hispanics has shown an increase, with 63% of older Hispanic Americans having completed high school and 18% having earned a bachelor's degree or higher (US Department of Health and Human Services, 2020). Sanchez-Soto and colleagues found that, as a group, Hispanics experience a lower return on higher education than do NHW (Sanchez-Soto et al., 2018). This may lead to fewer incentives to seek higher education as well as raising the overall relative cost, as Hispanics' income lags behind that of Non-Hispanic counterparts. This further leads to longer time to recover educational costs and/or pay off school loans for Hispanics. Policy programs to increase educational access for Hispanics would need to include addressing individual and systemic discrimination that occurs post- graduation.

9.4.3.3 Neighborhood and Built Environment

The Healthy People 2030 goal to reduce disparities in this area is to create neighborhoods and environments that promote health and safety. The neighborhoods in which many older Hispanics reside are subject to food insecurity. Food insecurity is defined as a lack of access to nutrient-rich foods. These neighborhoods have only 32% of the chain supermarkets available to primarily Caucasian neighborhoods. Of the available grocery stores, Latinos usually pay higher prices for their foods (Cordova, 2021; Powell et al., 2007; Chung & Myers, 1999). On the other hand, architectural features, such as front porches, that facilitate social interactions were positively associated with perceived social support among older Latinos (Brown et al., 2009). This perceived social support in turn was associated with reduced psychological distress.

9.4.3.4 Social/Community Context

Relationships and interactions with family, co-workers, and community can have a significant and beneficial impact on health. Foreign-born Latinos are more likely to live in segregated neighborhoods (Iceland & Scopilliti, 2008). These neighborhoods may offer advantages to new immigrants in the way of community and social support. They facilitate living among others with a familiar culture, shared primary language, established social and employment networks, and affordable housing (Iceland & Scopilliti, 2008).

9.4.3.5 Healthcare Access and Quality

As a group, Latinos are less likely to have health insurance coverage and access to healthcare services including preventative medical care (Velasco-Mondragon et al., 2016; Funk & Lopez, 2022). Even when Latinos have insurance, difficulty in obtaining transportation and quality of healthcare further contribute to health outcomes disparities. A 2013 study by Fennell, et al. found that the nursing homes in which older Hispanics were more likely to reside are characterized by "severe deficiencies in performance, understaffing, and poor care" (Fennell et al., 2010). Additional barriers to accessing quality health care faced by Latino are lack of transportation and low English language proficiency, compounded by a lack of Spanish-speaking employees or Spanish language health education materials in health care agencies (Rose Community Foundation, 2020; Garcia et al., 2019). To further exacerbate the issue of healthcare accessibility and quality, between 2014 and 2019, Spanish-language mental health services decreased in most US states (Pro et al., 2022).

9.4.4 Physical Health

Social, environmental, and biological forces have modified the epidemiologic profile of Hispanics in the US. There is growing recognition that different Hispanic subgroups demonstrate different incidences of disease, however, most available medical literature either focuses on one or two of the larger subgroups (Mexicans or Puerto Ricans, for example), or Latinos as a single group. As a result, there are almost no data on health and health behaviors of other Latino groups in the US (Chen, et al., 2020).

Both health risk factors and disease incidences are different for US Hispanics compared to NHW (CDC, 2022). Hispanics have 35% less heart disease and 49% less cancer. Overall, they exhibit lower mortality rates, but specifically have higher death rates from diabetes. Compared to NHW, Latinos have poorer blood pressure control, are less likely to complete colorectal cancer screening, and are more likely to be obese. In 2020, the leading causes of death, in order, for US Latinos were: COVID-19, heart disease and cancer (CDC, 2022).

9.4.4.1 Cardiovascular Disease

Despite having an increased prevalence of CVD, as well as several of the associated risk factors (diabetes, obesity, and hypertension), Hispanics are consistently found to have lower age-adjusted mortality rates than NHW, for all types of CVD (Khan et al., 2022; Dominguez et al., 2015; CDC, 2015). For example, Khan and colleagues examined 834,532 CVD deaths among Hispanics, and 14,288,611 CVD deaths in NHW. They found a statistically significant lower mortality rate among Hispanics (186 per 100,000) versus NHW (254 per 100,000) (Khan et al., 2022). These findings are consistent with the Hispanic Paradox described in more detail later in the chapter. Factors, such as strong family and social supports, genetics and protective dietary habits have all been proposed as mitigating the presence of CVD risk factors in Hispanics.

9.4.4.2 Cancer

In 2021, the American Cancer Society estimated that more than 176,000 new cancer cases, and 46,500 cancer death would occur among US Hispanics. (Miller et al., 2021). Latinos exhibit 25–30% lower incidence and mortality rates for all cancers combined, and for the most common cancers. Latinos have higher rates of infection-related cancers, with an almost double risk of liver and stomach cancer. Among Hispanic women, cervical cancer is 32% higher in the US, and 78% higher in Puerto Rico, compared to NHW women. The prevalence of localized (and therefore more treatable) breast cancer is lower for Hispanic women. Screening for many of these cancers is available, however, utilization of preventive healthcare services is lower among Hispanics. Successful strategies to address these disparities have been reported and include peer health advisors and patient navigators, community-based programs that encourage and facilitate access to screening, and the promotion of health behaviors.

9.4.4.3 Liver Disease

In 2019, chronic liver disease was the seventh leading cause of death for all Hispanics, but fourth for Hispanic men aged 45–64. Hispanics have a higher prevalence of chronic alcoholic liver disease and non-alcoholic fatty liver disease, a higher incidence of hepatocellular carcinoma, and higher mortality from hepatitis B and C infection (Atiemo et al., 2019). Atiemo et al. recently investigated the "Hispanic paradox" in a retrospective cohort of more than 20,000 patients in Chicago. The Hispanic patients had lower socioeconomic status (based on public insurance as payment source). In spite of this, this study found a survival advantage for Hispanic patients with cirrhosis over other racial and ethnic groups. However, compared with NHW, both Hispanic men and women are more likely to die from liver and intrahepatic bile duct cancer (US Department of Health & Human Services, 2021).

9.4.5 Mental Health

Studies have shown that foreign-born Latinos living in the US have lower rates of depressive disorders and other psychiatric problems than Latinos born in the US (Grant et al., 2004; Alegria et al., 2008). Garcia and colleagues, however, found that Mexican Americans, especially women, who migrated to the US in later life (after age 50) were at increased risk for chronic depression (García, et al., 2019). Suicide rates among Hispanics are consistently lower than those of the general population. For Latinos, aged 65–74 and 75+, the rates were 6.5 and 7.7 per 100,000 population versus 15.2 and 17.8 per 100,000 in the general population (CDC, 2021).

As a group, Hispanics underutilize mental health services for several reasons (Department of Health & Human Services, 2021; Bridges et al., 2012). These can include: lack of health insurance, stigma associated with mental health problems and services, low English proficiency and lack of Spanish-speaking providers, lack of knowledge regarding available services, and greater likelihood of using folk healers, *curanderos*, or seeking help from a religious leader. They may experience psychological distress as physical symptoms, and thus seek help from a primary care provider. One recent study identified that the existence of community mental health centers which served a higher proportion of older adults, increased MH service utilization among older Hispanics. Additionally, higher levels of education and more severe perceived MH needs were associated with higher MH service utilization by older Latinos (Kim, 2019).

9.5 Impact of Acculturation on Health of Hispanics

Acculturation is the process of learning and incorporating values, beliefs, and cultural and social patterns of the new country in which immigrants now reside. This process can impact both physical and psychological health, behaviors such as diet and physical activity, environmental exposures, and health outcomes. The extent to which an immigrant becomes acculturated is highly variable and multifactorial. For example, Latino immigrants who live in predominantly Latino neighborhoods, or *barrios*, may function daily with minimal to no interactions with the majority society (Schwartz et al., 2010). Decreased interaction with the host society can mitigate the impact of transition to a new culture and reduce the degree of exposure to discrimination. This has been suggested as one of the contributors to health advantages among older US Latinos, although this has been mainly studied in Mexican-Americans (Ostir et al., 2003; Eschbach et al., 2004).

Behaviors often change as part of acculturation. Data from Stimpson et al. suggests that immigrants' eating behaviors change the longer they reside in the US (Stimpson et al., 2020). Specifically, the researchers found that immigrants spend less time food shopping, preparing meals, and consuming food, and more time spent eating while engaging in other activities such as watching television. Less time spent on eating behaviors appears to coincide with greater consumption of processed foods and food eaten away from home. These changes are associated with a higher risk of obesity (Batis et al., 2011). Similarly, other high risk health behaviors and outcomes such as smoking tobacco, alcohol use, high body mass index, and decreased consumption of low-fat foods all increase with greater degree of acculturation (Abraido-Lanza et al., 2016). Ortega and colleagues found that acculturation seems to be associated with greater access to food, however, rather than a change in dietary risk (Ortega-Velez & Castañeda-Pacheco, 2017).

Health outcomes may be impacted too. The Women's Health Initiative examined the relationship between acculturation and cancer risk and mortality in 6484 postmenopausal Latinas (Lopez-Pentecost et al., 2022). They found that less acculturated Latina women had a 56% lower risk for any cancer and an 83% lower risk for cancer mortality when compared to more acculturated Latinas. Some studies have also reported a higher degree of acculturation to be associated with CV risk factors among middle-aged Latinos (Eamranond et al., 2009; Kandula et al., 2008). On the other hand, Lopez et al., however, found higher levels of acculturation were associated with lower blood pressure, better lipid profiles, and lower prevalence of CV disease in elderly Latinos (average age 69.8) (López et al., 2014).

Rates of mental health disorders tend to increase with length of residence in the US (Cook et al., 2009). Several reasons for this finding have been proposed. Living for longer periods of time in the US increases exposure to stressful living conditions and discrimination, and prolongs separation from family. This can increase the risk of developing depressive and anxiety disorders and reduce resiliency. Perreira, et al. evaluated how 6 specific factors (perceived discrimination, language and social acculturation, ethnic and family identity, social networks, and perceived U.S. social standing) vary with time residing in the US among 15,000 Latinos (Perreira et al., 2015). The results of the study showed a greater burden of psychological distress, depressive symptomatology, and anxiety with both duration of residence and younger age at migration. Latinos residing in the US 21 years or longer (compared to those living in US less than 10 years), had higher rates of moderate to severe symptoms of psychological distress (25% vs. 18%), depression (31% vs. 23%), and anxiety (30% vs. 23%). There were subgroup differences. Puerto Ricans had the highest rates of psychological distress (29%), depression (39%), and anxiety (37%). Central Americans had the lowest rates of psychological distress (17%), Mexicans the lowest rates of depressive symptoms (22%), and Cubans the lowest rates of anxiety symptoms (22%). Similarly, Jimenez and colleagues found that the prevalence of depression and anxiety in older Latinos who had spent more than half their lives living in the US was comparable to rates in older NHW (Jimenez et al., 2010).

9.6 The Hispanic Paradox

US Hispanics generally experience longer life expectancy despite having greater prevalence of chronic diseases, lower socioeconomic status and education, and fewer societal advantages than NHW counterparts. This is known as the Hispanic Paradox. Also referred to as the Immigrant Health paradox, Hispanic immigrants tend to report better self-reported physical and mental health than native born Americans (Jimenez et al., 2010; Markides & Rote, 2015; Casanova & Aguila, 2020) despite the stressors faced in the U.S., such as lower wages, undesirable work, language barriers, and discrimination (Hernandez et al., 2022). The use of large datasets, such as US national vital statistics, have consistently found a mortality advantage for Latinos compared to NHW (CDC 2015, 2022). Markides et al. compared vital statistics data and national community surveys linked to the National Death Index, as well as the Medicare-NUDIMENT data maintained in the Social Security Administration. The analyses of these large databases showed a mortality advantage for US Latinos, particularly for older Latinos, although the vital statistics method found a lower advantage (Markides & Eschback, 2005). Ruiz et al. conducted a meta-analysis of 58 studies with more than 4.6 million participants (Ruiz et al., 2013). They found that Hispanic populations have a 17.5% lower mortality risk, and this difference was greater among older adults, providing additional evidence that supports that this is a true phenomenon.

A large descriptive cross-sectional study used mortality data from the World Health Organization Mortality Database (Chen et al., 2020). Between 2001 and 2015, 22 million deaths occurred in persons aged 20–64 years. These deaths were examined to calculate all-cause, cause-specific and age-standardized mortality rates by age, sex, race/ethnicity and country. Premature mortality rates were lower for US Latinos and several Latin American countries than for NHW in US. Among women, US Latinas had the lowest premature mortality rates of the 16 populations studied. Among men, Peru had the lowest premature mortality rates.

Of interest is that this finding is not unique to the US. It has also been reported in Hispanics who migrate from Latin America and the Caribbean to many other countries, including, Australia, Canada, United Kingdom, the Netherlands, and several western European countries (Shor et al., 2017). Several reasons have been postulated as contributory to the Hispanic Paradox.

9.6.1 Underreporting Ethnicity

Some researchers have suggested the paradox is mainly caused by underestimates of mortality rates. Many years ago, the Bureau of Census used Spanish surnames as the method to identify people of Hispanic descent. This undercounted Latina women who married non-Hispanics and changed their last names, accordingly (Ellis, 1962). The US Census now specifically asks the person to self-identify their ethnicity as Hispanic or Latino. Additional reasons for ethnic misidentification, include missing social security numbers, and complex surnames, (all of which could lead to mistakes in matching death records to national databases), overstatement of age, or undocumented status of the Hispanic person (Smith & Bradshaw, 2006; Palloni & Arias, 2004). Many of these issues have been addressed by examining large databases and cross-matching community surveys with health indices. The Hispanic longevity advantage persists.

9.6.2 Healthy Migrant Hypothesis

This hypothesis speculates that immigrants who come to the US are overall healthier, such that there is a selection bias. For example, compared to NHW patients, a meta-analysis demonstrated that US Hispanics have lower rates of coronary heart disease events, and lower cardiovascular disease mortality (Cortes-Bergoderi et al., 2013). However, even when US Latinos develop illness, they exhibit lower mortality. Latinos had significantly lower mortality risk across the seven cancer types (breast, ovarian, prostate, colorectal, pancreatic, liver and lung) examined (Wang et al., 2022). This suggests that there are likely other forces at play.

9.6.3 Salmon Bias Hypothesis

Also described as "selective return" migration, this theory postulates that unhealthy migrants or migrants who experience deteriorating health have a greater tendency to return or move closer to their communities of origin than healthier immigrants (Turra & Elo, 2008). Turra et al. attempted to estimate whether mortality of foreign-born elderly Hispanics who have migrated from the United States is higher than among foreign-born elderly Hispanics remaining in the US. They did provide the first direct test of the salmon bias and the results were consistent with the hypothesis. Mortality was higher among foreign-born Hispanic primary social security beneficiaries living abroad than among foreign-born beneficiaries residing in the United States. This excess mortality was 12–25% for persons born in Puerto Rico and 15–20% for other foreign-born Hispanics. They also found a similar pattern of excess mortality for foreign-born NHW immigrants, showing an 8–10% higher death rates than native-born NHW living in the United States. These results suggest that the salmon bias hypothesis has more general applicability and it could also contribute to the lower mortality rate of foreign-born NHW elderly living in the United States. However, this theory does not fully explain the Hispanic Paradox.

9.7 Resilience Among Hispanics

Beyond the hypotheses for the Hispanic Paradox, there are several important sources of resilience among Hispanics that may also contribute to their health outcomes and mortality advantage.

9.7.1 Diet

Latinos consume legumes such as beans more frequently than NHW and preferences vary by acculturation level (Heer & Winham, 2020). Beans and legumes are rich in plant protein, fiber, B-vitamins, iron, folate, calcium, potassium, phosphorous, and zinc, while also being low in fat (US National Library of Medicine, n.d.). It is hypothesized that increased consumption as part of cultural practice is protective against inflammation and possibly cardiovascular disease. However, an associated contributor is that consumption of beans is associated with less consumption of animal proteins and fats. However, further research is needed.

9.7.1.1 Traditional/Alternative Medicine

The use of alternative medicine is common in Latino culture. Herbal self-care remedies are often part of cultural values and practices and are used more by women of Latino ethnicity than in other ethnic groups (Green et al., 2017). One 2004 study demonstrated that 63% of the Hispanic subjects used one or more types of alternative medicine (Mikhail et al., 2014). The majority were women, and the most reported types of alternative practices were herbs, prayer, and dietary supplements. Common characteristics of users included lower yearly income, less English proficiency, and lower educational level. *Curanderismo* is a traditional Mexican American healing system that holistically treats disorders through religious, spiritual, and health-related means (Tafur et al., 2009). *Curanderos* treat the individual on three levels- material, spiritual, and mental (Texas State Historical Association, 2022). They employ the use of symbols, objects, rituals, and herbs. Use of these health practitioners may be as high as 50–75% in some parts of the US (Tafur et al., 2009). An emerging group of health care providers who blend nursing and Hispanic folk healing has arisen to provide culturally competent care in the US (Luna, 2003). While use of alternative practices appears to be a differentiating factor among Latinos compared to other ethnic groups, further research is needed elucidate the contribution, if any, between its use and the Hispanic paradox.

9.7.1.2 Religion and Spirituality

Most Latinos report that religion is very important in their lives (Pew Research Center, 2014). Religiosity and spirituality have been found to play an important role in the health and well-being of Latinos (Campesino & Schwartz, 2006). Consoli et al. reported that, although limited, some studies have shown that resilience among Latinos is often associated with religion and spirituality (Consoli et al., 2011). More recently, Piedra and colleagues interviewed community workers who reported that after financial security, spirituality was most important for positive aging among older Latinos (Piedra et al., 2021). Noting the importance of religion and spirituality for Hispanics, more research on this potentially important contributor to health outcomes is warranted.

Familismo

Familismo is the Hispanic cultural value which emphasizes the importance of strong nuclear and extended family ties, loyalty, closeness and getting along with and contributing to the wellbeing of the family. A recent study of 255 Hispanic participants found that Latinos who endorsed strong *familismo* experienced less loneliness and in turn had better overall physical and mental health, and health practices (Gallegos & Segrin, 2022). However, a Hispanic community study that included more than 4000 subjects found little evidence of a link between familism and physical health, although they did find that strong attitudes toward family support were associated with fewer symptoms of depression and anxiety (Diaz & Niño, 2019). A meta-analysis assessing several mental health outcomes found small effect sizes in the relationship between familism and depression, suicide and internalizing behaviors, and no significant effect for substance abuse (Valdivieso-Mora et al., 2016). The authors proposed that moderator variables, such as family communication, variability in the Latino samples and the way in which outcomes were measured may explain the small and non-significant findings. In generally, however, the impact of *familismo*, while frequently cited as contributory to the Hispanic paradox has not been evaluated adequately.

Barrio Advantage

As previously noted, many US Latinos, especially seniors, reside in predominantly Latino neighborhoods, or *barrios*. One study of over 3000 Mexican Americans aged 65 and older found that those who lived in high-density Mexican-American neighborhoods had a lower 7-year mortality, as well lower prevalence of stroke, cancer and hip fractures (Eschbach et al., 2004; Abraído-Lanza et al., 2016). The *barrio* offers community institutions, kinship, and intact family structures, and provides greater social integration and social support, often in Spanish. This also facilitates the sharing of information regarding available resources, conferring additional health outcomes benefits. This advantage may be specific to urban areas, however, as Murillo found that there was no such disease prevalence advantage in segregated rural Hispanic communities (Murillo, 2017). This study did not examine mortality risk, however.

9.7.1.3 Optimism

Studies have found that optimism is associated with health benefits and can confer a survival benefit, even to the those of advanced age (Jacobs et al., 2021; Yue et al., 2022). A multivariate analysis found that among centenarians in Spain, optimism was the main predictor of physical and cognitive health, and higher quality of life (Montoro-Rodriguez et al., 2018). Many Latinos, especially recent immigrants, are reported to have a positive outlook. When comparing life in the United States with that of their countries of origin, most US Latinos report that the US provides more opportunities to advance socioeconomically, better conditions to raise children, better access to health care and even better treatment of the poor (Pew Research Center, 2022). The vast majority (84%) of Latino survey respondents would choose to come to the US if they had to make the choice again. These advantages of life in the US may also contribute to the Hispanic paradox. A related hypothesis is that features of the Spanish language itself facilitate optimism by allowing the individual to consider hypothetical situations by use of the subjunctive tense, and enable the ability to minimize or exaggerate expressions (Llabre, 2021).

A related concept is that of having purpose in life. Among the Nicoya people, for example, the term is *Plan de Vida*, or, literally, life plan. It contributes to a positive outlook where the key is to find a sense of purpose, even in doing simple tasks, such as going for a walk, doing household chores, or gardening. A cohort study of nearly 7000 US adults older than 50 found a strong sense of purpose in life was associated with decreased mortality (Alimujiang et al., 2019).

The various components that all contribute to better health outcomes, longevity and even successful aging have been poorly studied, and warrant concerted research. This will serve to not only improve the health of Latinos, the largest minority group in the US, but also will provide recommendations on how to improve the overall health of other US populations.

9.8 Summary

The Hispanic Paradox has been consistently demonstrated in multiple large dataset and meta-analyses. While several hypotheses for the Hispanic Paradox have been proposed, no single factor has been able to fully explain this phenomenon. As a group, Hispanics often face multiple adverse social determinants of health that should be associated with worse health outcomes and greater mortality, and yet, these are not the findings. Among the sources of resilience for Latinos are traditional practices and behaviors, religion and community support, *familismo*, and a positive, optimistic outlook that includes having a purpose in life. Further examination of the factors that contribute to the Hispanic Paradox will not only help elucidate this phenomenon, but may also provide valuable insights that will improve the overall health outcomes of other ethnic and racial groups, including the majority population.

Additional Resources

Population Reference Bureau. https://www.prb.org/

Kaiser Permanente. A Provider's Handbook on Culturally Competent Care. 2018. Available at: http://residency-ncal.kaiserpermanente.org/wp-content/uploads/2018/12/Latino-Handbook.pdf. Accessed November 19, 2022.

Blue Zones: Live Better Longer. https://www.bluezones.com/

What's the Secret to Latino Longevity? https://nutritionfacts.org/2019/06/11/whats-the-secret-to-latino-longevity/

Llorente MD. Culture, Heritage and Diversity in Older Adult Mental Health Care. APPI Press. Washington DC. https://doi.org/10.1176/appi.books.9781615372119

Multiple Choice Questions

1. Which of the following descriptions of the Salmon Bias Hypothesis to explain the Hispanic Paradox is accurate?

   A. Latinos eat more salmon than other groups.
   B. Latinos spend more time than other groups fishing
   C. As Latinos age and became ill, they are more likely to return to their country of origin
   D. Latinos are more likely than other groups to supplement their diets with fish oil
   Correct Response: C

2. Among Hispanic subgroups, which of the following regions has the largest number of centenarians per 100,000 population?
   A. San Juan, Puerto Rico
   B. Madrid, Spain
   C. Havana, Cuba
   D. Nicoya, Costa Rica
   Correct Response: D
3. All of the following are proposed contributors to greater longevity among Hispanics, except:
   A. Acculturation
   B. *Barrio* advantage
   C. *Familismo*
   D. Optimism
   Correct Response: A

References

Abraído-Lanza, A. F., Echeverría, S. E., & Flórez, K. R. (2016). Latino immigrants, acculturation, and health: Promising new directions in research. *Annual Review of Public Health., 37*(1), 219–236. https://doi.org/10.1146/annurev-publhealth-032315-021545

Alegria, M., Canino, G., Shrout, P. E., Woo, M., Duan, N., Vila, D., & Meng, X. L. (2008). Prevalence of mental Illness in immigrant and non-immigrant U.S. Latino groups. *American Journal of Psychiatry., 165*(3), 359–369.

Alimujiang, A., Wiensch, A., Boss, J., Fleischer, N. L., Mondul, A. M., McLean, K., Mukherjee, B., & Pearce, C. L. (2019). Association between life purpose and mortality among US adults older than 50 years. *JAMA Network Open, 2*(5), e194270. https://doi.org/10.1001/jamanetworkopen.2019.4270

Atiemo, K., Mazumder, N. R., Caicedo, J. C., Ganger, D., Gordon, E., Montag, S., Maddur, H., VanWagner, L. B., Goel, S., Kho, A., Abecassis, M., Zhao, L., & Ladner, D. (2019 Dec). The Hispanic paradox in patients with liver cirrhosis: Current evidence from a large regional retrospective cohort study. *Transplantation, 103*(12), 2531–2538.

Austin, G., & Johnson, D. (2012, August 17). Hispanic or Latino: Which is correct? *Diversity Journal.*

Batis, C., Hernandez-Barrera, L., Barquera, S., Rivera, J. A., & Popkin, B. M. (2011). Food acculturation drives dietary differences among Mexicans, Mexican Americans, and Non-Hispanic Whites. *The Journal of Nutrition, 141*(10), 1898–1906. https://doi.org/10.3945/jn.111.141473

Bendixen & Amandi International. (2021). *The use of 'LatinX among Hispanic Voters'*. Available at: https://www.politico.com/f/?id=0000017d-81be-dee4-a5ff-efbe74ec0000, Accessed 19 Nov 2022.

Bernstein, David. (2021, December 7). What do Americans of Latin American origin prefer to be called? Not LatinX. *The Volokh Conspiracy.*

Blakemore, Erin. (2022, February 10). Hispanic? Latino? Here's where the terms come from. *National Geographic.*

Bridges, A. J., Andrews, A. R., 3rd, & Deen, T. L. (2012). Mental health needs and service utilization by Hispanic immigrants residing in mid-southern United States. *Journal of Transcultural Nursing, 23*(4), 359–368. https://doi.org/10.1177/1043659612451259

Brown, S. C., Mason, C. A., Lombard, J. L., Martinez, F., Plater-Zyberk, E., Spokane, A. R., Newman, F. L., Pantin, H., & Szapocznik, J. (2009). The relationship of built environment to perceived social support and psychological distress in hispanic elders: The role of "eyes on the street". *The Journals of Gerontology: Series B, 64B*(2), 234–246.

Buchholz, K. (2021, February 5). *Where 100 is the New 80*. Available at: https://www.statista.com/chart/14931/where-100-is-the-new-80/. Accessed 19 Nov 2022.

Buettner, D., & Skemp, S. (2016). Blue zones: Lessons from the world's longest lived. *American Journal of Lifestyle Medicine, 10*(5), 318–321. https://doi.org/10.1177/1559827616637066

Campesino, M., & Schwartz, G. E. (2006). Spirituality among Latinas/os: Implications of culture in conceptualization and measurement. *Advances in Nursing Science., 29*, 69–81.

Casanova, M., & Aguila, E. (2020). Gender differences in cognitive function among older Mexican immigrants. *The Journal of the Economics of Ageing, 16*, 100226.

CDC. (2015, May). *Vital signs: Hispanic health*. Available at: https://www.cdc.gov/vitalsigns/hispanic-health/index.html. Accessed 15 Nov 2022.

CDC. (2022, October 19). *Saving llives, protecting people: Health of hispanic or latino population*. Available at: https://www.cdc.gov/nchs/fastats/hispanic-health.htm. Accessed 15 Nov 2022.

Centers for Disease Control and Prevention. (2021, September 30). *Social determinants of health*. Centers for Disease Control and Prevention. Available at: https://www.cdc.gov/socialdeterminants/index.htm. Accessed 27 October 2022.

Centers for Disease Control and Prevention, National Center for Health Statistics. (2021). 1999–2020 Wide Ranging Online Data for Epidemiological Research (WONDER), Multiple Cause of Death files [Data file]. Retrieved from http://wonder.cdc.gov/ucd-icd10.html

Chen, Y., Freedman, N. D., Rodriquez, E. J., Shiels, M. S., Napoles, A. M., Withrow, D. R., Spillane, S., Sigel, B., Perez-Stable, E. J., & Berrington de González, A. (2020). Trends in premature deaths among adults in the United States and Latin America. *JAMA Network Open, 3*(2). https://doi.org/10.1001/jamanetworkopen.2019.21085

Chung, C., & Myers, S. (1999). Do the poor pay more for food? an analysis of grocery store availability and food price disparities. *Journal of Consumer Affairs, 33*(2), 276–296. https://doi.org/10.1111/j.1745-6606.1999.tb00071.x

Clarin. (2020). *La avanzada centenaria: hay mas de 15 mil mayores de cien anos en el pais y podrian ser el triple en 2040*. Available at: https://www.clarin.com/sociedad/avanzada-centenaria-15-mil-mayores-cien-anos-pais-podrian-triple-2040_0_NPhPb8Ac.html. Accessed 19 Nov 2022.

Cohn, D'Vera. (2010, March 3). Census history: Counting hispanics. *Pew Research Center*.

Consoli, M. L. M., Lopez, S. A., Gonzales, N., Cabrera, A. P., Llamas, J., & Ortega, S. (2011). Resilience and thriving in the Latino/a population: Intersections and discrepancies. *Interamerican Journal of Psychology, 45*(3), 351–362.

Cook, B., Alegria, M., Lin, J. Y., & Guo, J. (2009). Pathways and correlates connecting Latinos' mental health with exposure to the United States. *American Journal of Public Health., 99*(12), 2247–2254.

Cordova, J. (2021). Los Desiertos Americanos: Food deserts and their impact upon Hispanic American health. *Public Health Review, 4*(1), 1–4.

Cortes-Bergoderi, M., Goel, K., Murad, M. H., & Alli, T. (2013). Cardiovascular mortality in Hispanics compared to non-Hispanic whites. *European Journal of Internal Medicine, 24*(8), 791–799.

Department of Health & Human Services. (2022). *Healthy People 2030*. Available at: https://health.gov/healthypeople/priority-areas/social-determinants-health. Accessed 19 Nov 2022.

Department of Health & Human Services, Office of Minority Health. (2021, May). https://minorityhealth.hhs.gov/omh/browse.aspx?lvl=4&lvlid=69. Accessed 15 Nov 2022.

Diaz, C. J., & Niño, M. (2019 Sep). Familism and the Hispanic health advantage: The role of immigrant status. *Journal of Health and Social Behavior, 60*(3), 274–290.

Dominguez, K., Penman-Aguilar, A., Chang, M. H., Moonesinghe, R., Castellanos, T., Rodriguez-Lainz, A., Schieber, R., & Centers for Disease Control and Prevention (CDC). (2015). Vital signs: leading causes of death, prevalence of diseases and risk factors, and use of health services among Hispanics in the United States – 2009-2013. *MMWR. Morbidity and Mortality Weekly Report, 64*(17), 469–478.

Eamranond, P. P., Legedza, A. T., Diez-Roux, A. V., Kandula, N. R., Palmas, W., Siscovick, D. S., & Mukamal, K. J. (2009). Association between language and risk factor levels among Hispanic adults with hypertension, hypercholesterolemia, or diabetes. *American Heart Journal, 157*, 53–59.

Ellis, J. M. (1962). Spanish surname mortality differences in San Antonio, Texas. *Journal of Health and Human Behavior., 3*(2), 125–127.

Eschbach, K., Ostir, G. V., Patel, K. V., Markides, K. S., & Goodwin, J. S. (2004). Neighborhood context and mortality among older Mexican Americans: Is there a barrio advantage? *American Journal of Public Health, 94*(10), 1807–1812. https://doi.org/10.2105/ajph.94.10.1807

Estrada, J. (2015). *LULAC and American GI Forum: History and Geography 1929–1988*. University of Washington.

Feldman, J. M., & Bassett, M. T. (2021). Variation in COVID-19 mortality in the US by race and ethnicity and educational attainment. *JAMA Network Open, 4*(11), e2135967. https://doi.org/10.1001/jamanetworkopen.2021.35967

Fennell, M. L., Feng, Z., Clark, M. A., & Mor, V. (2010). Elderly Hispanics more likely to reside in poor-quality nursing homes. *Health Affairs, 29*(1), 65–73. https://doi.org/10.1377/hlthaff.2009.0003

Funk, C., & Lopez, M. H. (2022, June). *2. Hispanic Americans' experiences with health care*. Pew Research Center Science & Society. Available at: https://www.pewresearch.org/science/2022/06/14/hispanic-americans-experiences-with-health-care. Accessed 27 Oct 2022.

Gallegos, M. L., & Segrin, C. (2022 Aug). Family connections and the Latino health paradox: Exploring the mediating role of loneliness in the relationships between the Latina/o cultural value of familism and health. *Health Communication, 37*(9), 1204–1214.

Gamboa, Suzanne. (2021, December 9). Latino civil rights organization drops 'Latinx' from official communication. *NBC News*. Available at: https://www.nbcnews.com/news/latino/latino-civil-rights-organization-drops-latinx-official-communication-rcna8203. Accessed 13 Nov 2022.

Garcia, M. E., Bindman, A. B., & Coffman, J. (2019). Language-concordant primary care physicians for a diverse population: The view from California. *Health Equity, 3*(1), 343–349. https://doi.org/10.1089/heq.2019.0035

García, C., Garcia, M. A., Chiu, C. T., Rivera, F. I., & Raji, M. (2019). Life expectancies with depression by age of migration and gender among older Mexican Americans. *The Gerontologist, 59*(5), 877–885. https://doi.org/10.1093/geront/gny107

Gimeno-Miguel, A., Clerencia-Sierra, M., Ioakeim, I., Poblador-Plou, B., Aza-Pascual-Salcedo, M., González-Rubio, F., Rodríguez Herrero, R., & Prados-Torres, A. (2019). Health of Spanish centenarians: A cross-sectional study based on electronic health records. *BMC Geriatrics, 19*(1), 226. https://doi.org/10.1186/s12877-019-1235-7

Grant, B., Stinson, F., Hasin, D., Dawson, D., Chou, S., & Anderson, K. (2004). Immigration and lifetime prevalence of DSM-IV psychiatric disorders among Mexican Americans and Non-Hispanic Whites in the United States. *Archives of General Psychiatry., 61*, 1226–1233.

Green, R. R., Santoro, N., Allshouse, A. A., Neal-Perry, G., & Derby, C. (2017). Prevalence of complementary and alternative medicine and herbal remedy use in Hispanic and Non-Hispanic white women: Results from the study of women's health across the nation. *The Journal of Alternative and Complementary Medicine, 23*(10), 805–811. https://doi.org/10.1089/acm.2017.0080

Harris, J. (1991). The Exponence of Gender in Spanish. *Linguistic Inquiry, 22*(1), 27–62.

Heer, M. M., & Winham, D. M. (2020). Bean preferences vary by acculturation level among latinas and by ethnicity with Non-Hispanic white women. *International Journal of Environmental Research and Public Health, 17*(6), 2100. https://doi.org/10.3390/ijerph17062100

Hernandez, C. M., Moreno, O., Garcia-Rodriguez, I., Fuentes, L., & Nelson, T. (2022). The Hispanic paradox: A moderated mediation analysis of health conditions, self-rated health, and mental health among Mexicans and Mexican Americans. *Health Psychology and Behavioral Medicine, 10*(1), 180–198. https://doi.org/10.1080/21642850.2022.2032714

Hummer, R. A., & Hayward, M. D. (2015). Hispanic older adult health & longevity in the United States: Current patterns & concerns for the future. *Daedalus, 144*(2), 20–30. https://doi.org/10.1162/DAED_a_00327

Iceland, J., & Scopilitti, M. (2008). Immigrant residential segregation in U.S. metropolitan areas, 1990–2000. *Demography, 45*, 79–94.

Instituto Nacional de Estadistica y Geografia (INEGI). (2020). *Población total por entidad federativa y grupo quinquenal de edad según sexo, serie de años censales de 1990 a 2020.* Available at: https://www.inegi.org.mx/app/tabulados/interactivos/?pxq=Poblacion_Poblacion_01_e60cd8cf-927f-4b94-823e-972457a12d4b. Accessed 19 Nov 2022.

Jacobs, J. M., Maaravi, Y., & Stessman, J. (2021). Optimism and longevity beyond age 85. *The Journals of Gerontology. Series A, Biological Sciences and Medical Sciences, 76*(10), 1806–1813.

Jimenez, D. E., Alegría, M., Chen, C.-N., Chan, D., & Laderman, M. (2010). Prevalence of psychiatric illnesses in older ethnic minority adults. *Journal of the American Geriatrics Society, 58*, 256–264. https://doi.org/10.1111/j.1532-5415.2009.02685.x

Kandula, N. R., Diez-Roux, A. V., Chan, C., et al. (2008). Association of acculturation levels and prevalence of diabetes in the multi-ethnic study of atherosclerosis (MESA). *Diabetes Care, 31*, 1621–1628.

Khan, S. U., Lone, A. N., Yedlapati, S. H., Dani, S. S., Khan, M. Z., Watson, K. E., et al. (2022). Cardiovascular disease mortality among Hispanic versus non-Hispanic white adults in the United States, 1999 to 2018. *Journal of the American Heart Association, 11*(7), 1–12.

Kim, K. (2019). County context and mental health service utilization by older Hispanics. *The Gerontologist, 59*(3), 456–464.

Llabre, M. M. (2021). Insight into the Hispanic paradox: The language hypothesis. *Perspectives on Psychological Science, 16*(6), 1324–1336. https://doi.org/10.1177/1745691620968765

Lopez Torregrosa, L. (2021, December 14). Many Latino/as say 'Latinx' offends or bothers them. Here's why. *NBC News.*

López, L., Peralta, C. A., Lee, A., Zeki Al Hazzouri, A., & Haan, M. N. (2014). Impact of acculturation on cardiovascular risk factors among elderly Mexican Americans. *Annals of Epidemiology, 24*(10), 714–719. https://doi.org/10.1016/j.annepidem.2014.07.011

Lopez-Pentecost, M., Crane, T. E., Garcia, D. O., et al. (2022). Role of dietary patterns and acculturation in cancer risk and mortality among postmenopausal Hispanic women: Results from the Women's Health Initiative (WHI). *Journal of Public Health (Berlin), 30*, 811–822. https://doi.org/10.1007/s10389-020-01342-8

Luna, E. (2003). Nurse-curanderas. *Journal of Holistic Nursing, 21*(4), 326–342. https://doi.org/10.1177/0898010103258574

Markides, K. S., & Eschback, K. (2005). Aging, migration and mortality: Current status of research on the hispanic paradox. *The Journals of Gerontology: Series B, 60*(2), S68–S75. https://doi.org/10.1093/geronb/60.Special_Issue_2.S68

Markides, K. S., & Rote, S. (2015). Immigrant health paradox. In *Emerging trends in the social and behavioral sciences* (pp. 1–15). Wiley.

McKinsey and Company. (2021, December 9). *The economic state of Latinos in America: The American dream deferred.* Available at: https://www.mckinsey.com/featured-insights/sustainable-inclusive-growth/the-economic-state-of-latinos-in-america-the-american-dream-deferred. Accessed 19 Nov 2022.

Merriam-Webster. (2022a). Hispanic. *In Merriam-Webster.com dictionary*. Retrieved October 15, 2022, from https://www.merriam-webster.com/dictionary/hispanic.
Merriam-Webster. (2022b). Latino. *In Merriam-Webster.com dictionary*. Retrieved October 15, 2022, from https://www.merriam-webster.com/dictionary/latino
Merriam-Webster. (2022c). Chicano. *In Merriam-Webster.com dictionary*. Retrieved October 15, 2022, from https://www.merriam-webster.com/dictionary/chicano.
Merriam-Webster. (2022d). Latinx. *In Merriam-Webster.com dictionary*. Retrieved October 15, 2022, from https://www.merriam-webster.com/dictionary/latinx.
Mikhail, N., Wali, S., & Ziment, I. (2014). Use of alternative medicine among Hispanics. *The Journal of Alternative and Complementary Medicine, 10*(5), 851–859. https://doi.org/10.1089/acm.2004.10.851
Miller, K. D., Ortiz, A. P., Pinheiro, P. S., Bandi, P., Minihan, A., Fuchs, H. E., Martinez Tyson, D., Tortolero-Luna, G., Fedewa, S. A., Jemal, A. M., & Siegel, R. L. (2021). Cancer statistics for the US Hispanic/Latino population, 2021. *CA: A Cancer Journal for Clinicians, 71*, 466–487. https://doi.org/10.3322/caac.21695
Montoro-Rodriguez, J., Pinazo-Hermandis, S., & Cordoba-Castillo, V.. (2018). *Why centenarians are so optimistic about the future? Inn in aging*. Available at: https://academic.oup.com/innovateage/article/2/suppl_1/49/5171199. Accessed 18 Nov 2022.
Murillo, M. G. (2017). *The hispanic health paradox: Does the Barrio advantage exist outside of Urban Enclaves?* Available at: https://scholar.colorado.edu/concern/undergraduate_honors_theses/44558d705. Accessed 18 Nov 2022.
Museo Virtual de Ecologia Humana. (2018, May). *Centenarians in Cuba and the "Study of Cuban Centenarians"*. Available at: https://museoecologiahumana.org/en/piezas/centenarians-in-cuba-and-the-study-of-cuban-centenarians/. Accessed 19 Nov 2022.
Noe-Bustamante et al. (2020, August 11). About One-in Four U.S. Hispanics have heard of Latinx, but Just 3% Use It. *Pew Research Center*.
Ortega-Velez, M., & Castañeda-Pacheco, P. (2017). Acculturation and dietary change in Mexican-American immigrant women. *Open Journal of Social Sciences., 5*, 211–243. https://doi.org/10.4236/jss.2017.57014
Ostir, G. V., Eschbach, K., Markides, K. S., & Goodwin, J. S. (2003). Neighbourhood composition and depressive symptoms among older Mexican Americans. *Journal of Epidemiology and Community Health, 57*(12), 987–992. https://doi.org/10.1136/jech.57.12.987
Palloni, A., & Arias, E. (2004). Paradox lost: Explaining the Hispanic adult mortality advantage. *Demography, 41*(3), 385–415.
Perreira, K. M., Gotman, N., Isasi, C. R., Arguelles, W., Castañeda, S. F., Daviglus, M. L., Giachello, A. L., Gonzalez, P., Penedo, F. J., Salgado, H., & Wassertheil-Smoller, S. (2015). Mental health and exposure to the United States: Key correlates from the hispanic community health study of Latinos. *The Journal of Nervous and Mental Disease, 203*(9), 670–678. https://doi.org/10.1097/NMD.0000000000000350
Pew Research Center. (2014). *The shifting religious identity of latinos in the United States*. Available at: https://www.pewresearch.org/religion/2014/05/07/chapter-1-religious-affiliation-of-hispanics/.
Pew Research Center. (2022, January 20). *Latinos see US as better than place of family's ancestry for opportunity, raising kids, health care access*. Available at: https://www.pewresearch.org/race-ethnicity/2022/01/20/latinos-see-u-s-as-better-than-place-of-familys-ancestry-for-opportunity-raising-kids-health-care-access/. Accessed 19 Nov 2022.
Piedra, L. M., Ridings, J., Howe, M. J. K., Smith, J. L., O'Brien, C., Howard, A., & Conrad, K. J. (2021). Stakeholders' ideas about positive aging for latinos: A conceptual map. *Journal of Applied Gerontology, 40*(10), 1342–1355.
Powell, L. M., Slater, S., Mirtcheva, D., Bao, Y., & Chaloupka, F. J. (2007). Food store availability and neighborhood characteristics in the United States. *Preventive Medicine, 44*(3), 189–195. https://doi.org/10.1016/j.ypmed.2006.08.008

Pro, G., Brown, C., Rojo, M., Patel, J., Flax, C., & Haynes, T. (2022). Downward national trends in mental health treatment offered in spanish: State differences by proportion of hispanic residents. *Psychiatric Services, 73*(11), 1232–1238.

Rose Community Foundation. (2020, April). *Transportation challenges for Latino older adults*. Available at: https://rcfdenver.org/blog/transportation-challenges-latino-older-adults/. Accessed 27 Oct 2022.

Rosero-Bixby, L., Dow, W. H., & Rehkopf, D. H. (2013). The Nicoya region of Costa Rica: a high longevity Island for elderly males. *Vienna Yearbook of Population Research, 11*, 109–136. https://doi.org/10.1553/populationyearbook2013s109

Ruiz, J. M., Steffen, P., & Smith, T. B. (2013). Hispanic mortality paradox: A systematic review and meta-analysis of the longitudinal literature. *American Journal of Public Health, 103*(3), e52–e60.

Sanchez-Soto, G., Bautista-Leon, A., & Singelmann, J. (2018). The return-on-education gap between Hispanics and non-hispanic whites. *Papeles de Poblacion, 24*(98), 245–268.

Schwartz Seth, J., Unger Jennifer, B., Zamboanga Byron, L., & José, S. (2010). Rethinking the concept of acculturation: Implications for theory and research. *American Psychologist., 65*(4), 237–251.

Shor, E., Roelfs, D., & Vang, Z. M. (2017). The "Hispanic mortality paradox" revisited: Meta-analysis and meta-regression of life-course differentials in Latin American and Caribbean immigrants' mortality. *Social Science & Medicine, 186*, 20–33.

Smith, D. P., & Bradshaw, B. S. (2006). Rethinking the Hispanic paradox: Death rates and life expectancy for US non-Hispanic White and Hispanic populations. *American Journal of Public Health, 96*(9), 1686–1692.

Stimpson, J. P., Langellier, B. A., & Wilson, F. A. (2020). Time spent eating, by immigrant status, race/ethnicity, and length of residence in the United States. *Preventing Chronic Disease, 17*. https://doi.org/10.5888/pcd17.200122

Tafur, M. M., Crowe, T. K., & Torres, E. (2009). A review of *curanderismo* and healing practices among Mexicans and Mexican Americans. *Occupational Therapy International., 16*(1), 82–88. https://doi.org/10.1002/oti.265

Texas State Historical Association. (2022). *Curanderismo*. Available at: https://www.tshaonline.org/handbook/entries/curanderismo. Accessed 27 Oct 2022.

Torres, L. (2018, September 24). Latinx? *Latino Studies, 16*, 283–285.

Turra, C. M., & Elo, I. T. (2008). The impact of salmon bias on the Hispanic mortality advantage: New evidence from social security data. *Population Research and Policy Review, 27*(5), 515–530.

U.S. Department of Commerce. (2022, April). About the hispanic population and its origin. *U.S. Census*. Available at: https://www.census.gov/topics/population/hispanic-origin/about.html. Accessed 15 Oct 2022.

U.S. National Library of Medicine. (n.d.). *Healthy food trends – Beans and legumes: Medlineplus medical encyclopedia*. MedlinePlus. Retrieved October 27, 2022, from https://medlineplus.gov/ency/patientinstructions/000726.htm.

US Department of Health & Human Services (2020). *The profile of older Americans*. Available at: https://acl.gov/sites/default/files/Profile%20of%20OA/HispanicProfileReport2021.pdf. Accessed 19 Nov 2022.

US Department of Health & Human Services Office of Minority Health. (2021, August 11). *Chronic liver disease and hispanic Americans*. Available at: https://minorityhealth.hhs.gov/omh/browse.aspx?lvl=4&lvlid=62. Accessed 15 Nov 2022.

Valdivieso-Mora, E., Casie, P. L., Garnier-Villareal, M., et al. (2016). A systematic review of the relationship between familism and mental health outcomes in Latino population. *Frontiers in Psychology, 7*, 1632.

Velasco-Mondragon, E., Jimenez, A., Palladino-Davis, A. G., Davis, D., & Escamilla-Cejudo, J. A. (2016). Hispanic health in the USA: A scoping review of the literature. *Public Health Reviews, 37*(1). https://doi.org/10.1186/s40985-016-0043-2

Wang, F., Shu, X., Pal, T., Berlin, J., Nguyen, S. M., Zheng, W., Bailey, C. E., & Shu, X. O. (2022). Racial/ethnic disparities in mortality related to access to care for major cancers in the United States. *Cancers (Basel).*, *14*(14), 3390.

Woolf, S. H., Masters, R. K., & Aron, L. Y. (2022). Changes in life expectancy between 2019 and 2020 in the US and 21 peer countries. *JAMA Network Open, 5*(4), e227067. https://doi.org/10.1001/jamanetworkopen.2022.7067

Xu, J. (2016, January). *Mortality among centenarians in the US, 200–2014*. Available at: https://www.cdc.gov/nchs/products/databriefs/db233.htm. Accessed 15 Nov 2022.

Yue, Z., Liang, H., Qin, X., Ge, Y., Xiang, N., & Liu, E. (2022). Optimism and survival: Health behaviors as a mediator-a ten-year follow-up study of Chinese elderly people. *BMC Public Health, 22*(1), 670.

Zaragoza, Cosme. (2017). Aztlán: "Essays on the Chicano Homeland. Revised and Expanded Edition." *University of New Mexico Press*, p. 137.

Chapter 10
Financial Planning for Centenarians

Adrian A. Llorente

Financial planning for retirement is an ongoing process. As people age, their needs and financial circumstances change. Even after retirement, your plans should be reviewed on a regular basis to make sure that they are still appropriate for your current situation. This includes making adjustments to your investment portfolio, as well as to your spending habits. If you are nearing retirement age, or if you have already retired, there are a number of resources available to help you with your financial planning including books and websites that offer advice on retirement planning, and financial planners who specialize in helping people with their retirement plans.

Key Take Away Points

1. It's never too early or too late to plan for retirement.
2. Retirement planning should take into account known expenses, sources of income and life expectancy.
3. Because life circumstances change over time, a financial plan is not static, and should be periodically reviewed.

10.1 Introduction

Financial planning for retirement is an important consideration for everyone, and ideally begins at an early age, but it is especially critical for those who are approaching or have already reached retirement age. There are a number of potential sources of income in retirement which can include Social Security benefits, pension plans, and personal savings. In addition to income, there are a number of other factors that

A. A. Llorente (✉)
Laguna Hills, CA, USA

R. E. Kheirbek, M. D. Llorente (eds.), *Current Perspectives on Centenarians*, International Perspectives on Aging 36,
https://doi.org/10.1007/978-3-031-30915-1_10

can affect retirement planning. These include inflation, health care costs, and longevity. Finally, the amount of money you will need to have saved by retirement will also depend on the age at which you want to retire. This chapter provides an overview of these key factors to consider when planning for financial needs in retirement, with particular attention to the likely financial needs of living to or past 100 years.

10.2 Retirement Planning for Centenarians

The number of people who are expected to live past 100 is increasing rapidly. In 2021, the UN reported the number of centenarians worldwide was expected to grow to approximately 573,000 (United Nations, 2022). In 2015, the United States had the largest total number of centenarians, with nearly 72,000 (Stepler, 2016). That number is projected to grow to 378,000 by 2050. This rapid growth is being driven by a number of factors, including the use of antibiotics to combat infections, advances in medical care, and increases in healthier lifestyle choices. As the number of centenarians continues to increase, there will be significant implications for retirements for individuals, and for society and fiscal policy makers. Although poverty rates have generally declined among older adults, certain subgroups still exhibit higher poverty (Congressional Research Service, 2022). Approximately 12.8% of seniors aged 80 years and older experience poverty, compared with 9.5–9.7% among those between the ages of 65 and 79. Among those 80 and older, women, regardless of race and ethnicity, experience the highest poverty rates, averaging 14.7% in 2021. Poverty rates for seniors aged 65 and older also vary by race and ethnicity as follows: 18.7% among Hispanics of any race; 17.8% among non-Hispanic Blacks, and 8.0% among non-Hispanic Whites.

10.2.1 Longevity of Retirement Periods

As people live to be centenarians, retirements are necessarily lasting for longer periods of time. In 1950, the average life expectancy at birth for Americans was 68 years (US Department of Health, Education and Welfare, 1954). This means that if the individual retired at age 65, the average retirement duration was about 3 years. But by 2021, average life expectancy grew to 76 years (Arias et al., 2022). If retirement still occurs at age 65, the average retiree can now expect to spend 11 years in retirement. A centenarian, however, would have to plan for at least 35 years in retirement, approximately one-third of their life. As a result of living longer, Americans are now having to work longer and retire at later ages than in the past. A recent Gallup poll found that the average age of retirement in 2022 is now 61, compared to age 57 in 1991 (Jones, 2022).

10.2.2 Inflation

Inflation is the gradual increase in the prices of goods and services over time and has a significant impact on retirement accounts. When inflation increases, the purchasing power of fixed income, such as Social Security benefits or pension payments, decreases. This can result in retirees having to reduce their expenditures in order to make ends meet. In addition, inflation can eat away at the value of savings and investments, which can make it difficult to maintain one's lifestyle in retirement, and thus lower standards of living. Following the COVID-19 pandemic, inflation in the US rose, hitting a peak in June 2022 of 9.1%, and an annual rate of 8.3%, the highest rate since 1981 (Statista, 2022). To illustrate the impact of inflation on retirees, AARP found that 1% inflation over 20 years, based on a $1341 monthly fixed income, would result in approximately $34,000 loss of buying power (AARP, 2022a, b). Using this same calculation, the impact of the current annual rate of inflation of 8.3% would increase that loss of buying power to more than $400,000 for the average retiree. It would be a much higher number for centenarians, possibly even double. As a result, many older retirees are returning to the workforce. A recent Joblist survey found that 27% of retired job seekers were "unretiring" due to financial reasons, and 21% specifically mentioned inflation worries (Joblist, 2022).

10.3 What Are the Typical Costs in Retirement?

10.3.1 Housing Costs

Housing is often the single largest expected expense, and if the person owns their own home, the biggest asset. However, as people age and their needs change, predicting and possibly reducing housing costs are part of retirement planning. As children move away, a large home may become increasingly challenging and costly to maintain. One option is to take in boarders, such as college students, who can pay rent to offset expenses. Another option is to downsize to a smaller home. The existing equity in the home may cover the costs of buying a new home, so that a mortgage is not needed. Maintenance costs and property taxes will also likely be lower, thus further reducing housing costs.

10.3.2 Income Tax on Social Security and Pensions

When total annual income exceeds $25,000 for an individual, Social Security (SS) income is subject to federal income tax (AARP, 2022a, b). Persons who work, even part time, or who draw distributions from pension or IRA plans will likely be required to pay federal income taxes on their SS income. Further, as of the 2022 tax year, 11 states also tax some, or all, of their residents' SS benefits. These include: Connecticut, Kansas, Minnesota, Missouri, Montana, Nebraska, New Mexico, Rhode Island, Utah, Vermont and West Virginia. Some state policies follow the federal regulations. Others offer state-specific deductions, exemptions based on age, income or disabled veteran status. None of this applies to Supplemental Security Income (SSI) because to be eligible for this program, persons must be very low income, and SSI is not subject to income tax. Similarly, nine states don't tax retirement incomes because they have no state income taxes (Waggoner, 2020). These are: Alaska, Florida, Nevada, New Hampshire, South Dakota, Tennessee, Texas, Washington, and Wyoming. Three others, Illinois, Mississippi, and Pennsylvania, don't tax distributions from 401(k) plans and IRAs. Thirty-four states don't tax military retirement income at all, and 13 states have partial allowances for military pay.

10.3.3 Real Estate, Property and Sales Tax

There are additional taxes that should be considered when planning for retirement (Niedt et al., 2022). While some states do not have state income tax, they often generate revenue through other types of taxes, including property and sales taxes. For example, New Jersey has the highest median property tax rate in the country and imposes a tax on inherited property worth $500 or more (Muhlbaum & Mengle, 2022). Forty-five states and the District of Columbia have state sales tax, and 38 states have local sales taxes that can add significant costs to a fixed income level. As an example, the average combined state and local sales tax in Louisiana is 9.5%, which is a large additional cost each time a senior needs to make a purchase.

10.3.4 Health Care Costs

Health care costs can have a significant, and at times, unexpected impact on retirement and finances. Healthier seniors have been found to have more wealth than those with health problems, and as medical problems develop, wealth tends to decline (Johnson, 2016; Poterba et al., 2012). Poterba et al. further found that 46% of seniors die with less than $10,000 in assets and rely almost entirely on SS benefits for support. Of note is that this group is disproportionately in poor health.

According to a study by Royal Bank of Canada, at age 65, the average retiree can expect to spend $6100 per year on health care costs (Royal Bank of Canada, 2021). This report found that nearly 80% of respondents reported worry about their ability to cover health care expenses, but only 56% had factored health care costs into their retirement planning. A recent study examined mean per capita medical spending in 9 countries in the last 12 months of life (based on insurance data) (French et al., 2017). Total costs were highest in the United States, with the highest cost categories being hospital expenses, long-term care and professional services. Since centenarians can spend up to three times longer in retirement than the average retiree, over the course of retirement, they will likely spend more on healthcare. A recent study examined hospitalization costs among centenarians, and found that overall, US centenarian hospital admissions cost significantly more than those for other younger aged US seniors (2.7 times more than those 85+, and 2.1 times more thank those 65–84 years) (Twersky & Davey, 2022). Nearly a third of these hospital admissions were due to potentially preventable conditions. Of note is that even among centenarians, healthcare disparities are seen. Black, Hispanic, Asians/Pacific Islanders and other race centenarians had higher hospitalization costs compared to Whites. Black and Hispanic centenarians had significantly longer mean lengths of stay. This suggests that minorities may have higher health-related costs into older age.

10.3.5 Long Term Care Costs

The average cost of living in an assisted living facility (ALF) can vary depending on the location, type of facility, and the level of care required. In general, ALFs provide housing, personal care, medication management, support services, such as light housekeeping, and often meals, laundry and transportation, to individuals who need assistance with activities of daily living, but do not require skilled nursing care. The average monthly US cost of ALF was $4500 in 2021 (Genworth, 2022). Costs of assisted living are typically paid for by out-of-pocket personal funds, as they are not covered by insurance or federal programs.

According to the Administration on Aging, a 65 year old has an almost 70% chance of needing long term care in their lifetime, either through home health services, assisted living or nursing home (US Department of Health and Human Services, 2020). Women need care longer than men, and approximately 35% will need nursing home care. Here too, the cost varies by location and level of care needed, but median monthly US costs in 2021 for a private room in a nursing home were $9034 (Genworth, 2021).

Medicare typically covers nursing home care for the first 100 days. After that period, Medicare no longer covers nursing home costs. Medicaid does cover these costs, but only for those who are eligible. The criteria for Medicaid eligibility are state-specific, and financially based, usually for persons with very limited income and few financial assets (American Council on Aging, 2021). In general, a 65 year old single person must have income less than $2742 per month to qualify for nursing home Medicaid. The individual must also pass the "asset test". One must determine which assets count towards the limit, and which are exempt (American Council on Aging, 2022a, b), but in general, the person is only allowed no more than $2000 in countable assets to qualify for nursing home Medicaid. Further, asset transfers made by the Medicaid applicant within the previous 5 years are scrutinized. This is referred to as the Medicaid Look-Back Period (American Council on Aging, 2022a, b). If countable assets were transferred, a penalty period of Medicaid ineligibility will be applied. The limits are higher for married couples, but the asset rules are more complex.

In the US, Medicaid currently covers nearly 50% of the total nursing home costs. In 2021, the average annual costs of a shared room in a nursing home was $94,900, but vary greatly, ranging from a low of $61,503 in Texas to the highest national costs of $378,000 in Alaska (American Council on Aging, 2022a, b). Many individuals have health and disability insurance, but these polices offer limited nursing home benefits, and none cover ALFs. Costs of long-term care are usually paid for through personal funds and can include savings, income and proceeds from sale of assets. There are government programs that can assist with covering costs, but persons must meet eligibility criteria, which are financial/income based. Examples of these programs include the Program of All-Inclusive Care for the Elderly (PACE) (Centers for Medicare & Medicaid Services, 2021), State Health Insurance Assistance Program (SHIP) (Administration for Community Living, 2022), and the Department of Veterans Affairs for eligible veterans (US Department of Veterans Affairs, 2022).

10.4 What Are the Common Sources of Retirement Income?

10.4.1 Social Security

Social Security (SS) is the main source of income for most retired workers (Social Security Administration, 2022a, b, c, d). Nearly 90% of people 65 and older were receiving a SS benefit. Among beneficiaries, 37% of men and 42% of women receive 50% or more of their income from SS. Social Security is a pay-as-you-go system, meaning that benefits are funded and paid for through current workers' payroll taxes. If you do not contribute into the system and obtain the required number of credits, you will not be entitled to the benefits. A maximum of 4 credits can be earned per year, and for individuals born after 1928, 40 credits are needed to qualify for a retirement income benefit (Social Security Administration, 2022a, b, c, d). Credits are earned based on wages, and the amount of earnings to earn a credit can change each year. In 2022, for example, one Social Security credit is earned for each $1510 in covered earnings. If you are self-employed or have a small business, in order to qualify for Social Security, you will need to pay the combined employee and employer Social Security taxes (Social Security Administration, 2022a, b, c, d). For many people, Social Security benefits will be the primary source of income in retirement. It is important to understand how these benefits are calculated and what factors can affect them. For example, delaying the start of benefits can often result in a higher monthly payment because the social security benefits are calculated based on the average indexed monthly earnings. The calculation process starts with the highest 35 years of earnings. Then, those years are averaged and divided by 12 to get the average monthly earnings. After that, the Social Security Administration applies a benefit formula to calculate your primary insurance amount, which is the amount you would receive if you retire at full retirement age. Full retirement age historically was 65 years. Starting in 1983, however, Congress passed a law that raises this age as a result of people living longer (Social Security Administration, 2022a, b, c, d). For those born in 1938, the retirement age gradually increases by a few months for each year, reaching 67 for people born in 1960 and later.

10.4.2 SSI

There are also a number of programs, such as the Supplemental Security Income (SSI) program, which provide cash assistance to low-income individuals who are aged, blind, or disabled. SSI benefits are based on need and are intended to supplement the beneficiary's other income and resources. The Social Security Administration (SSA) uses a two-step process to determine if an applicant is eligible for the Supplemental Security Income (SSI) program. First, the SSA determines if the applicant is disabled or blind according to their guidelines. If the applicant is determined to be disabled or blind, the SSA then considers whether the applicant has limited income and resources; this level is different for each state but is generally based on the federal poverty level.

10.4.3 Pensions

Pension plans can be an important source of income in retirement. However, 32% of the current US workforce in private industry has no access to private pension coverage (Social Security Administration, 2022a, b, c, d). Most pension plans require that employees work for a certain number of years before they become eligible to receive benefits. There are also a number of different types of pension plans, including defined benefit plans and defined contribution plans. A defined benefit plan provides a retirement income based on a fixed formula (Internal Revenue Service, 2022a, b). The biggest advantage of this type of plan is that the benefit amount is predictable, employers can contribute more than in other plans, and benefits are not dependent on asset returns. Disadvantages include the cost of administering these plans, their complexity, and if minimum or maximum contribution requirements are not met or exceeded, excise taxes may apply. Defined contribution plans are those in which the employee and/or employer contribute, and usually, the contributions and earnings are taxed at distribution. Examples of this type of plan include 401(k), 403(b), employee stock ownership plans, and profit-sharing. The IRS requires individual account holders to start taking a required minimum distribution (RMD) at age 72 (Internal Revenue Service, 2022a, b).

10.4.4 Personal Savings

Personal savings are an additional safety net for retirement, and help to cover unexpected costs, such as medical bills, and home and auto repairs. Long-term savings can facilitate a new car payment, or cover costs of travel or unexpected increased inflation. In addition, for those have reached their maximum contribution limits on retirement accounts, additional ways to supplement retirement saving can be through investments, such as certificates of deposit (CDs).

10.5 How Much Should I Save for Retirement? It Depends

Planning for retirement is necessarily an informed calculation based on known expenditures, factoring in possible unexpected expenditures, understanding income, and then planning for "extras", such as the costs of travel or hobbies. There are a number of different ways to think about and make these calculations. Historically, a very general rule of thumb was that you needed around $1 million to retire comfortably. Another way of thinking about this is to calculate the amount of income you currently live on, and then you would need savings that would produce 80% of income annually for at least 20 years. Another common way is the 50/30/20 rule. This is a personal finance guideline that suggests allocating only 50% of your income towards your needs, 30% towards your wants and 20% towards savings or debt repayment. This simple rule can help you make better financial decisions and get on track to reaching your long-term financial goals. Another easy way to think about saving for retirement is the 70/10/20 rule. In this rule, 70% is for monthly expenses including *EVERYTHING* you spend money on, including bills, utilities, emergency, etc. The next 10% goes to donation/tithing, or investments, retirement, saving for college, etc. The last 20% goes into savings, unless you have pressing debt in which case it should go towards paying off the debt first.

10.6 Employer Sponsored Retirement Plans

A 401(k) is a tax-deferred retirement savings account that is sponsored by an employer. Employees can choose to have a certain percentage of their paycheck withheld and deposited into their 401(k) account. Most employers will also match a portion of the employee's contribution, up to a certain percentage. For example, an employer may match 50% of the employee's contribution, up to 6% of the employee's salary. Additional employer sponsored plans include 457(b) and 403 (b). The main difference between these plans is that 401(k) plans are sponsored by private employers, 403(b) are accounts for schools and universities, churches and non-profits, and 457(b) are accounts for state and local governments. At a minimum, you should contribute the amount your employer matches. Ideally, you would contribute more than that, up to the maximum contribution allowed. For 2023, participants can contribute up $22,500. People over 50 can contribute an additional $7500 as a "catch-up" contribution.

10.7 Individual Retirement Accounts (IRA)

A traditional IRA is an account that anyone can open and contribute to. Contributions are made with pretax dollars, which reduces the taxable income for that year. The money in a Traditional IRA grows tax-deferred, meaning you won't pay income taxes on the account until you begin to withdraw funds at retirement.

A Roth IRA is an individual retirement account that offers tax-free growth and tax-free withdrawals in retirement. Unlike a traditional IRA, contributions to a Roth IRA are made with after-tax dollars. The primary benefit of a Roth IRA is that the contributions and the earnings on those contributions can grow tax-free and be withdrawn tax-free after the age 59½ assuming the account has been open for at least 5 years. In other words, you pay taxes on money going into your Roth IRA, and then all future withdrawals are tax-free. The amount you can contribute to a Roth IRA is limited by your income and tax filing status. As of 2023, a single filer can't contribute to a Roth IRA if they earn more than $153,000. There are no required minimum distributions for a Roth IRA, like there are for 401(k) plans and traditional IRAs.

In 2023, for both the traditional and Roth IRAs, the maximum contribution limit is $6500. If you are age 50 or older, you can make catch-up contributions of an additional $1000. These limits apply across all such accounts, so even if you have multiple accounts, you can't contribute more than the maximum.

10.8 Conclusions

In retirement, you will no longer have the benefit of a regular paycheck to cover unexpected expenses. Therefore, it's important to have a plan in place to cover unexpected costs. This may include having an emergency fund, long-term care insurance, or both. Housing is typically the biggest expense in retirement. Health care costs can be a significant expense in retirement, and there will likely be some out-of-pocket costs such as premiums, deductibles, and copays. Many Americans are finding that working past "typical" retirement age or part-time post retirement can facilitate having more financial security. Careful planning is essential for retirement, and that should include an accurate assessment of likely costs and sources of income.

Additional Resources (Readings, Media, etc.)

Retirement

Many investment companies offer retirement calculators, seminars and online courses.

American Association of Retired Persons. AARP Retirement Calculator: Are you Saving Enough. Available at: https://www.aarp.org/work/retirement-planning/retirement_calculator.html. Accessed January 14, 2023.

Fiscal Policy

Aaron HJ. The Centenarian Boom: Providing for Retirement in a Long-Lived America. March 2000. Available at: https://www.brookings.edu/articles/the-centenarian-boom-providing-for-retirement-in-a-long-lived-america/. Accessed January 14, 2023.

Auerback AJ. Societal Aging: Implications for Fiscal Policy. April 2012. Available at: https://www.imes.boj.or.jp/en/conference/2012/Session2_out.pdf. Accessed January 14, 2023.

Bogetic Z, Onder H, Onal A, Skrok E, Schwartz A, Winkler H. Fiscal Policy Issues in the Aging Societies. March 9, 2015. Available at: https://openknowledge.worldbank.org/bitstream/handle/10986/21782/952660NWP0MFM000Box385292B00PUBLIC0.pdf?sequence=1&isAllowed=y. Accessed January 14, 2023.

Multiple Choice Questions

1. If one lives to 100, what is the average number of years one would spend in retirement?

   A. 20
   B. 25
   C. 30
   D. 35
   Correct Answer: D

2. For 2023, what is the maximum contribution one can make to a 401(k) plan?

   A. $500
   B. $6500
   C. $22,500
   D. There's no limit
   Correct Answer: C

3. Which of the following retirement savings plans allows you to withdraw the contributions and the earnings on those contributions tax-free?

   A. Traditional IRA
   B. Roth IRA
   C. 401(k)
   D. 403(b)
   Correct Answer: B

References

Administration for Community Living. (2022, August). *SHIP*. Available at: https://acl.gov/programs/connecting-people-services/state-health-insurance-assistance-program-ship. Accessed 29 Dec 2022.

American Association of Retired Persons. (2022a, May). 5 *Unexpected reasons retirees are returning to work*. Available at: https://www.aarp.org/retirement/planning-for-retirement/info-2022/returning-to-work.html. Accessed 29 Dec 2022.

American Association of Retired Persons. (2022b). *Which states tax social security benefits?* Available at: https://www.aarp.org/retirement/social-security/questions-answers/which-states-do-not-tax-social-security-benefits.html. Accessed 28 Dec 2022.

American Council on Aging. (2021, March). *State specific medicaid eligibility requirements*. Available at: https://www.medicaidplanningassistance.org/state-specific-medicaid-eligibility/. Accessed 28 Dec 2022.

American Council on Aging. (2022a, March). *2021 nursing home costs by state and region*. Available at: https://www.medicaidplanningassistance.org/nursing-home-costs/. Accessed 28 Dec 2022.

American Council on Aging. (2022b, December). *Understand Medicaid's look-back period; penalties, exceptions & state variances*. Available at: https://www.medicaidplanningassistance.org/medicaid-look-back-period/.

Arias, E., Tejada-Vera, B., Kochanek, K. D., & Ahmad, F. B. (2022, August). *Provisional life expectancy estimates for 2021*. Available at: https://www.cdc.gov/nchs/data/vsrr/vsrr023.pdf. Accessed 29 Dec 2022.

Centers for Medicare & Medicaid Services. (2021, December). PACE. https://www.cms.gov/Medicare-Medicaid-Coordination/Medicare-and-Medicaid-Coordination/Medicare-Medicaid-Coordination-Office/PACE/PACE. Accessed 29 Dec 2022.

Congressional Research Service. (2022, December 6). *Poverty among the population aged 65 and older*. https://sgp.fas.org/crs/misc/R45791.pdf. Accessed 23 Jan 2023.

French, E. B., McCauley, J., Aragon, M., Bakx, P., Chalkley, M., Chen, S. H., et al. (2017, Jul 1). End-of-life medical spending in last twelve months of life is lower than previously reported. *Health Affairs, 36*(7):1211–1217. https://doi.org/10.1377/hlthaff.2017.0174. PMID: 28679807.

Genworth. (2021, November). *Cost of care survey*. Available at: https://www.genworth.com/aging-and-you/finances/cost-of-care.html. Accessed 28 Dec 2022.

Genworth. (2022). *Cost of care survey*. Available at: https://www.genworth.com/aging-and-you/finances/cost-of-care.html. Accessed 29 Dec 2022.

Internal Revenue Service. (2022a, September). *Retirement plan and IRA required minimum distributions FAQs*. Available at: https://www.irs.gov/retirement-plans/retirement-plans-faqs-regarding-required-minimum-distributions. Accessed 28 Dec 2022.

Internal Revenue Service. (2022b, November). https://www.irs.gov/retirement-plans/plan-participant-employee/definitions#:~:text=Defined%20Contribution%20Plan%20is%20a,any%20investment%20and%20administrative%20fees. Accessed 28 Dec 2022.

Joblist. (2022, July). *Q2 2022 US Job Market Report*. Available at: https://www.joblist.com/jobs-reports/q2-2022-united-states-job-market-report. Accessed 29 Dec 2022.

Johnson, Richard W. (2016). *Later-life household wealth before and after disability onset*. Urban Institute. Available at: https://aspe.hhs.gov/reports/later-life-household-wealth-after-disability-onset. Accessed 29 Dec 2022.

Jones, J. M. (2022, July 22). More in US retiring, or planning to retire. *Later*. Available at: https://news.gallup.com/poll/394943/retiring-planning-retire-later.aspx. Accessed 28 Dec 2022.

Muhlbaum, D., & Mengle, R. (2022, December). *10 least tax-friendly states for retirees*. Available at: https://www.kiplinger.com/retirement/601815/least-tax-friendly-states-for-retirees.

Niedt, B., Muhlbaum, D., & Mengle, R. (2022, November). *States tax retirees*. Available at: https://www.kiplinger.com/retirement/602202/taxes-in-retirement-how-all-50-states-tax-retirees. Accessed 28 Dec 2022.

Poterba, J. M., Venti, S. F., & Wise, D. A.. (2012). *Were they prepared for retirement? Financial status at advanced ages in the HRS and AHEAD cohorts*. NBER Working Paper 17824. Cambridge, MA: National Bureau of Economic Research. http://www.nber.org/papers/w17824.pdf

Royal Bank of Canada. (2021). *Taking control of health care in retirement*. Available at: https://www.rbcwealthmanagement.com/_assets/documents/insights/taking-control-of-health-care-in-retirement.pdf). Accessed 14 Jan 2023.

Social Security Administration. (2022a, January). *If you are self-employed*. Available at: https://www.ssa.gov/pubs/EN-05-10022.pdf. Accessed 28 Dec 2022.

Social Security Administration. (2022b). *Fact sheet*. Available at: https://www.ssa.gov/news/press/factsheets/basicfact-alt.pdf. Accessed 14 Jan 2023.

Social Security Administration. (2022c). *Retirement age calculator*. Available at:https://www.ssa.gov/benefits/retirement/planner/ageincrease.html. Accessed 28 Dec 2022.

Social Security Administration. (2022d). *Social security credits*. Available at: https://www.ssa.gov/benefits/retirement/planner/credits.html. Accessed December 28, 2022.

Statista. (2022, November). *Monthly 12-month inflation rate in the US from January 2020 to November 2022*. Available at: https://www.statista.com/statistics/273418/unadjusted-monthly-inflation-rate-in-the-us/. Accessed 29 Dec 2022.

Stepler, R. (2016). *World's centenarian popoulation projected to grow eightfold by 2050*. Available at: https://www.pewresearch.org/fact-tank/2016/04/21/worlds-centenarian-population-projected-to-grow-eightfold-by-2050/. Accessed 14 Jan 2023.

Twersky, S. E., & Davey, A. (2022). National hospitalization trends and the role of preventable hospitalizations among centenarians in the United States (2000–2009). *International Journal of Environmental Research and Public Health, 19*(2), 795. https://doi.org/10.3390/ijerph19020795

United Nations. (2022). *Department of economic and social affairs*. Available at: https://population.un.org/wpp/. Accessed 14 Jan 2023.

US Department of Health, Education and Welfare. (1954, November). *Life tables for 1949–51*. Available at: https://www.cdc.gov/nchs/data/lifetables/life49-51.pdf. Accessed 29 Dec 2022.

US Department of Health and Human Services. (2020, February). *How much care will You need?* Available at: https://acl.gov/ltc/basic-needs/how-much-care-will-you-need. Accessed 28 Dec 2022.

US Department of Veterans Affairs. (2022, September). *Geriatrics and extended care*. Available at: https://www.va.gov/GERIATRICS/pages/Paying_for_Long_Term_Care.asp. Accessed 29 Dec 2022.

Waggoner, J. (2020). *12 states that won't tax your retirement distributions*. Available at: https://www.aarp.org/money/taxes/info-2020/states-that-dont-tax-retirement-distributions.html. Accessed 28 Dec 2022.

Chapter 11
Religion, Spirituality and Longevity

Jeni Cook, Caitlyn Gudmundsen, and Ray Furr

Key Take Away Points

1. A Decades of research have demonstrated that religion and spirituality (R/S) are critical factors supporting physical and mental health as well as longevity. Elderly patients and those at the end of life say R/S is especially important to them and should be respected and integrated into their medical treatment.
2. Therapeutic care for the R/S needs of patients and families is a health care specialty. The Joint Commission Standards of Care and the National Consensus Project for Quality Palliative Care require spiritual assessments be conducted in health care facilities.
3. Professional chaplains should be employed to competently assess and address the R/S needs of patients and families.

Vignette: Rev. Dr. Dave deFreese serves as the VP of Church Relations at Mosaic, a Lutheran-founded organization in Omaha, Nebraska that provides whole-person healthcare to seniors. Dave observes that the spiritual services Mosaic incorporates can make a big difference in individual lives. He recalled a retired businessman who had been professionally successful, but once he retired, he lacked meaning

Pew Research Center bears no responsibility for the analysis or interpretations of the data presented here. The opinions expressed herein, including any implications for policy, are those of the author and not Pew Research Center.

J. Cook (✉)
Retired, Board Certified Healthcare Chaplain, Canyon Lake, TX, USA

C. Gudmundsen
CDC Foundation, Fairfax, VA, USA

R. Furr
Retired Minister, Canyon Lake, TX, USA

R. E. Kheirbek, M. D. Llorente (eds.), *Current Perspectives on Centenarians*, International Perspectives on Aging 36,
https://doi.org/10.1007/978-3-031-30915-1_11

in his life. He shared with Dave, "I climbed the ladder, and I climbed it well. After I climbed it, I realized I probably put my ladder against the wrong building."

The retired businessman recognized in his advanced age that though society deemed him to be a successful person, he had neither a community nor a deeper purpose beyond his career. He understood this to be a spiritual problem and sought Dave, a religious leader. Dave witnessed the elderly man change emotionally, mentally, and physically once he found a deep sense of spirituality and felt he had purpose in his life. He was liberated, happier, more connected to others, and more involved with service in his local community. Even late in life, the man's faith and connection to his religious community supported his health, enabling him to live a long, purpose-filled, high-quality life.[1]

11.1 Religion, Spirituality, and Health: A Well-Founded Connection

The connection between religion/spirituality and physical health has long been recognized[2] and researchers have found benefits across a variety of health outcomes,[3] including improved mental health[4] and reduced risk for multiple chronic psychotic disorders,[5] improved cardiovascular health such as lower blood pressure,[6] improved immune functioning,[7] and overall lower mortality risk.[8] Health benefits are not confined to individuals who adhere to institutionalized religion, but are also found

[1] deFreese, Dave. Mosaic, Omaha, Neb. Interview. Conducted by Caitlyn Gudmundsen. 23 September 2022.

[2] Idler, E. L. (2014). Religion: The invisible social determinant. In Ellen L. Idler (Ed.), *Religion as a Social Determinant of Public Health.* Oxford Academic. pp. 1–24.

[3] Zimmer, Z., Jagger C., Chiu, C.T., Ofstedal, M. B., Rojo, F., Saito, Y. (2016). Spirituality, religiosity, aging and health in global perspective: A review. *SSM Population Health*, 10(2), 373–381. https://doi.org/10.1016/j.ssmph.2016.04.009. PMID: 29349154; PMCID: PMC5758000.

[4] Koenig, H. G. (2009). Research on religion, spirituality, and mental health: A review. *Canadian Journal of Psychiatry,* 54, 283–291.

[5] Koenig, H. G. (2012). Religion, spirituality, and health: The research and clinical implications, *International Scholarly Research Notices*, 2012, Article ID 278730. https://doi.org/10.5402/2012/278730. PMID: 23762764; PMCID: PMC3671693.

[6] Sørensen, T., Danbolt, L. J., Lien, L., Koenig, H. G., Holmen, J. (2011). The relationship between religious attendance and blood pressure: the HUNT Study. *International Journal of Psychiatry in Medicine,* 42(1), 13–28. https://doi.org/10.2190/PM.42.1.b. PMID: 22372022.

[7] Maselko, J., Kubzansky, L., Kawachi, I., Seeman, T., Berkman, L., (2007). Religious service attendance and allostatic load among high-functioning elderly. *Psychosomatic Medicine,* 69(5), 464–472. https://doi.org/10.1097/PSY.0b013e31806c7c57

[8] Hummer, R. A., Ellison, C. G., Rogers, R. G., Moulton, B. E., Romero, R. R. (2004). Religious involvement and adult mortality in the United States: Review and perspective. *Southern Medical Journal,* 97, 1223–1230.

among people with looser affiliations, many of whom consider themselves to be "spiritual, not religious."

The terms "religion" and "spirituality" are often conflated but can have distinct meanings. Spirituality refers to an individual's search for a higher meaning or purpose beyond oneself. It involves an effort to transcend biological surroundings, connect with the divine, and live in harmony with one's environment. Though religion can be practiced individually, it usually includes corporate meaning and involves participation in a community with an agreed upon set of beliefs and moral code. The rituals and communal practices within a religion can also provide a way to make meaning and express a sense of spirituality.[9]

Though "religion" and "spirituality" have different meanings, both are associated with positive health outcomes and will be referred to in the collective throughout this chapter as "R/S." Religious and spiritual practices are diverse globally, but studies have found health benefits across R/S traditions. Specific R/S practices will be mentioned in this chapter, but R/S will refer to a wide array of religious and spiritual traditions across the globe.

An early peer-reviewed study that found an independent correlation between R/S and health was the famous Alameda County, California longitudinal study which began in 1965. Over 6000 participants in Alameda County responded to survey questions about their health and lifestyle, and five subsequent data collections took place over the following three decades. The survey collected data on religious service attendance, including frequency of attendance, and found that religious involvement was associated with lower death rates from all causes. The results were particularly strong among women, with weekly religious service attendance supporting health at similar levels as never smoking cigarettes and regular physical exercise.[10]

Multiple studies since Alameda County have confirmed the correlation between R/S and health, though the strength of the protection varies. The Nurses' Health Study found that attending a religious service more than once per week was associated with 33% lower all-cause mortality compared with women who had never attended religious services,[11] while other research using data from the Third National Health and Nutrition Examination Survey (NHANES III) indicates that frequent churchgoers had a 55% reduction for all-cause mortality.[12]

---

[9] White, M. S., Addison, C. C., and Jenkins, B. W. (2022). Beliefs and practices regarding spirituality as a healthcare strategy. *Open Journal of Preventive Medicine*, 12, 59–72. https://doi.org/10.4236/ojpm.2022.123004

[10] Housman, J.; Dorman, S. The Alameda County Study: A systematic, chronological review. *American Journal of Health Education*, 36(5), 302–308.

[11] Shanshan, L., Meir, J. S., Williams, D. R., VanderWeele, T. J. (2016). Association of religious service attendance with mortality among women. *JAMA Internal Medicine,* 176(6), 777–785. https://doi.org/10.1001/jamainternmed.2016.1615

[12] Bruce, M. A., Martins, D., Duru, K., Beech, B. M., Sims, M., Harawa, N., et al. (2017). Church attendance, allostatic load, and mortality in middle aged adults. *PLoS ONE,* 12(5), e0177618. https://doi.org/10.1371/journal.pone.0177618

The correlation between R/S and health is well-documented, but there is skepticism that the data is self-reported and based on volunteer samples. As an alternative measure of religious involvement, a recent study analyzed obituaries and found that the mention of religiosity in the obituary was associated with longer life up to 9.45 years.[13]

Demographic trends indicate that as people age, they tend to become more religious and more interested in connecting to the transcendent.[14] Rev. Dr. Dave deFreese has anecdotally noticed this trend, saying that the elderly people in his line of work tend to ask more serious questions and are concerned with whether their lives remain purposeful. It is important then, that those who provide healthcare for the aging understand the impact of R/S on health and the mechanisms through which it can provide support.

11.2 How R/S Supports Health and Longevity

There are various ways that R/S contributes to health and longevity, including the *social connections* that involvement in a religious community offers. French sociologist Emile Durkheim first noticed the importance of social ties when he identified that suicide rates were unequally distributed across Europe and aimed to understand the social factors that contribute to suicide. He found social influences, with religion being a key example, were protective factors against suicide.[15] Modern studies have found social ties are critically important to health, including protecting against cognitive decline[16] and mortality in older adults.[17] Institutionalized religion can provide important social ties throughout an individual's life, and unlike other avenues for social ties (sports teams, social hobbies, country clubs, etc.), is not dependent on the individual's physical ability level or economic status. These social ties are stable over time and may contribute to the strength of the relationship between physical health and frequency of religious service attendance.

[13] Wallace, L. E., Anthony, R., End, C. M., Way, B. M. (2019). Does religion stave off the grave? Religious affiliation in one's obituary and longevity. *Social Psychological and Personality Science, 10*(5), 662–670. https://doi.org/10.1177/1948550618779820

[14] Atchley, R. C. (2009). *Spirituality and Aging*. The John Hopkins University Press.

[15] Durkheim, E. *(1897). Suicide, a study in sociology* (1951 Edition, J. A. Spaulding, & G. Simpson, Trans.). Routledge.

[16] Crooks, V. C., Lubben, J., Petitti, D. B., et al. (2008). Social network, cognitive function, and dementia incidence among elderly women. *American Journal of Public Health,* 98, 1221–1227. https://doi.org/10.2105/AJPH.2007.115923.

[17] Kauppi, M., Kawachi, I., Batty, G. D., et al. (2018). Characteristics of social networks and mortality risk: evidence from 2 prospective cohort studies. *American Journal of Epidemiology,* 187, 746–753. https://doi.org/10.1093/aje/kwx301.

Within those important religious social networks, R/S exerts *social control* over individuals in ways that benefit health.[18] For example, many religious traditions discourage alcohol and drug use. Recent studies have found that people claiming not to be religious had higher patterns of alcohol consumption,[19] and the highest levels of smoking compared to Christians and Muslims.[20] Religious groups can reinforce healthy behaviors and these trends have significant implications at a population level.

Finding meaning through R/S has positive impacts that are physiological, mental, and emotional. Psychological stress impacts psycho-neuro-endocrine-immune pathways specifically interfering with the functional actions of the hypothalamic-pituitary-adrenocortical and sympathetic-adrenal-medullary axes. R/S engagement and practices have been shown to modulate these systems and *reduce stress*.[21] Beliefs, attitudes, and practices give meaning to a patient's suffering which seems to relieve the psychological stressors and make pain more bearable. Many spiritual leaders perform rituals, such as an imam reciting chapters from the Qur'an or communion in the Christian tradition, at a hospital bedside. These sacraments and rituals provide grounding that can reduce stress and offer peace and healing, affecting the mind and even body chemistry. Regular spiritual practices such as meditation are also shown to reduce stress and have a wide array of health benefits including enhanced immune function,[22] and emotional benefits for those in social isolation, which has particular implications for older populations.[23]

At the age of 100+, centenarians have outlived most if not all their contemporaries and lost many family members and friends throughout their lifetimes. *Finding meaning and purpose* in life is crucial and R/S contributes to centenarians' *resilience*, and there is evidence that R/S helps elderly patients cope with adversity and isolation.[24] One centenarian who participated in a qualitative study shared,

---

[18] Ko, S. (2015). Religion as a Social Determinant of Public Health, Ellen Idler, Ed, Oxford University Press, 2014. *Christian Journal for Global Health*, 2(2), 76–77. https://doi.org/10.15566/cjgh.v2i2.88.

[19] Ponce, T. D., Picciano, A. P., de Vargas, D. (2021). Women's alcohol consumption in a primary health care service. *Rev Esc Enferm USP*. 25;55: e20200458. English, Portuguese. https://doi.org/10.1590/1980-220X-REEUSP-2020-0458. PMID: 34448803.

[20] Hussain, M., Walker, C., Moon, G. (2019). Smoking and religion: Untangling associations using English survey data. *Journal of Religion and Health*, 58(6), 2263–2276. https://doi.org/10.1007/s10943-017-0434-9. PMID: 28667475; PMCID: PMC6842333.

[21] Saad, M., Medeiros, R. (2017). Implications for public health of the religiosity-longevity relation. *Revista da Associacao Medica Brasileira,* 63 (10), 837–841. https://doi.org/10.1590/1806-9282.63.10.837. PMID: 29267484.

[22] Ngô, T. L. (2013). Review of the effects of mindfulness meditation on mental and physical health and its mechanisms of action. *Santé mentale au Québec*, 38(2), 19–34. French. https://doi.org/10.7202/1023988ar. PMID: 24719001.

[23] Lindberg, D. A. (2005). Integrative review of research related to meditation, spirituality, and the elderly. *Geriatric Nursing*, 26(6), 372–377. ISSN 0197–4572, https://doi.org/10.1016/j.gerinurse.2005.09.013

[24] Balducci, L. (2019). Geriatric oncology, spirituality, and palliative care. *Journal of Pain and Symptom Management*, 57(1), 171–175. https://doi.org/10.1016/j.jpainsymman.2018.05.009. Epub 2018 Jun 19. PMID: 29772281.

> I read the Bible every morning. After they get me dressed or when I'm able to dress myself, that's the first thing I do. After my breakfast I get the Bible and read the lesson and then I'm ready for the day and I feel like it's my strength. It gives me strength to do the things that I need to do.[25]

In contrast to the retired businessman who had lost meaning in his life, Rev. Dr. Dave deFreese shared the story of a local children's television program host in Omaha named Miss Jean. The television program taught children about religion and even after Miss Jean retired, she remained involved in the television programming. Though she was retired from her full-time career, she often said, "You never retire from your calling from God." Even toward the end of her life, Miss Jean had a reason to get out of bed in the morning – she had purpose and meaning because of her faith,[26] which contributed to her resilience.

In addition to supporting longevity, patients report that R/S increases their quality of life and helps them cope with adversity and illness.[27] A study of cancer patients found that positive religious coping mechanisms, including feeling God's presence and finding strength in religion, were associated with higher quality of life measures.[28] Another study found that quality of life associated with R/S extends to cancer survivors and even caregivers of those fighting cancer.[29]

According to Howard Friedman, professor of psychology at the University of California and co-author of the book, *The Longevity Project*, it is "the values drawn from religious tradition–such as respect, compassion, gratitude, charity, humility, harmony, meditation and preservation of health–that seem to predict longevity, not the dogma preached at the altar."[30] Though world religions teach different practices and have varying beliefs, there are often common threads and central tenants shared across religions. Most religions teach believers to have *hope*, and most religious followers place their confidence in their understanding of a "higher power's" promises, whether that's healing, safety, life beyond earth, justice, or any number of other hopes. During the COVID-19 pandemic, a study in Turkey found that elderly people with lower levels of spiritual well-being had higher levels of hopelessness,[31] which

[25] Manning, L. K., Leek, J. A., Radina, M. E (2012). Making sense of extreme longevity: Explorations into the spiritual lives of centenarians. *Journal of Religion, Spirituality and Aging*, 24(4), 345–359. https://doi.org/10.1080/15528030.2012.706737. Epub 2012 Sep 27. PMID: 23139646; PMCID: PMC3489187.

[26] See footnote 1.

[27] Fitchett, G. (2017). Recent progress in chaplaincy-related research. *Journal Pastoral Care and Counseling*, 71(3), 163–175. https://doi.org/10.1177/1542305017724811. PMID: 28893170.

[28] Tarakeshwar, N., Vanderwerker, L. C., Paulk, E., Pearce, M. J., Kasl, S. V., Prigerson, H. G. (2006). Religious coping is associated with the quality of life of patients with advanced cancer. *Journal of Palliative Medicine*, 9(3), 646–657.

[29] Peteet, J. R., Balboni, M. J. (2013). Spirituality and religion in oncology. *CA: A Cancer Journal for Clinicians*, 63(4), 280–289. https://doi.org/10.3322/caac.21187. Epub 2013 Apr 26. PMID: 23625473.

[30] Ducharme, J. (2018, Feb 15). You asked; Do religious people live longer? *Time* https://time.com/5159848/do-religious-people-live-longer/

[31] Durmuş, M., Öztürk, Z. (2022). The effect of COVID-19 outbreak on older adults' hopelessness, loneliness, and spiritual well-being in Turkey. *Journal of Religion and Health*, 61(1), 851–865. https://doi.org/10.1007/s10943-021-01494-1. Epub 2022 Jan 7. PMID: 34997453; PMCID: PMC8740876.

can have immense negative implications for their physical, mental, and emotional health. Many religions also strongly emphasize *forgiveness and reconciliation*, and since social ties are important for health while interpersonal stress is harmful, the ability to forgive and maintain positive relationships is important for healthy aging.[32]

Despite the varying practices and beliefs, health protection is common across major world religions[33] and it is important for clinicians to recognize the role R/S can play in a patient's health, regardless of their religious identity. To some providers, R/S and healthcare may appear to be unrelated, but their goals are often well-aligned. Caring for the sick and elderly has long been a value for many religious groups, and many of the first hospitals established in the United States were and still are faith-based groups.[34] Holistic health and well-being are often at the core of the practices and tenants of R/S; understanding the intersection of religion and health and supporting centenarians' spiritual well-being can have important implications for their health outcomes.

11.3 Blue Zones: Areas in the World Where People Live longer, Healthier Lives

Dan Buettner, a National Geographic Fellow, and author discovered locations in the world where people live the longest and enjoy the healthiest lives. He labeled these areas as Blue Zones. Nine factors were identified as contributing to their longevity, three are directly related to R/S. The centenarians interviewed in the Blue Zones all had a deep sense of purpose, placed a high priority on family relationships, and belonged to and were active in a faith-based community.[35]

One of the Blue Zones included the Japanese island of Okinawa which has one of the largest populations of centenarians in the world. Scientists observed these senior adults lived not only long lives, but healthy, active, and productive ones. The Okinawa Centenarian Study (OCS) is the world's longest, continuous study of more than 3000 centenarians.[36] Okinawans embrace a spirituality that gives a deep sense of purpose in their lives – "ikigai." Translated, "ikigai" means "why I wake up in the morning." It is an approach to life that finds meaning in daily activities, such as gardening, fishing, or weaving. They make each task a prayerful activity.

---

[32] Webster, N. J., Ajrouch, K. J., Antonucci, T. C. (2021) Towards positive aging: Links between forgiveness and health. *OBM Geriatrics*, 4(2). https://doi.org/10.21926/obm.geriatr.2002118. Epub 2020 May 12. PMID: 34296188; PMCID: PMC8293913.

[33] VanderWeele, T. J. (2017). Religion and health in Europe: Cultures, countries, context. *European Journal of Epidemiology,* 32(10), 857–861. https://doi.org/10.1007/s10654-017-0310-7. Epub 2017 Sep 7. PMID: 28884408; PMCID: PMC5681407.

[34] Cilliers, L., Retief, F. P. (2002). The evolution of the hospital from antiquity to the end of the Middle Ages. *Curationis*, 25(4), 60–66. https://doi.org/10.4102/curationis.v25i4.806. PMID: 14509111.

[35] https://www.bluezones.com/

[36] https://orcls.org/about/

Unlike most places of the world, Okinawa is a contemporary society in which women lead the mainstream religion. Some researchers speculate that the elderly women's active engagement in religious roles and communities may be an important factor in reducing their depression and associated rates of suicide. Rates of suicide for elderly Okinawan women have, for many years, been among the lowest in East Asia, a region known for high rates of suicide among older women.[37]

11.4 When R/S Gets Sick

While the empirical evidence regarding the positive aspects of R/S is extensive, it is also clear that some theological beliefs and practices are counterproductive to good health. Religious/Spiritual *toxicity* is defined here as religious or spiritual beliefs, practices and interventions that result in harmful rather than healing effects for the patient.

Case Study Larry was in his late forties when he was diagnosed with a malignancy behind his eye. His physicians recommended surgery, radiation and chemotherapy but the diagnosis was bleak. Larry's immediate reactions were disbelief and denial, and he focused his anger on his doctors. He turned to a faith healer for a miracle cure who assured Larry that he had been healed and said if he had an unwavering faith, he would make a complete recovery. As the cancer progressed, the pain intensified, it became evident there was no miraculous intervention. Depression set in and Larry returned to medical professionals for relief. He died only a few months after the original diagnosis. Desperate people often resort to desperate measures including toxic religious belief. In his denial and subsequent decisions, Larry did not receive the benefits of medical or spiritual interventions that might have given him more time and a higher quality of life.

11.5 Religious/Spiritual Struggles as a Predictor of Mortality

Patients who experience spiritual struggles or distress tend to have higher levels of mortality. Researchers have categorized religious/spiritual struggles into six groups.[38]

[37] Pritchard C, Baldwin, D.S. (2002) Elderly suicide rates in Asian and English-speaking countries. *Acta Psychiatrica Scandanavica*, 105(4):271–5. https://doi.org/10.1034/j.1600-0447.2002.1014.x. PMID: 11942931.

[38] Exline, J. J., Pargament, K. I., Grubbs, J. B., Yali, A. M. (2014). The Religious and spiritual struggles scale: Development and initial validation. *Psychology of Religion and Spirituality*, 6(3), 208–222.

1. Divine Struggles: The patients feel anger or disappointment with God as though God no longer loves them, has abandoned or is punishing them.
2. Demonic Struggles: The patients believe an external, evil force has attacked and/or is torturing them with illness.
3. Doubt-related Struggles: The patients are confused about their religious beliefs and feel guilty about theological doubts.
4. Moral Struggles: The patients feel guilt and shame resulting from a toxic belief that moral failure has contributed to their illness.
5. Ultimate Meaning Struggles: The patients struggle with whether their life has meaning or makes a difference.
6. Internal Personal Struggles: The patients may perceive or experience conflicts with others or institutions about issues that are sacred to them.

Some of these struggles are rooted in the theological teachings of the faith group. For example, some faith groups advocate a toxic belief referred to as "prosperity theology" that equates health, economic, and social status as evidence for their standing with the divine. If a person is healthy and wealthy, they are thought to be blessed by God. Being poor or ill then becomes a sign that the person is not living up to the expectations of the deity and is being punished or disciplined by the higher power.

Another example of toxic teachings emerged in the early stages of the HIV/AIDS epidemic. Some church leaders identified the disease as God's judgment against homosexuality which created anger, guilt and shame for both patients and their families. This toxic theology is still prevalent in many circles and continues to create stigmas that hinders public health from ending the HIV/AIDS epidemic.

11.6 Unhealthy R/S Intervention and Public Health

Though it was previously mentioned that social control can support individual health, unhealthy social control or religious community influences can also work against well-being. The growing reluctance to vaccines is often influenced by religious communities, though religious reasons behind vaccine hesitancy are varied and span different religions and sects.[39] During the COVID-19 outbreak, a group of Christians with extreme views, opposed public health restrictions and negated the necessity of public vaccination.[40] However, extremism is not the only reason for faith-based vaccine hesitancy. Timing is an important consideration for vaccinations among Muslims, as many Muslims believe vaccination should not be allowed

[39] Perry, S. L., Whitehead, A. L., Grubbs, J. B. (2020). Culture wars and COVID-19 conduct: Christian Nationalism, religiosity, and Americans' behavior during the Coronavirus pandemic. *Journal for the Scientific Study of Religion*, 59, 405–416. https://doi.org/10.1111/jssr.12677

[40] See footnote 39.

during the annual period of fasting called Ramadan.[41] In addition, many people of faith, including some Christians, Jews, and Muslims, believe that one's destiny is determined by God's will and that nothing should interfere with this divine providence.[42]

Fortunately, most religious groups are not in conflict with sound advice from public health authorities and see no theological or social ambiguities in following public health guidance. In fact, many see it as aligned with their mission to ensure their community has access to health promoting resources. Clear, direct communications with patients and enlisting the help of faith-based communities are critically important and effective in overcoming vaccine hesitancy[43] and other faith-based resistance to health measures.

11.7 Science, R/S and Holistic Healthcare

Religious groups built the first hospices to shelter migrants and pilgrims in the first century and by the fourth century, they were operating modern-type hospitals. In fact, infirmaries became an established part of every monastery.[44] In the era of Enlightenment, scientific and medical approaches made necessary advances to treat and cure disease. As medical approaches were appropriately prioritized, R/S was unfortunately sidelined, perhaps resulting in an overcorrection. Silos and a degree of animosity between the disciplines developed[45] and are often evident in both fields.

Today, some zealous religious leaders promote anti-science rhetoric and criticize public health,[46] and some healthcare professionals believe that religion and spirituality do not belong in healthcare facilities.[47] Nevertheless, many others in both fields acknowledge that these two helping professions need not be antithetical, and

---

[41] Peiffer-Smadja, N., Ouedraogo, R., D'Ortenzio, E., Cissé, P. N., Zeggani, Z., Beavogui, A. H., et al. (2017). Vaccination and blood sampling acceptability during Ramadan fasting month: A cross-sectional study in Conakry, Guinea. *Vaccine*, 35(25), 69–74. https://doi.org/10.1016/j.vaccine.2017.03.068

[42] Williams, J. T. B., O'Leary, S. T. (2019). Denver religious leaders' vaccine attitudes, practices, and congregational experiences. *Journal of Religion and Health*, 58(13), 56–67. https://doi.org/10.1007/s10943-019-00800-2

[43] Viskupič, F., Wiltse, D. (2022). The messenger matters: Religious leaders and overcoming COVID-19 vaccine hesitancy. *PS: Political Science & Politics, 55*(3), 504–509. https://doi.org/10.1017/S104909652200004X

[44] See footnote 34.

[45] See footnote 5.

[46] Brown, S. J. (2015, September 22). Are evangelicals anti-science? National Association of Evangelicals. https://www.nae.org/evangelicals-anti-science/

[47] Hummer, R. A. (2005). Commentary: Understanding religious involvement and mortality risk in the United States: Comment on Bagiella, Hong, and Sloan. *International Journal Epidemiology*, 34(2), 452–3. https://doi.org/10.1093/ije/dyi037. Epub 2005 Mar 3. PMID: 15746207.

certainly not hostile.[48] Sixty-eight percent of American adults see no conflict between their personal religious beliefs and science,[49] and *holistic* healthcare cannot be provided for many elderly patients without incorporating both medicine and R/S in a complete treatment plan.

Decades of research have identified that the oldest U.S. generations consistently practice R/S more frequently and value it more highly than those that follow.[50]

Exhibit 11.1

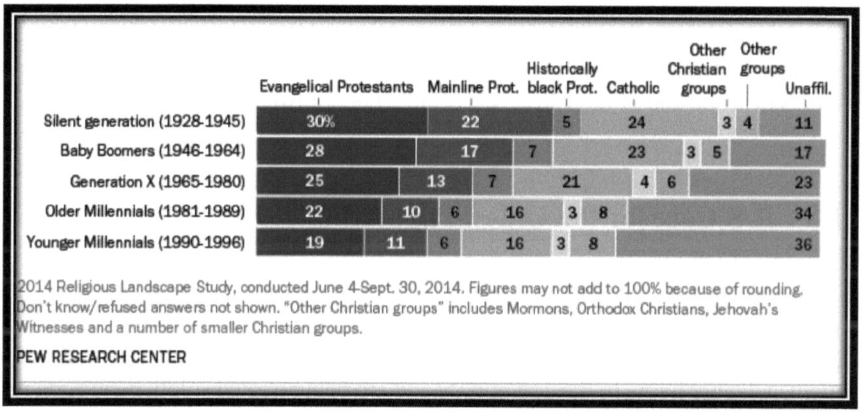

Exhibit 11.1 is from the Pew 2014 Religious Landscape Study and measures only *formal* religious participation. It does not indicate how individuals value spirituality in other forms. The exhibit identifies the faith groups most likely encountered in the patient population of U.S. healthcare facilities. While these faith group sizes may be useful to clinicians practicing in U.S. healthcare settings, no matter how small a minority faith group may be in the U.S., the *individual* patient's religious preference must be identified, respected and their R/S needs addressed.

Even as formal religious participation continues to decline, 81% of Americans *believe in God,* and among those 65 years and older, 87% find this belief important.[51] Yet a narrow understanding of the healing process, on the part of some providers, may marginalize R/S in the delivery of healthcare.

Vignette: Late one afternoon, a young professional chaplain was caring for an elderly, male patient in a teaching hospital. She had been referred to him by the

[48] Mason, G. (2022, October 31). Religion, science must join forces. *The Dallas Morning News.* https://www.dallasnews.com/opinion/commentary/2022/11/01/religion-and-science-must-come-together-to-fight-climate-challenges/

[49] https://www.pewresearch.org/science/2015/10/22/perception-of-conflict-between-science-and-religion/

[50] https://www.pewresearch.org/fact-tank/2015/05/12/millennials-increasingly-are-driving-growth-of-nones/

[51] https://news.gallup.com/poll/393737/belief-god-dips-new-low.aspx

supervisory nurse, as the patient had just received more bad news. Over 10 min into a solemn visit, a team of residents and student doctors charged into the room, interrupting the visit, with the question, "And who are you?" The head resident said, "You'll need to excuse yourself, Chaplain. We have some important work to do now."

The chaplain reentered the room when the procedure was complete, but the patient was sedated and barely lucid. At the patient's request, they prayed together and ended the visit. The patient died unexpectedly in the early morning hours of the next day.

All healthcare work is important. For patients who value R/S, it too should be honored at all times. There is value in mutual respect among all disciplines, and patients near the end of their lives, especially, benefit from this recognition.

11.8 R/S Care for the Oldest Population

In considering the best ways to provide R/S care for centenarians, the following discussion will focus on residential facilities, including assisted living, long-term care, rehabilitation, skilled nursing, hospice care, and hospitalization. Elderly patients who are living in the community and are being treated solely in physicians' offices, generally have other R/S resources available to them. R/S care in each setting mentioned above may need to take different forms and will require different levels of resources. For example, some long-term care facilities may need to provide a modified but regular worship service, whereas in some settings, patients might not be able to participate in group activities. All settings should find ways to integrate R/S in a meaningful way for patients who want this type of intervention. As mentioned above, the vast majority of gerontology patients have indicated this is a high priority for them.

11.8.1 R/S Guiding Documents

There are three documents that can support clinicians in understanding how to care for the R/S needs of seniors in residential care.

1. **The First Amendment to the U.S. Constitution** – This amendment allows those living in the U.S. to practice their chosen faith as they wish, and no one is allowed to impose any form of religion upon them. Given that residential healthcare treatment usually does not enable patients to travel to community religious resources, "free exercise" of religion must be honored and provided, as long as it is not contra-indicated in the treatment plan or disruptive to others in the facility. On the other hand, the first amendment also protects patients from the imposition

of religion. The priority must be given to the *patient's* R/S preferences and needs – not those of the visitor or provider. This includes well-meaning, local R/S representatives, and staff members who would proselytize, such as trying to sway the patient to their own religious position or belief system.

2. **The National Consensus Project (NCP) for Quality Palliative Care**, 4th Edition, **Domain 5: Spiritual, Religious and Existential Aspects of Care** – These guidelines recognize R/S as an essential part of holistic healthcare, stating "Spirituality is recognized as a fundamental aspect of compassionate, patient and family-centered palliative care. Palliative care interdisciplinary teams (IDT) serve each patient and family in a manner that respects their spiritual beliefs and practices. Teams are also respectful when patients and families decline to discuss their beliefs or accept spiritual support."[52]
3. **The Joint Commission (TJC) Standards of Care –** In Provision of Care, Treatment, and Services (PC). Element 1 for PC.02.02.13, this standard states, "To the extent possible, the hospital provides care and services that accommodate the patient's and his or her family's comfort, dignity, psychosocial, emotional, and spiritual end-of-life needs."[53] The (TJC) standard for Advanced Certification for Palliative Care states that the core palliative care team should include a chaplain with specialized training.[54]

As healthcare standards and guidelines, both of the latter two resources require spiritual *assessments,* though neither identifies which member of the interdisciplinary team (IDT) is qualified to create or select them. Some form of spiritual assessment is now suggested and encouraged (or required) by nursing, social work, and counseling professions,[55] and by 2012, nearly 90% of US medical schools had included R/S in their academic curriculum.[56] This attention among a variety of professionals highlights the important role that R/S plays in how patients respond spiritually to disease and to healthcare. While identifying the importance of R/S is a positive advancement, the roles and responsibilities among various disciplines have become unnecessarily confused,[57] given that there is no widely recognized and qualified provider responsible for this assessment.

---

[52] National Consensus Project for Quality Palliative Care. Clinical Practice Guidelines for Quality Palliative Care, 4th edition. Richmond, VA: National Coalition for Hospice and Palliative Care; 2018. http://www.nationalcoalitionhpc.org/ncp/

[53] Part-2.-Body-Mind-Spirit-JC-*The-Source*-Feb.2018-Vol.16.2. p.4.

[54] Joint Commission Resources. Palliative care certification manual 2015–2016, cited in Few Hospital Palliative Care Programs Meet National Staffing Recommendations Joanne Spetz, Nancy Dudley, Laura Trupin, Maggie Rogers, Diane E. Meier, and Tamara Dumanovsky Health Affairs 2016 35:9, 1690–1697.

[55] Nelson-Becker, H. (2018) Spirituality, Religion, and Aging: Illuminations for Therapeutic Practice. SAGE Publications, Inc.

[56] See footnote 5.

[57] de Diego-Cordero, R., Lopez-Gomez, L., Lucchetti, G., Badanta, B. (2022). Spiritual care in critically ill patients during COVID-19 pandemic. *Nursing Outlook*, 70(1), 6477. https://doi.org/10.1016/j.outlook.2021.06.017

Table 11.1 Collected and condensed NCP spiritual, religious and existential aspects of care

Guideline 5.1	Patient and family spiritual beliefs and practices are assessed and respected. Palliative care professionals acknowledge their own spirituality as part of their professional role and are provided with education and support to address each patient's and family's spirituality
Criteria	
5.1.1	The IDT has policies and processes in place to ensure spiritual care is respectful
5.1.2	Either directly, through referral, or in collaboration with the professional chaplain, the IDT facilitates spiritual cultural rituals or practices as desired by the patient and family
5.1.3	IDT members never impose their individual beliefs on others
5.1.4	Spiritual needs of families may differ from patients and are also recognized and supported
5.1.6	In all settings, the IDT includes professional chaplains who have evidence-based training to assess and address spiritual issues
5.1.7	The professional chaplain is the spiritual care specialist, conducting the assessment and addressing the spiritual aspects of the care plan
5.1.8	Professional chaplains develop community partnerships when needed/requested. Community representatives are supervised by a trained, professional chaplain who coordinates services
5.1.10	Led by the professional chaplain, opportunities are provided to engage staff in self-care and self-reflection regarding their own spirituality
5.1.11	Every member of the IDT is trained in spiritual care and recognizes the importance of the spiritual aspects of care
5.1.12	Members of the IDT receive training to cultivate openness to spirituality through empathetic listening
Guideline 5.2	The spiritual assessment process includes spiritual screening, spiritual history, and a full spiritual assessment
Criteria	
5.2.1	All aspects of screening, history, and assessment are conducted using standardized tools
5.2.2	Spiritual screening is completed as part of every clinical assessment to identify spiritual distress and the need for urgent referral to a professional chaplain
5.2.4	A spiritual assessment is triggered based on the results of the screening and history
Guidelines 5.3; 5.4	
5.3; 5.4	Guidelines for R/S treatment and ongoing care through transitions of patient health and/or care settings

Of the above resources, the NCP Guidelines are the most comprehensive in outlining what is expected and needed related to R/S in healthcare settings. The NCP identifies the explicit need for *chaplains* who have "evidence-based training to assess and address spiritual issues…" For a condensed reference from the NCP spiritual care guidelines, see Table 11.1.

The NCP guidelines also define the terms spiritual screening, spiritual history, spiritual assessment, spiritual distress, and professional chaplain. For reference, this chapter provides definitions for these terms, and others, in the Appendix.

11.8.2 Limitations of The Joint Commission R/S Standards

The Joint Commission (TJC) Standards have required spiritual assessments of patients since 2004 but have offered no guidance on who is best qualified to create, select or conduct them. This has likely created the confusion mentioned above, and the multiple disciplines which have developed R/S assessments for their own use.[58,59] As a result, there are some professionals in each discipline who want to be responsible for spiritual matters, while others do not. Holistic healthcare is an essential concept, but it becomes counterproductive when it centers on the turf of clinicians rather than the needs of patients.

There is some indication TJC (like NCP) is moving toward acknowledging spiritual *screening*, as well as the need for spiritual *assessments*,[60] which would be helpful for all IDT members. True assessments require significantly more time than screenings and consider the patient's R/S strengths, resources and distress. Spiritual assessments also require an evaluator who understands the theological implications of the patients' responses, and how they contribute to or conflict with the healthcare treatment plan.

Current TJC standards allow local management to determine who will be assigned to conduct these spiritual assessments, just as TJC allows management to decide the level to which disciplines will be staffed. Such management determinations are often based upon budgetary concerns and who can be assigned R/S as a *collateral* duty, rather than who is best trained and would provide the most competent care for these needs. Furthermore, assuming that R/S needs are identified in spiritual assessments, TJC does not require R/S providers or interventions to address these important patient needs.

In comparison, NCP is specific and direct, stating, "Specialist-level palliative care programs include salaried professional chaplains and related programmatic expenses."[61] NCP recognizes the need for professional chaplains and comprehensive, integrated R/S care.

11.9 How Spiritual Care Is Best Accomplished

Comprehensive R/S care (screenings, assessments, and interventions) requires teamwork, but not every clinician is best equipped to *assess and address spiritual needs*.

---

[58] Drury, C., Hunter, J. (2016). The hole in holistic patient care. *Open Journal of Nursing*, 6(Jan-Feb) 776–792. https://doi.org/10.4236/ojn.2016.69078

[59] See footnote 55.

[60] Part-1.-Body-Mind-Spirit-JC-*The-Source*-Feb.2018-Vol.16.1. p 6.

[61] https://www.nationalcoalitionhpc.org/ncp/ Clinical Practice Guidelines for Quality Palliative Care, 4th Edition, Domain 5: Spiritual, Religious, and Existential Aspects of Care; Clinical and Operational Implications.

11.9.1 *Who Should Not Be Required to Conduct Spiritual Assessments?*

Based upon first amendment rights, no staff member who is uncomfortable discussing R/S concepts should be assigned to perform this duty. During the height of the COVID-19 pandemic, many nurses were required to provide R/S care and were uncomfortable in this role.[62] Requiring this on a routine basis of a reluctant employee may result in less-than-optimal patient care and damage employee morale.

11.9.2 *Who Should Not Be Allowed to Conduct Spiritual Assessments?*

Again, the answer is based upon first amendment rights and respectful patient care. Those who feel compelled by their faith to convert or persuade patients to their religious belief system (proselytize) and those who are intolerant or less than respectful of other faiths or religion in general, should not be allowed to interact with patients for this purpose.

11.9.3 *The Best Option for Conducting R/S Assessments*

Many hospitals and palliative care programs employ professional chaplains who have the responsibility for R/S care. Professional chaplains are clinical specialists with the expertise to address the patient's complicated theological and spiritual distress and support their R/S strengths and coping. However, it is not necessary for a chaplain to conduct the *spiritual screening*. A spiritual screening tool is as simple as a few questions about religious preference, religious affiliation, and the patient's desire to see a chaplain. A screening checklist could include questions that trigger a chaplain referral and can be conducted by clinical or administrative staff. However the screening tool is best created with input from a chaplain.

Though professional chaplains are best suited to conduct spiritual assessments, some healthcare facilities do not employ chaplains and the responsibility for spiritual assessments is assigned to staff members who are untrained in R/S. They often request more training to assist them in this collateral duty, and while this request should be honored, a brief continuing education class in religious sensitivities does not substitute for theological and clinical pastoral education (CPE), nor does it prepare staff members as R/S professionals. Many staff members, eager to alleviate pain for patients and families, offer their own theological beliefs that actually create

[62] See footnote 57.

or amplify spiritual distress in patients and families. "It's all in God's will." "God wants you to fight this evil disease and be a testimony to his ability to heal." "God needed your loved one more than you did." While, such messages may be meaningful to the speaker, the patient and families may find these comments hurtful and toxic.

Effective spiritual assessments and follow-up spiritual interventions involve extensive time for which collateral duty assignments do not allow. Medical team members are subject to being called to an urgent physical need, interrupting a conversation that a patient or family may deem "sacred." Rushing R/S visits implies that the spiritual aspect of the patient is not important.

11.9.4 Professional and Board-Certified Chaplains

A professional chaplain has (1) graduate and post-graduate degrees from accredited theological institutions, (2) training in clinical pastoral education, (3) pastoral experience, and (4) a current letter of endorsement/support from a nationally recognized faith group. Upon meeting these requirements, one might qualify for board certification.

A seminary is graduate school for a minister working in any setting and though theological education differs among faith groups, there are many similarities. Most Protestant seminaries in the U.S. offer a Master of Divinity (M.Div.) as the standard degree. This is a *three-year post graduate degree.* The curriculum includes theology, philosophy, church history, pastoral care and counseling (akin to psychological counseling), the study of ancient traditions and texts, communication and preaching, education about non-Christian world religions, and often supervised pastoral experience. However, a seminary degree does not fully prepare the graduate to be a professional chaplain in a clinical setting.

Beyond the academic degrees, the designation of professional chaplain requires *Clinical Pastoral Education.* A professional chaplain has at least 2000 h of supervised training in a clinical setting conducted by a nationally recognized training organization, such as the Association for Clinical Pastoral Education (ACPE). In addition to this supervised clinical training, at least another year of work experience in a pastoral role is required for board certification.

Finally, a current letter of endorsement from a nationally recognized faith group must be obtained. Many of these faith groups have established processes and timelines that candidates must complete before a letter of endorsement from their faith group will be issued.

A professional chaplain must apply to be board certified. Board certification requires the four elements listed above and includes an additional screening process through a national organization, such as the Association of Professional Chaplains (APC), the National Association of VA Chaplains (NAVAC), the National Association of Catholic Chaplains (NACC) and the National Association of Jewish Chaplains (NAJC). These organizations have identified necessary competencies for chaplains and how they should be assessed. In addition to basic board certification, some of these organizations have developed advanced certifications in specialty areas, including palliative care.

Extensive qualifications for a professional chaplain are why the NCP states that,

> The chaplain is the spiritual care specialist on the interdisciplinary teams, and is trained to address spiritual and religious concerns of all patients and caregivers, regardless of their spiritual or religious beliefs and practices. The chaplain is also an emotional care generalist, and interfaces closely with the social worker and other mental health providers to provide psychosocial-spiritual care as a unified domain.[63]

11.10 Addressing Spiritual Distress

A holistic approach to patient care understands that patients who have physical or mental crises or challenges are also likely to have spiritual struggles. This is most easily identified in the nearly universal question, "Why is this happening (to me)?" This and many other conflicts are identified in the literature as spiritual distress, spiritual struggle, spiritual needs, spiritual pain or sometimes spiritual injury. One study of 203 religious patients with cancer found that 72% acknowledged having spiritual needs that went wholly or mostly unmet by the medical system.[64] In a clinical setting, examples of spiritual distress include a sense of guilt, doubting one's faith, feeling punished by or alienated from God and/or others, suffering, a sense of hopelessness or brokenness, fear, grief/bereavement, etc. As identified above, these struggles are theological in nature and patients often need someone who is professionally trained to assist them.

Such spiritual distress has been demonstrated to affect overall health, to include greater depression, lower physical functioning, lower life satisfaction, and more hospitalized nights.[65] Most significantly, R/S distress has been identified as a predictor for increased mortality among older medical patients, even after controlling for demographic, physical and mental health factors.[66]

---

[63] https://www.nationalcoalitionhpc.org/ncp/ Clinical Practice Guidelines for Quality Palliative Care, 4th Edition, Appendix I: Glossary.

[64] Balboni, T. A., Vanderwerder, L. C., Block, S. D., Paulk, M. E., Lathan, C. S., Peteet, J. R., Prigerson, H. G. (2007). Religiousness and spiritual support among advanced cancer patients and associations with end-of-life treatment preferences and quality of life. *Journal of Clinical Oncology*, 10; 25(5), 555–560.

[65] Park, C. L., Wortmann, J. H., Edmondson, D. (2011). Religious Struggle as a Predictor of Subsequent Mental and Physical Well-being in Advanced Heart Failure Patients. *Journal of Behavioral Medicine,* 34, 426–436.

[66] Park, C. L., Aldwin, C. M., Choun, S., Suresh, D. P., Bliss, D. (2016). Spiritual peace predicts 5-year mortality in congestive heart failure patients. *Health Psychology*, 35(3), 203–210.

11.11 Patients Say Their R/S Needs Are Important

Balboni has suggested that as physical health wanes, spiritual health may play an even more prominent role in determining patient well-being.[67] Park and associates found that congestive heart failure patients who reported high levels of religious behavior, support, and commitment exhibited higher levels of adherence to medical advice from their physicians.[68]

In a study with cancer patients, seven factors were ranked by patients in order of importance to their end-of-life (EoL) decision making process. Faith in God ranked only slightly behind patients' highest priority, the oncologist's treatment recommendations.[69] In another study of patients with advanced illness, out of nine attributes ranked in order of importance, being at peace with God ranked second, just marginally behind pain control.[70] A study of 191 patients with congestive heart failure found that a self-reported sense of *spiritual peace* was associated with reduced mortality risk by 20% after controlling for health status, health behaviors and demographics.[71] Later life and centenarian studies point to the many benefits of experiencing spiritual peace in later life, which improves mental and physical resilience, quality of life, and has been demonstrated to increase longevity.[72,73]

Many patients believe their R/S has sustained them significantly during adversities, which has been referred to as *spiritual resilience.*[74] Manning defines this as "the ability to sustain one's sense of self and purpose through a set of beliefs, principles or values while encountering adversity, stress and trauma by using internal and external spiritual resources."[75] Patients report that R/S coping contributes to their ongoing sense of physical, mental, and emotional well-being, and that ongoing spiritual growth and development, especially during advancing years, allows them to maintain hope. For example, patients have shared the following:

---

[67] See footnote 64.

[68] Park, C. L., Moehl, B., Fenster, J. R., Suresh, D. O., Bliss, D. (2008). Religiousness and Treatment Adherence in Congestive Heart Failure Patients. *Journal of Religion, Spirituality and Aging,* 20(4), 249–266.

[69] Silvestri, G. A., Knittig, S., Zoller, J. S., Nietert, P. J. (2003). Importance of Faith on Medical Decisions Regarding Cancer Care. *Journal of Clinical Oncology,* 21(7), 1379–82.

[70] Steinhauser, K. E., Christakis, N. A., Clipp, E. C., McNeilly, M., McIntyre, L., Tulsky, J. A. (2000). Factors considered important at the end of life by patients, family, physicians, and other care providers. *Journal of the American Medical Association,* 284(19), 2476–2482.

[71] See footnote 66.

[72] Manning, L., Ferris, M., Narvaez Rosario, C., Prues, M., Bouchard, L. (2019). Spiritual resilience: Understanding the protection and promotion of well-being in later life. *Journal of Religion Spirituality and Aging*, 31(2), 168–186.

[73] See footnote 25.

[74] Ramsey, J. L., Blieszner, R. (2012). Understanding spiritual resiliency and aging. In J. Hendricks (Ed.), *Spiritual resilience and aging: hope, relationality, and the creative self. Society and Aging Series,* (3–21). Routledge.

[75] See footnote 72.

> You learn that you got through that, and you can get through this. Keep praying, keep trusting that the Lord will work it out…the Lord has gotten you through that and He will get you through this.[76]

> My relationships embody compassion and empathy and justice. Those kinds of things are common elements to all great religions, and then there's the whole social side. I find that people in church, not just the ministers or priests, but also many of the people who attend church…are often caring…I have been supported by these people in my faith community and have depended on them over the years. I take comfort in knowing they are there.[77]

A survey of patients at the Mayo Clinic hospitals found that 70% of respondents wanted to see a chaplain at least once during their hospital stay. Over a third of those surveyed wanted the chaplain to visit every few days.[78] Especially those religious patients who may not have regular visits from family or their faith group community, chaplains offer social and spiritual support and can often speak in the patient's religious language.

Estimates are that the chaplain workforce is able to visit 20% (+/– 10%) of hospitalized patients.[79] While patients say that R/S is very important, they receive very little, if any support for it during inpatient healthcare treatment.

A 2016 survey of over 410 US palliative care programs identified funded chaplains in only 38% of them, most of which were approximately half-time positions. The most commonly reported unfunded positions were chaplains, which represented about 43% of the chaplain workforce in the palliative care programs surveyed.[80] These unfunded positions are "volunteer chaplains" who often do not have adequate training or experience to provide competent treatment.

11.12 Professional Chaplains' Contributions to Healthcare

When treated in an inpatient setting, patients may feel that the primary focus is on measurements, procedures and protocols. While those are essential to treatment and healing, chaplain interventions help to reaffirm patients' uniqueness, self-worth and ability to make informed but self-determined decisions.

---

[76] See footnote 72.

[77] See footnote 72.

[78] Piderman, K. M., Marek, D. V., Jenkins, S. M., Johnson, M. E., Buryska, J. F., Shanafelt, T. D., O'Bryan, F. G., Hansen, P. D., Howick, P. H., Durland, H. L., Lackore, K. A., Lovejoy, L. A., Mueller, P. S. (2010). Predicting patients' expectations of hospital chaplains: a multisite survey. *Mayo Clinic Proceedings,* 85(11), 1002–10. https://doi.org/10.4065/mcp.2010.0168. PMID: 21037043; PMCID: PMC2966363.

[79] Flannelly, K. J. Galek, K., Handzo, G. F. (2005). To what extent are the spiritual needs of hospital patients being met? *International Journal of Psychiatry in Medicine*, 35(3), 319–323. https://doi.org/10.2190/9X2X-QQEU-GDE9-VUXN. PMID: 16480247

[80] Spetz, J., Dudley, N., Trupin, L., Rogers, M., Meier, D. E., Dumanovsky, T. (2016). Few hospital palliative care programs meet national staffing recommendations. *Health Affairs (Millwood),* 35(9), 1690–1697. https://doi.org/10.1377/hlthaff.2016.0113. PMID: 27605652.

In the Mayo Clinic survey of over 1500 patients, reasons for wanting to see a chaplain were: "Remind me of God's care and presence" (78%), "Offer support to family and friends" (71%), "Be with me during times of particular anxiety or uncertainty" (69%), and "Pray and/or read scripture or sacred texts" (62%). Thirty-nine percent also ranked as important, "Counsel me regarding moral/ethical concerns or decisions."[81] These are interventions that professional chaplains are educated and trained to provide.

Chaplains assess, respect and provide or find ways to meet the religious and spiritual needs that patients and families identify as their own. Religious or spiritual *rituals*, such as prayer, reading sacred scriptures, serving communion, conducting baptisms, or reciting a declaration of faith (such as the Shahadah or Shema), play an important role in grounding patients and families in familiar, comforting and transcendent experiences. Some of these rituals, such as the Sacrament of the Sick (in the Catholic tradition), can only be performed by clergy. Many rituals are more meaningful when conducted by clergy, because for religious patients the chaplain may be viewed as a representative of God.

Chaplains are also trained to provide emotional support for people in crisis, which describes many patients in healthcare facilities. In addition to interventions such as empathetic listening, chaplains help patients and families in crisis find courage, strength and hope, and utilize their own belief and value system to make important healthcare, especially EoL decisions. Amy Greene, Director of Spiritual Care at the Cleveland Clinic says:

> Chaplains tend to be good in a crisis – if people are sad, upset, or angry/we have a high tolerance for those emotions…Chaplains help people find their own way back to courage…When everything goes wrong and they didn't get the outcome they wanted, patients and family members can still feel cared for.[82]

Chaplains can accept and "bless" tears and other emotional expressions that often make some clinicians uncomfortable. This is likely one reason nurses make the most referrals to chaplains.[83] Chaplains can sometimes attend to an overwrought and unruly family or patient and return a chaotic treatment area to a more tranquil setting for all.

White et al. have identified a number of spiritual interventions that counter distress and benefit health. They include allowing the patient to explore issues of guilt, forgiveness and reconciliation, clarifying values, meaning and purpose and reframing goals.[84] Through training and/or experience, many chaplains incorporate into their ministries the use of guided imagery, meditation, music, poetry and art, all of which can contribute to the patient's well-being, quality of life and sense of purpose. The chaplain's role in assisting patients and families who are making

---

[81] See footnote 78.

[82] See footnote 60.

[83] Fogg, S. L., Flannelly, K. J., Weaver, A. J., & Handzo, G. F. (2004). An analysis of referrals to chaplains in a community hospital in New York over a seven Year Period. *Journal of Pastoral Care and Counseling*, *58*(3), 225–235. https://doi.org/10.1177/154230500405800307

[84] See footnote 9.

choices about palliative care, hospice or EoL care is substantial. Balboni's research found that when patients facing EoL choices received spiritual care from a team that included chaplains, the patients had a higher quality of life at the end of life and were more likely to choose comfort care rather than aggressive care.[85] Likewise, more hospitalized patients chose home hospice in settings that included chaplains on the IDT.[86]

The largest body of research related to chaplain care has studied the relationship between chaplain visits and patient satisfaction. It demonstrates that chaplain care is associated with greater patient/family satisfaction, not just with spiritual care, but with their overall hospital experience.[87] In one study of 1440 patients in 14 US hospitals, patients stated that chaplain visits helped them recover quicker, ready themselves to return home, and cope with hospitalization easier. Many said the chaplain visits helped them find strength, the ability to cope, and feel more hopeful.[88] Johnson found that when patients died in ICU, families gave higher overall satisfaction ratings for ICU care when they and their patients had received care from qualified spiritual providers.[89]

Chaplains further contribute to multidisciplinary teamwork by helping to align the patient's treatment plan with the patient's self-identified goals and values, and communicating with team members the patient's spiritual resources, distress levels, and spiritual treatment plan. For these reasons, chaplains should be invited and expected in treatment team meetings. Chaplains also help multidisciplinary teams meet accreditation standards for spiritual care without adding collateral duties to other professionals.

Finally, for those staff members who wish to avail themselves of it, chaplains understand care for staff as an important part of their role. This requires the building of trusted relationships and demonstrated commitment to teamwork. Chaplains can help staff members who feel abused by patients and/or families, support staff members who experience a family crisis or transition, and offer pastoral/spiritual care during religious or spiritual struggles.

---

[85] Balboni, T. A., Paulk, M. E., Balboni, M. J., Phelps, A. C., Loggers, E.T., Wright, A. A., Block, S. D., Lewis, E. F., Peteet, J. R., Prigerson, H. G. (2010). Provision of spiritual care to patients with advanced cancer: associations with medical care and quality of life near death. *Journal of Clinical Oncology*, 20;28(3), 445–52. https://doi.org/10.1200/JCO.2009.24.8005. Epub 2009 Dec 14. PMID: 20008625; PMCID: PMC2815706.

[86] Flannelly, K. J., Emanuel, L. L., Handzo, G. F., et al. (2012). A national study of chaplaincy services and end-of-life outcomes. *BMC Palliative Care,* 11(10), 1–6. https://doi.org/10.1186/1472-684X-11-10

[87] See footnote 27.

[88] VanderCreek, L. (2004). How satisfied are patients with the ministry of chaplains? *Journal of Pastoral Care and Counseling*, 58(4), 335–342.

[89] Johnson, J. R., Engelberg, R. A., Nielsen, E. L., Kross, E. K., Smith, N. L., Hanada, J. C., Doll O'Mahoney, S. K., Curtis, J. R. (2014). The association of spiritual care providers' activities with family members' satisfaction with care after a death in the ICU*. *Critical Care Medicine*, 42(9), 1991–2000. https://doi.org/10.1097/CCM.0000000000000412. PMID: 24797373; PMCID: PMC4134753.

11.12.1 Reasons Not to Use Local Clergy (or Others) as Volunteer Chaplains

Utilizing volunteer chaplains, including local clergy, is a common practice used to keep facility costs to a minimum. Local clergy and volunteer chaplains come from a variety of faith groups and educational backgrounds. Some have little or no theological training, and most will have no experience providing pastoral care in a clinical setting, in contrast to professional chaplains. More than a few may be uncomfortable and feel out of place in a healthcare setting. Furthermore, local volunteers have difficulty knowing how to integrate their work into the overall treatment plan as NCP recommends, and should not participate in interdisciplinary team (IDT) meetings according to the Health Insurance Portability and Accountability Act (HIPAA).

Generally, those who wish to volunteer as chaplains either want to conduct worship services or visit patients indiscriminately at the bedside. Allowing such interventions by volunteers can be risky because there is little or no quality control of the volunteer's message (which might conflict with the patient's treatment plan), and they can also violate patient privacy. A patient's pastor or clergy person (from his/her faith group) should be encouraged to visit if the patient desires, but not clergy who are unknown to the patient, unless specific and prior patient consent has been given.

Balboni found that 42% of advanced cancer patients reported receiving little or no spiritual care from either the medical facility or their local religious community. A reasonable expectation would be that advanced cancer patients would need and receive the highest levels of spiritual care.[90]

11.12.2 Reluctance to Employ Professional Chaplains Could Be Costly

A facility is not prohibited from employing a high school or college graduate with no clinical or pastoral experience for a much lower salary than a professional chaplain. However, there are many ways this may be a very costly decision. Without a professional chaplain, the patient's religious objections to medical procedures and dietary requirements could be easily overlooked, creating anger and resentment on the part of the patient and/or family. A professional chaplain salary is minimal compared to the cost of a lawsuit.

Multiple studies have found that patients and individuals in the community support R/S integration in medical treatment,[91] and good public relations are essential

[90] See footnote 64.

[91] See footnote 64.

for hospitals. A news story about a patient who had his/her faith insulted and first amendment rights violated by a naïve, uneducated/untrained volunteer, or employee can cause negative publicity for the hospital and staff.

11.13 Recommendations for Clinicians to Improve the R/S Care of Their Oldest Patients in Treatment Facilities

1. Advocate for the inclusion of professional or board-certified chaplains on the healthcare team.
2. Advocate for the inclusion of a R/S screening, assessment, and referral process.
3. Refer to a professional chaplain when screenings indicate it would be helpful and when there is a significant change in health status. Other good referral triggers are: the patient is tearful or anxious, lacks family support, expresses excessive anger, families are struggling, etc.
4. Listen patiently and respectfully when patients want to talk about their R/S without imposing personal beliefs.
5. If a patient requests that you pray aloud with them and you feel comfortable in doing so, it may provide comfort and support. Do not do so unless you ask in advance what the patient wants to pray about, and unless you can genuinely join in that prayer. If not, refer to a chaplain.
6. Allow for religious expression without unnecessary constraints (i.e., ensure halal and kosher meal options are available, allow baptism by immersion unless there is an open wound or other contraindication, etc.).
7. Don't allow patients to be subjected to proselytizing (by anyone).
8. Don't assume that every patient is a member of the area's most predominate faith group. Respect the religious diversity of the patients and families you serve.
9. Invite and expect professional chaplains to attend team meetings. Seek their input.
10. Include professional chaplains in end-of-life discussions with patients and families.
11. Invite professional chaplains to provide R/S training for IDT when needed.
12. Remember that R/S care for staff by a professional chaplain is free and confidential, when desired.

11.14 From Clinician to Administrator: How to Improve R/S Care at the Organizational Level

1. Establish an institutional policy that ensures patients' free expression of religion and prohibits proselytizing of patients, families and staff.
2. Consider research findings concerning the health benefits of professional R/S care, and how professional chaplains help staff and institutions.

3. Recognize and weigh legal exposure and possible negative public relations associated with failure to provide professional R/S care.
4. Hire an adequate number of professional chaplains for the patients served.
5. Consider that one major, nation-wide healthcare network requires that professional chaplains conduct all spiritual assessments and provide spiritual interventions.[92]

11.15 Summary

Religion and Spirituality play a significant role in the well being of people around the world and are especially important to the elderly according to a plethora of studies. The literature supporting the connections between R/S and health continues to grow. Centenarians are among the most diligent in the practice of their faith including prayer, meditation, rituals, and participation in faith group communities. Centenarians with strong R/S ties are often healthier, more content and find meaning and purpose in life. Patients with R/S distress experience higher levels of depression, diminished physical functioning, longer hospital stays and have higher mortality rates than those who have a sense of spiritual peace. Assessments and interventions by clinically trained professional chaplains are therapeutic for patients, and provide essential support for families, staff, and healthcare organizations.

Comprehensive and holistic healthcare requires understanding the nature of humanity as well as the physical being. If a primary goal of gerontology is to avoid the patient's *expiration,* healthcare may need to give more attention and support to the patient's *inspiration*. Many elderly patients identify R/S as a critical and ongoing source of such inspiration, providing their lives with meaning, purpose, hope, peace and a connection with someone or something that transcends them.

Viktor Frankl, psychiatrist and holocaust survivor, observed his fellow prisoners in German prison camps and found that feelings of dehumanization, hopelessness and meaninglessness resulted in loss of health and eventually, death.[93] Frankl is also frequently quoted as saying, "Those who have a 'why' to live, can bear with almost any 'how'."[94]

While most U.S. centenarians have not experienced the suffering of a death camp, they have survived considerable pain and tremendous loss. For many of them, R/S is a primary source of coping, comfort and peace. This search for a sense of peace, amidst all the loss, is best described by this patient:

---

[92] Department of Veterans Affairs, Veterans Health Administration Directive 1111, Spiritual Care, July 21,2021.

[93] Frankl, V. E. (1959). *Man's search for meaning: An introduction to logotherapy.* Beacon Press.

[94] https://www.goodreads.com/quotes/315385-those-who-have-a-why-to-live-can-bear-with

> The key is having peace of mind. I would like to think [about] peace on earth, but there will never be peace on earth. Fortunately, though, you can have peace of mind even when there's no peace on earth.[95]

Acknowledgments Chaplain Jeni Cook, M.Div, D.Min. and Board Certified Chaplain, a retired federal healthcare chaplain who served at all levels of a national healthcare system for Chaplain Service; Caitlyn Gudmundsen, MPH and M.Div., Senior Program Officer, CDC Foundation, who has also served previous public health positions in other non-profit organizations, and Ray Furr, M.Div, APR, who has served many denominational and church leadership positions.

Multiple Choice Questions

1. How does religion and spirituality contribute to health and longevity in elderly patients?
   A. Increases social connections
   B. Reduces risky health behaviors
   C. Provides meaning that helps individuals cope with suffering, adversity and isolation.
   D. Helps individuals find and maintain hope and purpose in life.
   E. All of the above.
2. Why do inpatients need professional care for their R/S needs?
   A. Toxic R/S beliefs and practices are common and may complicate or impede the healing process.
   B. Most elderly patients say that R/S is important to them and should be included as part of their medical treatment.
   C. It's easy and cost effective to find local clergy to meet the R/S needs for any patient.
   D. Members of the IDT don't have time or adequate education to competently care for these deeply personal and theological needs.
   E. All of the above
   F. A, B, D
3. What benefits do professional chaplains provide to patients and families?
   A. Help align patients' personal goals with their overall treatment plan.
   B. Provide emotional and spiritual support during crises, especially during end-of-life care.

[95] Cherry, K. E., Marks, L. D., Benedetto, T., Sullivan, M. C., Barker, A. (2013). for the Louisiana Healthy Aging Study. Perceptions of longevity and successful aging in very old adults. *Journal of Religion, Spirituality and Aging,* 25(4). https://doi.org/10.1080/15528030.2013.765368. PMID: 24353480; PMCID: PMC3864892.

C. Provide rituals of comfort and meaning such as prayer, worship services, communion, etc.
D. Address issues of spiritual distress and help patients recognize and utilize spiritual resources in the healing process.
E. Assist patients and families in understanding and coping with their medical status and treatment.
F. All of the above.

Answers: 1. E, 2. F, 3. F.

Appendix

Glossary of Terms

Interdisciplinary Team (IDT)

In the interdisciplinary model, each team member possesses unique expertise and skills. Team members from various disciplines are in close and frequent communication and collaborate with information and ideas about the patient's care. Leadership of team activities is determined by the situation and the area of expertise required. Professional chaplains should be part of the interdisciplinary team which include physicians, nurses, social workers, dietitians, sometimes therapists, and depending upon diagnosis mental health professionals.

Professional Chaplain

The professional chaplain holds a Master of Divinity Degree (or the equivalent), has successfully completed at least 2000 h of supervised clinical pastoral education and has been endorsed by their faith group to minister in a healthcare setting. The professional chaplain participates on the interdisciplinary team as the spiritual care specialist, with the expertise to address spiritual and religious needs of patients and families, regardless of the particular faith group, beliefs and practices. Professional chaplains work closely with the social workers and other mental health providers to deliver psychosocial-spiritual care.

Board Certified Chaplain

In addition to the Master of Divinity degree (or equivalency), the 2000 h of clinical pastoral education, and faith group endorsement, a board-certified chaplain has undergone a peer-review process to be board certified. This process begins with certification as a healthcare chaplain, however, certified chaplains can also obtain specialized certifications, such as in palliative care.

Religion

Religion is an organized set of beliefs, practices, rituals and moral codes aimed at connecting oneself and the community with each other and the sacred or divine. Religion may be practiced within a community or in private. A person can practice and express their spirituality through their religious preference.

Spirituality

Spirituality refers to an individual's search for a higher meaning or purpose beyond oneself. It involves an effort to transcend biological surroundings, connect with the divine, and live in harmony with one's environment. Spirituality can be expressed in ways not usually defined as religious, such as music, art, literature, caring for others or nature, etc.

Spiritual Assessment

A spiritual assessment requires an extensive, open-ended conversation, involving active listening to what the patient identifies as important life events, transitions in his/her life, and how those are understood by the patient. A spiritual assessment should be conducted by a professional chaplain who has the training to listen for theological and spiritual themes, spiritual resources, and spiritual distress. As an outcome of this patient visit, the professional chaplain summarizes the patient's religious/spiritual needs and resources and how they may affect the overall treatment plan. The professional chaplain formulates a *spiritual* care plan of treatment to pursue, with expected outcomes.

Spiritual Distress

Spiritual Distress is a disturbance in the person's religious/spiritual belief system that interferes with the overall health and well-being of the patient. It often develops as a result of some form of suffering, interpersonal conflict, or dissonance between what one believes and what he/she thinks they *should* believe. People experiencing spiritual distress often lose a sense of peace, purpose and connections to others who give their lives meaning. Those experiencing spiritual distress have higher risk levels for morbidity.

Spiritual History

A spiritual history is usually conducted as part of a comprehensive medical examination by the physician (usually in a medical office) to understand how spiritual issues may impact the patient's overall care. The clinician may include this spiritual history as a potential resource in the patient's treatment plan, and to help guide them when making referrals. The spiritual history questions delve deeper in understanding the patient's life goals, hopes and resources than does a spiritual screening. Clinicians conducting a spiritual history should have some education/training for the process, comfort with issues that might arise, and the ability to engage patients in such discussions.

Spiritual Screening

A spiritual screening is conducted at intake in a healthcare facility and can be assigned to a variety of employees. The screening should quickly determine important religious/spiritual data about the patient and/or family. The spiritual screening uses a few simple questions that help all team members identify potential patient and family needs. Most spiritual screenings ask about the patient/family religious preference, whether they belong to a faith group organization, how important religion or spirituality is to them, and whether they have any religious or spiritual needs/concerns at intake. This process screens for the need to promptly refer the patient to a professional chaplain.

Chapter 12
Whole Health, Wellness and Longevity

Mary Gallagher-Seaman

Key Take Away Points

1. Whole health in centenarians encompasses the physical, mental, spiritual and social well-being and includes maintaining a healthy diet, regular exercise, proper management of chronic health conditions, social connections, cognitive stimulation, emotional support, community engagement, and support networks.
2. Community engagement and support networks appear to play a crucial role in promoting a sense of purpose and fulfillment in centenarians.
3. The environment plays a critical role in promoting healthy aging for centenarians, as it can provide access to resources such as nutritious food, opportunities for physical activity, and social connections, as well as a sense of safety and security, which can all contribute to their overall well-being.

Illustrative Vignette

Jim was a Korean War Veteran, 102 years of age, lived in an accessory dwelling unit next to his 74-year-old daughter's home. Jim has a medical history that includes PTSD, arthritis, congestive heart failure (well managed as evidenced by no hospitalization in 7 years), hearing loss and hypertension (recently elevated). Jim was in conflict with his daughter about her safety concerns of his living situation (not allowing assistance) and his blood pressure was found elevated at his last routine visit. Jim expressed anxiety that "they're going to put me in a home if I don't do what they want". Jim used the local VA for his healthcare and participated in a Whole Health visit with his Primary Care Geriatric team to co-create a plan of care.

M. Gallagher-Seaman (✉)
Veterans Health Administration, Office of Patient Centered Care & Cultural Transformation, Washington, DC, USA
e-mail: mary.gallagher-seaman@va.gov

R. E. Kheirbek, M. D. Llorente (eds.), *Current Perspectives on Centenarians*, International Perspectives on Aging 36,
https://doi.org/10.1007/978-3-031-30915-1_12

Despite his advanced age and medical conditions, Jim was still active and engaged in the community. He attended church regularly. Jim was cognitively intact and used to play cards with "the guys" he had come to know from the local Veterans of Foreign War (VFW) hall of which he had been member of for more than 50 years. He is unable to get to the VFW mid-week and his apartment is not "in shape" to have visitors.

His whole health visit at the local VA began with a review of the Circle of Health, during which Jim shared his mission, aspiration, and purpose (MAP). His faith and family were core values. Jim reported that he experienced joy when spending time with his grown children, grand and great grandchildren. His long held religious practices and beliefs mattered greatly to him, as did his desire to attend weekly church services. During the pandemic, he had attended services virtually with the technologic support of his grandson.

By focusing on his MAP and using the Circle of Health as a self-inventory tool to look at where Jim was now and where he wanted to be, in each of the 8 areas of self-care, medical and CIH approaches to care, the team and Jim with his daughter started planning over the next 2 visits.

During the visit the team used coaching techniques to assist Jim in planning around his MAP: Maintain spiritual practices, engage with family, live independently, and maintain social connections by playing cards while managing his medical conditions. Jim adamantly wanted to continue to live in his home. His daughter, who also attended the visits, shared that she had concerns about his ability to clean and eat well. In the past, there had been some challenges with Jim accepting assistance. Jim shared that he didn't want to burden his family. After discussion with all parties and focus on Jim's MAP, Jim agreed to accept assistance with meal prep and housekeeping. The impact on Jim's physical health was seen in a decrease of his blood pressure, likely due to decreasing prepared and convenience foods that Jim had been consuming previously. Mapping care to Jim's MAP turned the conversation from "should do" to "helping Jim align with his MAP' and allow change.

Jim was able to play cards with his "guys" at his home, newly "company ready" thanks to Jim's willingness to allow weekly housekeeper services. Jim kept attending church in person, and virtually as needed) with a rotating group of family members who created a weekly routine that included post-service breakfast at a local restaurant. This increase in social contact was an added benefit to Jim.

As a result of this family's commitment to whole health, Jim was able to continue to enjoy his favorite activities, seeing family, attending church, and playing cards with his friends. He also found that his mood and overall well-being had improved significantly.

Jim's story is a testament to the importance of whole health in aging, and the role that families can play in supporting their loved ones through the VA healthcare system. By recognizing the interconnectedness of all aspects of health and actively working to address them, Jim and his family were able to help him live a fulfilling and satisfying life beyond his 102 years.

Jim's example also serves as an inspiration for other veterans and their families to prioritize their health and well-being, and to take an active role in their care, even at an advanced age.

12.1 Introduction

The United Nations Decade of Healthy Aging (2021–2030) global collaborative noted that in the span from 2019–2030, the number of persons aged 60 years or over is projected to grow by 38% worldwide, from 1 to 1.4 billion (World Health Organization, 2019). This increase will be greatest and most rapid in the developing world. While this "silver tsunami" will have impacts on many levels, the personal impact is likely to reverberate strongly in the healthcare arena.

The factors that can contribute to successful aging are complex. Physiologic issues such as aches and pains of osteoarthritis, often plague many older adults. Socio-economics issues of living on an income that may or may not grow at a rate that keeps pace with changing economic needs is also a concern for many seniors. There are additional psychological considerations, which can manifest as loneliness as similar-aged friends, family and partners die and/or other family members move into busier periods of their own lives. As Mae West (and sometimes Anthony Hopkins) is credited with saying 'getting old isn't for the faint of heart".

While successful aging can be challenging at times, we understand that all lives end at some time. Many of us spend considerable time planning for when we are no longer alive by creating wills, financial planning, making final arrangements. While this type of planning can be a gift to those left behind, time spent planning for our wellness, at more than a perfunctory level is often overlooked.

12.1.1 Successful Aging and Centenarians

Studies have shown that longevity is only partly influenced by genetics. Much greater contributions occur from lifestyle factors, such as physical activity, dietary and other lifestyle choices, management of physical and mental health, and life satisfaction. (Hao et al., 2019). A related concept is that of having a purpose in life, the sense that one's life has meaning and that one has a clear sense of direction in one's life. Purpose in life has been associated with lower mortality, and reduced risk of disease, disability and cognitive impairment. (Marone et al., 2020; Cohen et al., 2016; Musich et al., 2018)

Many factors may contribute to successful aging in centenarians, many of which have yet to be studied adequately or identified as core elements (Borras et al., 2020). Additionally, simply living a long time is not synonymous with successful aging. In addition to the factors noted above, social connectedness, emotional support, community engagement and support networks, and cognitive stimulation have all been identified as key factors in aging successfully. Living with family or friends, personal optimism, less disease/chronic illness, and access to social activities, (Cheung & Lau, 2015) strong connection to religious beliefs, (Archer et al., 2005) and emotional vitality (Araújo et al., 2016) were also associated with successful aging. Aspects of one's personality such as low scores on neuroticism and high scores on extraversion, openness to experience, agreeableness, and conscientiousness are also components of successful aging (Baek et al., 2016).

Given the magnitude of factors, some within one's control and others outside their control, how does one plan for a rich and vivid lifespan? One such model is that of Whole Health, a holistic approach to care being delivered in the United States Veterans Health Administration (VHA), which addresses both self-care and clinical care, while acknowledging the role of community and social determinants of health, which can provide a path to enjoying a long health span, which this chapter will review.

12.1.2 Planning for Successful Aging: The VA Whole Health Model

Whole Health is an approach to healthcare that empowers and equips people to take charge of their health and well-being and to live their life to the fullest (Kligler et al., 2022). Whole Health acknowledges that the patient is an expert on themselves and what matters most to them, while clinicians are the experts on health, disease and treatment.

The goal of VA's Whole Health approach starts with understanding the person's life mission, aspiration, and purpose (MAP), often described as "what matters most to you" and providing care to improve overall health and well-being (US Dept of Veterans Affairs, 2022). The Whole Health approach begins with connecting care and self-care to one's MAP. This link to MAP has been shown to have a positive impact on overall well-being. Blue Zones are identified geographic areas where large clusters of centenarians reside. In the Blue Zone studies, knowing one's sense of purpose in life was associated with up to 7 years of extra life expectancy (Buettner & Skemp, 2016).

To illustrate the application of the Whole Health initiative towards improved healthcare outcomes, we turn to the management of chronic pain, one of the most challenging clinical situations routinely encountered in health care. Reducing opioid use, while effectively managing chronic pain, is often a very difficult balance and the subject of much discussion in the literature over the past decade (Roth et al., 2020). VHA's Whole Health approach, which includes complimentary and integrative health practices, was employed with patients who were experiencing chronic pain. The outcomes of a 2022 study of Whole Health in VHA indicated that opioid use decreased 23% (31.5–6.5) to 38% (60.3–14.4) among Veterans using a Whole Health approach, (depending on level of Whole Health use), compared to an 11%

(12.0–9.9) decrease among Veterans using traditional care (Bokhour et al., 2022). Whole Health users reported greater improvements in perceptions of care (SMD = 0.138), engagement in health care (SMD = 0.118) and self-care (SMD = 0.1), life meaning and purpose (SMD = 0.152), pain (SMD = 0.025), and perceived stress (SMD = 0.191) when compared to Veterans using a traditional care.

The Whole Health approach puts the patient at the center of their care and empowers and equips them to engage in their well-being and starts with MAP. A 2019 non-VA research study of 6985 older adults and their partners indicated that stronger purpose in life was associated with decreased mortality (Alimujiang et al., 2019) Kim et al. in 2013 studied more than 6000 American adults over age 50 and found that greater purpose in life is correlated with a lower risk of stroke (Kim et al., 2013). This correlates to the findings in the Blue Zone findings of centurions.

Mission, Aspiration & Purpose Discovering one's MAP begins with mindful awareness of what matters most. Our values are unique to each of us guide and act as a compass to provide direction to where we find meaning and purpose. Our values guide our daily decisions. Every decision we make is an opportunity to live, moment by moment, according to our values. Ultimately the choices we make influence our self-care, such as choices about what food and drink we consume, our relationships with our family, friends and co-workers, and the movement we provide our body and how we recharge ourselves. Those choices we make, informed by our values, impact our well-being, satisfaction with the quality of our lives and our health span (US Dept of Veterans Affairs, 2022). Values can shift over time, as life events begin and end. A review of MAP is helpful periodically throughout one's lifetime.

Life span is the number of how many days/years one lives; health span is the number of days/years one is living life with well-being. Having a long life span can include long years of pain and suffering or loss of independence due to disease. A long health span, which includes years of vitality, social engagement and high satisfaction quality of life, is the true goal of life. Many of one's daily self-care choices impact health span and are outside medical care, such as our movement, food choices, sleep patterns and connection to others. Aligning one's values, or their MAP to one's self-care goals and actions can have a powerful impact on improving health span.

The Circle of Health The Circle of Health was developed by the VHA as a tool to guide self-exploration of one's values and self-care choices.

The Circle of Health (Fig. 12.1) starts in the center with "me", the user. With mindful awareness, there is exploration and recognition of one's values and MAP. The "me" includes consideration of the unique social determinants of health that impact one's well-being. One's MAP can be used outside of clinical care to independently set health goals aimed at improving health span or incorporated into medical care by clinicians co-creating goals and plans of with patients.

A simple inquiry using "the big questions", is most often enough to begin exploration of one's MAP. The "big questions" include:

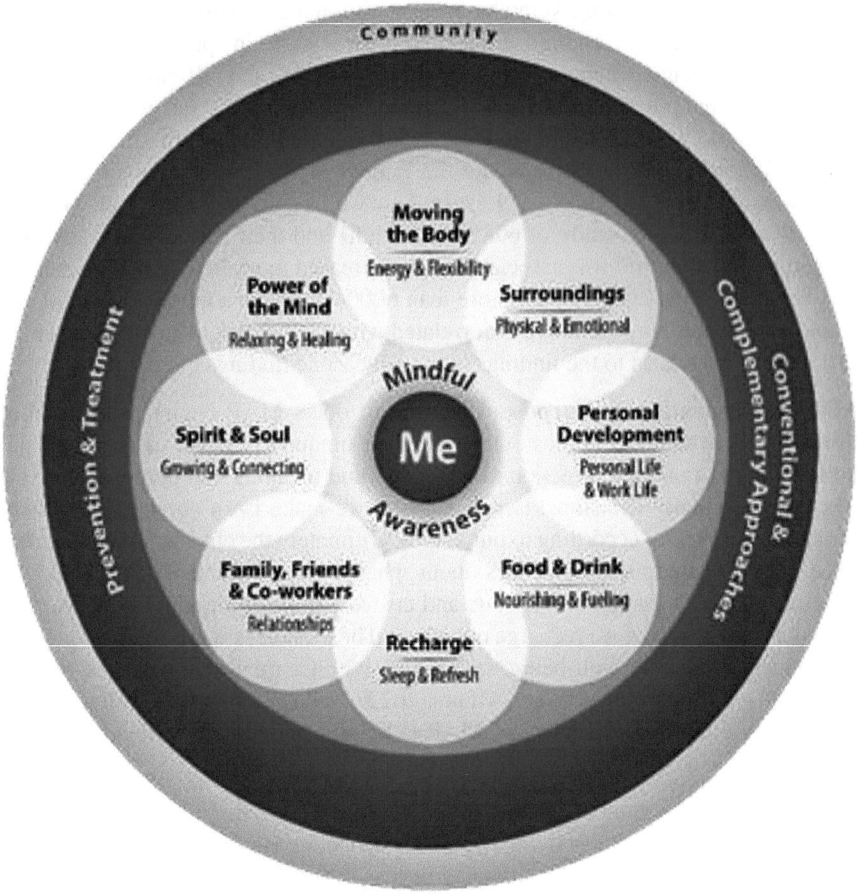

Fig. 12.1 Circle of Health (Source: The Circle of Health - Whole Health (va.gov))

- What do you live for?
- What matters most to you?
- What brings you a sense of joy or happiness?[1]

Identifying MAP is more than a quick thought: the power of the Whole Health approach comes from uncovering one's values and MAP via self-exploration.

There are eight areas of self-care in the green area of the Circle of Health (Figure One). One reflects on the current state and the desired state for each area. The areas of self-care are described in depth in the Personal Health Inventory (PHI), developed in VHA, which offers a structured deeper dive through the Circle of Health (US Dept of Veterans Affairs, 2022). There is a rating system in the PHI used to indicate where one is now and what is desired. This allows for a quick view of

[1] PHI-long-May22-fillable-508.pdf (va.gov) Page 3.

strengths and opportunities for consideration of goal setting, as well as progress over time.

The eight self-care areas are graphically represented as overlapping to acknowledge the interconnectedness of the areas. For example, moving the body impacts rest and sleep. If movement is limited, sleep can be more challenging. Moving the body can impact family, friends and co-workers' area as well. If one isn't able to participate in movement based activities there can be challenges to connection to those who matter. The overlap and potential impact vary by individual and will be explored while using the Circle.

The PHI offers the following explanation of each area of the Circle of Health below. Additional alignments from other sources specific to older adults are included (Haslam et al., 2015; Buettner & Skemp, 2016).

- Moving the Body "*Energy and Flexibility*"
  Our physical, mental, and emotional health are impacted by the amount and type of movement we do. Activity gives you energy and strength and is also good for your mind. Movement can promote flexibility. Regular activity can help with many issues affecting one's health, for example it can help lower blood pressure and cholesterol and reduce the risk for heart disease. Movement is available at every stage of life and level of ability. Examples of activity and movement include walking, gardening, dancing, chair yoga, or lifting weights.

- Surroundings "*Physical and Emotional*"
  Surroundings include where we live, work, learn, play, and worship—both indoors and out. Safe, stable, and comfortable surroundings have a positive effect on our health, particularly as you age. Aging can require, and be supported by, additions and revisions to your environment that support safety and ease of movement: chair lifts, raised seating, removal of small rugs, grab bars, etc. Your environment can affect your health. You may have issues with safety, or things like clutter, noise, bad smells, poor lighting, or water quality. You may be able to change some of these factors, but you may not be able to change them all. It starts with paying attention to the influences of your environment on your life and health. Improve what you can for a safe, comfortable, and healthy space.

- Personal Development "*Personal Life and Work Life*"
  Our health is impacted by how we spend our time. We feel best when we can do things that really matter to us or bring us joy. How do you spend your time and energy during the day? Do things give you energy or make you tired? Do you spend time doing what matters most to you? How do you feel about your finances and how are they affecting your life? These factors affect not only your happiness, but also your health.

- Food and Drink "*Nourishing and Fueling*"
  What we eat and drink can have a huge effect on how we experience life, both physically and mentally. Choose healthy eating habits that fit your lifestyle. A healthy diet can help prevent disease and promote healing, especially from chronic conditions such as arthritis, heart disease, diabetes, and depression. Learn which

foods and drinks support your health and life goals. Keep your body and mind properly fueled and hydrated. One of the shared characteristics of the Blue Zones, geographic regions that are home to some of the world's oldest people. is semi-vegetarianism – the majority of food consumed is derived from plants and consumption of legumes (Buettner, 2022)

- Recharge "*Sleep and Refresh*"

Our bodies and minds need rest in order to optimize our health. Recharging also involves activities that replenish your mental and physical energy.

- Family, Friends, and Co-workers "*Relationships*"

Our relationships, including those with pets, have as significant an effect on our physical and emotional health as any other factor associated with well-being. Feeling alone can sometimes make you get sick or keep you sick. Positive social relationships are healthy. Healthy relationships with a life partner, friends, neighbors, or co-workers can be a source of strength. Studies have shown that social connectedness is particularly important for the life expectancy of people aged over 70 years. Those with the lowest social network index scores had a 50% greater risk of mortality than those with the highest scores (Haslam et al., 2015). Blue zone inhabitants had common lifestyle characteristics including being socially active and integrated into their communities as well as a "family first" approach (Buettner & Skemp, 2016).

- Spirit and Soul "*Growing and Connecting*"

Connecting with something greater than ourselves may provide a sense of meaning and purpose, peace, or comfort. Spiritual connection can take many forms. When things are hard, where do you turn for strength and comfort? Some people turn to spiritual or religious faith. Some people find comfort in nature. Some connect with art, music or prefer quiet time alone. Some want to help others. You may express this as a guide to living fully. Blue zone findings showed that attending faith-based services, of any denomination, 4 times per month can add 4–14 years of life expectancy (Buettner & Skemp, 2016)

- Power of the Mind "*Relaxing and Healing*"

Our thoughts are powerful and can affect our physical, mental, and emotional health. Changing our mindset can aid in healing and coping. Your mind can affect your body. Sometimes when you think about stressful things, your heart rate and blood pressure go up (without you even recognizing it). You can use the power of your mind to lower blood pressure or control pain. Mind-body practices tap into the power of the mind to heal and cope and can help us advance what we want most in life (US Dept of Veterans Affairs, 2022).

Once an individual's MAP has been self-identified, self-care goals can begin. To further the Whole Health approach, MAP can be taken into a clinical encounter. The patient brings their expertise on their MAP and the clinician brings their expertise on health, disease and treatment. Together they co-create a plan to support the patient's well-being. Both patient and clinician will have action steps.

The clinician's action steps may include prescribing medication, lifestyle guidance and additional supports such as referrals to physical therapists, further medical/surgical consultation, or possibly mental health services to address the patient's needs. Self-care steps can include exercise, dietary changes, or complimentary and integrative health (CIH) modalities focused on well-being.

Next in the Circle of Health is the dark blue area. This allows reflection on where one is with traditional, as well as complimentary and integrative health approaches, of well-being. The next outer light blue circle represents the power of community all of which are inclusive of the social determinants of health.

Complimentary and integrative health (CIH) modalities can be therapeutic as well as solely well-being focused. Yoga is used as a therapeutic, evidence-based approaches for low back pain (Park et al., 2020) Yoga can be used for effective management of the pain of knee osteoarthritis (Wang et al., 2018) Yoga is used as a fall prevention strategy in older adults, particularly those living in a community setting (Youkhana et al., 2016; Tiedemann et al., 2013). This same CIH approach, yoga, can also be used stress reduction or as a gentle exercise program to provide support for the physical and/or emotional strains of aging (Tulloch et al., 2018; Madhivanan et al., 2021). Other CIH approaches that offer benefits as well. Acupuncture, yoga, tai chi/qi gong, massage, meditation, guided imagery, clinical hypnosis and biofeedback are in use well-being (meditation, guided imagery, tai chi/qi gong, yoga) and as treatment approaches (acupuncture, biofeedback, clinical hypnosis, massage) within VHA (Farmer et al., 2021; Elwy & Taylor, 2020). CIH approaches use in older adults has a wide body of evidence regarding efficacy (NIH, 2019). Aligning MAP to action/care planning is a powerful step that can improve quality of life for older adults. It empowers one to take charge of one's health and to take steps to facilitate a longer health span.

Components of the whole health approach can also be found in several cultures. *Ikigai* is a Japanese concept that refers to the sense of purpose or meaning in one's life. It is often associated with Okinawans in the Blue Zones. The concept of *ikigai* is believed to play a significant role in the longevity of these individuals. *Ikigai* is rooted in the idea that everyone has a unique purpose or passion in life, and that finding and pursuing this purpose can lead to greater happiness and well-being. For many of the centenarians living in the Blue Zones, their *ikigai* is deeply connected to their community and cultural practices. For example, the Okinawans have a strong sense of community and a deep connection to their traditional culture, which provides them with a sense of purpose and belonging. Many of them find their *ikigai* in their daily activities such as gardening, socializing with friends, and participating in traditional cultural practices. Additionally, research suggests that having a sense of purpose in life is associated with lower levels of stress, better mental and physical health, and reduced risk of cognitive decline. People who have a strong sense of *ikigai* tend to have a more positive outlook on life and are more likely to engage in healthy behaviors such as regular physical activity, healthy eating, and social engagement.

It's important to note that the concept of *ikigai* is not limited to the Blue Zones and can be applied to people of all ages and cultures. Finding one's *ikigai* can be a lifelong journey, and it can change and evolve over time. It's not only about having a job or a career but also about having a sense of purpose in everyday life, such as caring for loved ones, volunteering, or pursuing a hobby.

12.2 Conclusion

The Whole Health approach and such cultural concepts as *ikigai,* play a significant role in promoting not only longevity but also well-being. By understanding those approaches to health we can gain insight into how to promote healthy aging and longevity for people of all ages and cultures.

Additional Resources (Readings, Media, Etc.)

- https://www.bluezones.com/the-purpose-checkup-2/
- https://www.va.gov/wholehealth/
- https://www.va.gov/WHOLEHEALTH/professional-resources/clinician-tools/Evidence-Based-Research.asp
- https://www.va.gov/wholehealthlibrary/
- https://www.va.gov/WHOLEHEALTHLIBRARY/self-care/index.asp
- https://www.va.gov/WHOLEHEALTH/veteran-handouts/index.asp
- https://blogs.va.gov/VAntage/71858/whole-health-approach-centers-around-matters-you/
- https://www.wholehealth.org/
- https://www.youtube.com/watch?v=fgNzmQBGehU
- https://www.va.gov/WHOLEHEALTH/phi.asp
- https://www.va.gov/WHOLEHEALTH/docs/PHP-WalletCard-May22-fillable-508.pdf
- https://www.va.gov/WHOLEHEALTH/docs/Live-Whole-Health-App-Fact-Sheet-508_Nov2020.pdf
- https://mobile.va.gov/app/mindfulness-coach
- https://www.va.gov/WHOLEHEALTHLIBRARY/tools/index.asp
- https://www.va.gov/WHOLEHEALTHLIBRARY/docs/Values.pdf
- https://wheelofhealth.dukehealth.org/
- United Nations, Resolution. Dec 2020. https://documents-dds-ny.un.org/doc/UNDOC/GEN/N20/363/87/PDF/N2036387.pdf?OpenElement Yoga also ha

Multiple Choice Questions

1. Why are values important to healthcare?
    (a) What we value guides where we find meaning and purpose. Values are age group specific and they rarely change over time.
    (b) What one values makes one happy. Happy people are healthier.
    (c) They make people feel better to share with their care team.
    (d) Greater sense of purpose in life is linked with decreased mortality.
    CORRECT ANSWER: D
2. The best way to learn one's meaning, aspiration and purpose is:
    (a) Refer the patient to a health coach for deep exploration
    (b) Hand a personal health inventory to the patient to complete
    (c) Ask the patient directly "what brings you a sense of joy and happiness to you" and one or two follow-up questions using therapeutic communication techniques
    (d) Ask the care giver/family member what they believe matters most to the patient
    CORRECT ANSWER: C
3. What do you do with the information on mission, aspiration and purpose (MAP) once received?
    (a) Use MAP to co-create a plan of care or personal health plan including self-care goals.
    (b) Write it in the chart.
    (c) Acknowledge the sharing of information.
    (d) Use MAP to assist in getting the patient to do what the provider believes is best for them.
    CORRECT ANSWER: A

References

Alimujiang, A., Wiensch, A., Boss, J., Fleischer, N. L., Mondul, A. M., McLean, K., Mukherjee, B., & Pearce, C. L. (2019). Association between life purpose and mortality among US adults older than 50 years. *JAMA Network Open, 2*(5), e194270. https://doi.org/10.1001/jamanetworkopen.2019.4270. PMID: 31125099; PMCID: PMC6632139.

Araújo, L., Ribeiro, O., Teixeira, L., & Paúl, C. (2016). Predicting successful aging at one hundred years of age. *Research on Aging, 38*(6), 689–709. https://doi.org/10.1177/0164027515603771. Epub 2015 Sep 2.

Archer, S., Brathwaite, F., & Fraser, H. (2005). Centenarians in Barbados: The importance of religiosity in adaptation and coping and life satisfaction in the case of extreme longevity. *Journal of Religion, Spirituality & Aging, 18*, 3–19.

Baek, Y., Martin, P., Siegler, I. C., Davey, A., & Poon, L. W. (2016). Personality traits and successful aging: Findings from the Georgia centenarian study. *The International Journal of Aging and Human Development., 83*(3), 207–227. https://doi.org/10.1177/0091415016652404

Bokhour, B. G., Hyde, J., Kligler, B., Gelman, H., Gaj, L., Barker, A. M., Douglas, J., DeFaccio, R., Taylor, S. L., & Zeliadt, S. B. (2022). From patient outcomes to system change: Evaluating the impact of VHA's implementation of the whole health system of care. *Health Services Research, 57 Suppl 1*(Suppl 1), 53–65. https://doi.org/10.1111/1475-6773.13938. Epub 2022 Mar 4. PMID: 35243621; PMCID: PMC9108226.

Borras, C., Ingles, M., Mas-Bargues, C., Dromant, M., Sanz-Ros, J., Román-Domínguez, A., Gimeno-Mallench, L., Gambini, J., & Viña, J. (2020). Centenarians: An excellent example of resilience for successful ageing. *Mechanisms of Ageing and Development., 186*, 111199. ISSN 0047–6374.

Buettner, D. 2022. Blue zones diet: Food secrets of the world's longest-lived people. https://www.bluezones.com/2020/07/blue-zones-diet-food-secrets-of-the-worlds-longest-lived-people/

Buettner, D., & Skemp, S. (2016). Blue zones: Lessons from the World's longest lived. *American Journal of Lifestyle Medicine, 10*(5), 318–321. https://doi.org/10.1177/1559827616637066. PMID: 30202288; PMCID: PMC6125071.

Cheung, K. S., & Lau, B. H. (2015). Successful aging among Chinese near-centenarians and centenarians in Hong Kong: A multidimensional and interdisciplinary approach. *Aging & Mental Health., 20*, 1314–1326. https://doi.org/10.1080/13607863.2015.1078281

Cohen, R., Bavishi, C., & Rozanski, A. (2016). Purpose in life and its relationship to all-cause mortality and cardiovascular events: A meta-analysis. *Psychosomatic Medicine, Feb-Mar;78(2):122-33*, 122–133. https://doi.org/10.1097/PSY.0000000000000274. PMID: 26630073).

Elwy, A. R., & Taylor, S. L. (2020). Progress of veterans health administration complementary and integrative health research along the quality enhancement research initiative implementation roadmap. *Med Care, 58*(Suppl 2 9S), S75–S77. https://doi.org/10.1097/MLR.0000000000001382

Farmer, M. M., McGowan, M., Yuan, A. H., Whitehead, A. M., Osawe, U., & Taylor, S. L. (2021). Complementary and integrative health approaches offered in the veterans health administration: Results of a National Organizational Survey. *Journal of Alternative and Complementary Medicine, 27*(S1), S124–S130. https://doi.org/10.1089/acm.2020.0395

Hao, Z., Chen, L., Li, Y., Zou, X., Li, H., Feng, Z., et al. (2019). Characteristics of centenarians' lifestyles and their contribution to life satisfaction: A case study conducted on Hainan Island. *Archives of Gerontology and Geriatrics, 83*, 20–27. https://doi.org/10.1016/j.archger.2019.03.022

Haslam, C., Cruwys, T. S., Haslam, A., & Jetten, J. (2015). Social connectedness and health. *Encyclopedia of Geropsychology.* https://doi.org/10.1007/978-981-287-080-3_46-1

Kim, E. S., Sun, J. K., Park, N., & Peterson, C. (2013). Purpose in life and reduced incidence of stroke in older adults: 'The health and retirement Study'. *Journal of Psychosomatic Research, 74*(5), 427–432. https://doi.org/10.1016/j.jpsychores.2013.01.013. Epub 2013 Feb 28.

Kligler, B., Hyde, J., Gantt, C., & Bokhour, B. (2022). The whole health transformation at the veterans health administration: moving from "What's the Matter With You?" to "What Matters to You?". *Medical Care, 60*(5), 387–391. https://doi.org/10.1097/MLR.0000000000001706

Madhivanan, P., Krupp, K., Waechter, R., & Shidhaye, R. (2021). Yoga for healthy aging: Science or hype? *Adv Geriatr Med Res, 3*(3), e210016. https://doi.org/10.20900/agmr20210016. Epub 2021 Jul 13. PMID: 34368806; PMCID: PMC8341166.

Marone, S., Bloore, K., Sebastiani, P., Flynn, C., Leonard, B., Whitaker, K., Mostowy, M., Perls, T. T., & Andersen, S. L. (2020). Purpose in life among centenarian offspring. *The Journals of Gerontology. Series B, Psychological Sciences and Social Sciences, 75*(2), 308–315. https://doi.org/10.1093/geronb/gby023. PMID: 29522128; PMCID: PMC7179803.

Musich, S., Wang, S. S., Kraemer, S., Hawkins, K., & Wicker, E. (2018). Purpose in life and positive health outcomes among older adults. *Popul Health Management, 21*(2), 139–147. https://doi.org/10.1089/pop.2017.0063. Epub 2017 Jul 5. PMID: 28677991; PMCID: PMC5906725.

National Institute of Health. NCCIH Clinical digest for health professional. Mind and Body Practices for Older Adults: What the Science Says. August 2019. Available at: https://www.nccih.nih.gov/health/providers/digest/mind-and-body-practices-for-older-adults-science. Accessed 26 Jan 2023.

Park, J., Krause-Parello, C. A., & Barnes, C. M. (2020). A narrative review of movement-based mind-body interventions: Effects of yoga, tai chi, and qigong for Back pain patients. Holist. *Nursing Practice, 34*(1), 3–23. https://doi.org/10.1097/HNP.0000000000000360. PMID: 31725096.

Roth, A. R., Lazris, A., Haskell, H., & James, J. (2020). Appropriate use of opioids for chronic pain. *American Family Physician, 102*(6), 335–337. Erratum in: Am Fam Physician. 2021 Jan 1;103(1):8.

Tiedemann, A., O'Rourke, S., Sesto, R., & Sherrington, C. (2013). A 12-week Iyengar yoga program improved balance and mobility in older community-dwelling people: A pilot randomized controlled trial. *The Journals of Gerontology. Series A, Biological Sciences and Medical Sciences, 68*(9), 1068–1075. https://doi.org/10.1093/gerona/glt087. Epub 2013 Jul 2.

Tulloch, A., Bombell, H., Dean, C., & Tiedemann, A. (2018). Yoga-based exercise improves health-related quality of life and mental Well-being in older people: A systematic review of randomised controlled trials. *Age and Ageing, 47*(4), 537–544. https://doi.org/10.1093/ageing/afy044

US Dept of Veterans Affairs. Whole Health Basics. (2022). Available at: https://www.va.gov/WHOLEHEALTH/veteran-resources/whole-health-basics.asp. Accessed 26 Jan 2023.

Wang, Y., Lu, S., Wang, R., Jiang, P., Rao, F., Wang, B., Zhu, Y., Hu, Y., & Zhu, J. (2018). Integrative effect of yoga practice in patients with knee arthritis: A PRISMA-compliant meta-analysis. *Medicine (Baltimore), 97*(31), e11742. https://doi.org/10.1097/MD.0000000000011742. PMID: 30075589; PMCID: PMC6081169.

World Health Organization. Ageing – Demographics. (2019). Available at: https://platform.who.int/data/maternal-newborn-child-adolescent-ageing/ageing-data/ageing%2D%2D-demographics. Accessed 26 Jan 2023.

Youkhana, S., Dean, C. M., Wolff, M., Sherrington, C., & Tiedemann, A. (2016). Yoga-based exercise improves balance and mobility in people aged 60 and over: A systematic review and meta-analysis. *Age and Ageing, 45*(1), 21–29. https://doi.org/10.1093/ageing/afv175. Epub 2015 Dec 25.

Chapter 13
Oral Health and Longevity Geriatric Dentistry, Care Pathways, Oral Health Epidemiology

Pierre M. Cartier

Key Take Away Points

1. The oral cavity is a complex organ that is highly susceptible to the effects of aging due to the multiple functions that its tissues perform.
2. The pathway for attainment of optimal oral health later in life begins at birth and is modified positively and negatively by social, environmental, and biological factors encountered throughout life.
3. Supporting optimal oral health attainment throughout life requires interdisciplinary collaboration between clinicians, public health professionals, policymakers, health educators, and researchers.
4. The Seattle Care Pathways provide a tool for both clinicians and public health professionals to support optimal oral health attainment as individuals age.

13.1 Introduction

The oral cavity is a unique organ system due to the direct interaction that individuals have with it on a day-to-day basis, as well as its key functions in digestion, speech, and esthetics. Consequently, its tissues are highly susceptible to the direct effects of aging. Further, the oral cavity is susceptible to the effects of systemic diseases associated with aging and can provide a "mirror" to one's overall health.

Healthcare providers must be familiar with the expected effects of aging on oral health, as well as the interaction between these phenomena and overall physical and psychological health. Further, both healthcare providers and public health

P. M. Cartier (✉)
Department of Veterans Affairs, Washington, DC, USA
e-mail: pierre.cartier@va.gov

R. E. Kheirbek, M. D. Llorente (eds.), *Current Perspectives on Centenarians*, International Perspectives on Aging 36,
https://doi.org/10.1007/978-3-031-30915-1_13

professionals play key roles in advocating for optimal oral health attainment throughout the human lifespan; fluency in the principles of research, policy development, education, and program implementation is integral to these efforts.

13.2 Definition of Oral Health

Oral health is not solely the absence of oral diseases or injuries. Rather, it is an ongoing process of mitigating physical, chemical, and biological challenges to maintain the normal functioning of the oral cavity. This process begins at birth, continues throughout the human lifespan, and is modified by social, environmental, and biological factors.

The concept of *optimal oral health* varies between individuals. Efforts to assess oral health attainment individually are largely subjective and influenced by culture, life experiences, and other norms. Consequently, individuals may have varying inclinations to pursue preventive or comprehensive oral healthcare. For example, attrition of the teeth that causes esthetic and functional concerns for one individual may not present concerns for another. This subjectivity in oral health norms often presents concerns not only for clinicians, but also for public health professionals, third-party payers, and other stakeholders that have an interest in reducing morbidity from oral disorders and the associated financial and social implications related to them.

In 2016, the FDI World Dental Federation conceptualized oral health in a manner that cites the importance of physiological and psychosocial constructs in oral health, in addition to the traditional criterion of oral disease status (Fig. 13.1) (FDI World Dental Federation, 2022). The contemporary FDI definition states that "Oral health is multi-faceted and includes the ability to speak, smile, smell, taste, touch, chew, swallow, and convey a range of emotions through facial expressions with confidence and without pain, discomfort, and disease of the craniofacial complex." The 2016 FDI definition of oral health demonstrates that oral health is an integral component of one's overall health attainment, with significant implications for physical and psychological health, as well as one's overall quality of life. This definition also counters the notion that dental medicine and oral health are "siloed" with respect to other areas of medicine and public health, providing an impetus for interprofessional collaboration.

The 2016 FDI definition for oral health also redefines the role of dental medicine as a field not only treats oral diseases, but also collaborates with other disciplines to mitigate non-clinical factors that may prevent attainment of optimal oral health. It provides a universal definition of oral health that can be referenced by clinicians, public health workers, policy makers, and other stakeholders throughout the world. Further, this definition cites the importance of non-clinical factors in oral health attainment. Driving determinants include biological factors, social constructs, behaviors, social and physical environments, and care access (Glick et al., 2016). The definition also cites the important role of individuals' age, experiences, perceptions, expectations, and resiliency as dynamic "moderating factors" that influence

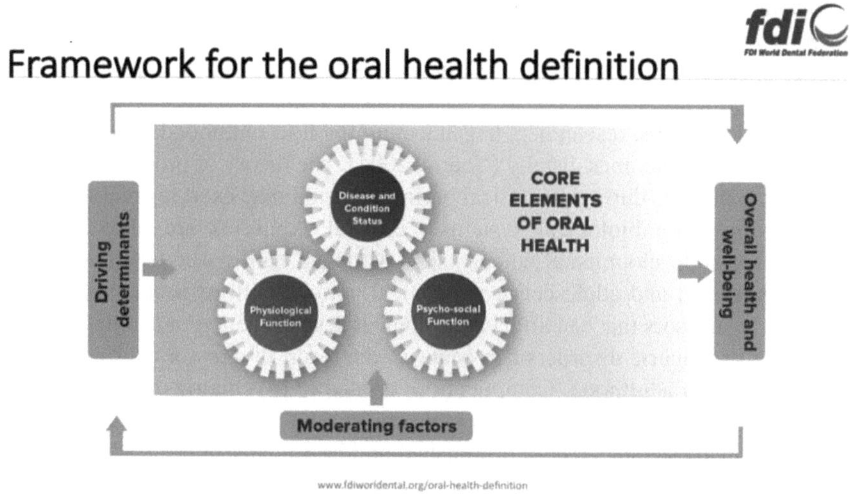

Fig. 13.1 FDI World Dental Federation definition of oral health. The FDI states that "Oral health is multi-faceted and includes the ability to speak, smile, smell, taste, touch, chew, swallow, and convey a range of emotions through facial expressions with confidence and without pain, discomfort, and disease of the craniofacial complex." The core components of oral health are (1) Disease and Condition Status (severity of oral disease, as well as presence or absence of discomfort); (2) Physiological Function (ability to chew food, swallow, speak, smile, and other actions); and (3) Psycho-Social Functioning (ability to carry out physiological, social, and occupational functions without being psychologically or socially uncomfortable). The core components of oral health are influenced by the 5 principal driving determinants of health (biological factors, social environment, physical environment, behaviors, and care access), as well as moderating factors (such as life experiences, resiliency, and age) that influence how an individual rates their own oral health. All of these factors in turn influence overall wellness. A bidirectional relationship exists between overall health and wellness and the driving determinants

how an individual may assess their own overall oral health. Insights provided by this definition guide not only clinical care, but also guide efforts to design research, public health programs, and policies that support oral health attainment across the human lifespan.

13.3 Life Course Development of Oral Health

The ongoing process of maintaining oral health and the factors that influence it are best described applying life course development principles. These principles provide not only a basis for understanding the factors that influence oral health development, but also provide a framework for modeling the influence of these factors in oral health maintenance. As seen in the 2016 FDI definition of oral health, overall wellness can bi-directionally influence the driving determinants of health. This relationship may influence both biological and non-biological determinants of health in a dynamic fashion. While it is challenging to forecast the impact of these relationships for individuals, health determinants are often known for specific populations and can be analyzed using life course principles to guide the development of programs and policies.

In the early 1980s, researchers began examining how childhood exposures may influence health outcomes distally (Young, 2004). The theory of programming suggests that exposures during the critical perinatal period may exert reversible or irreversible effects on biological systems. Perinatal exposures are often cited as contributors to developmental defects, such as dental hard tissue agenesis or oral clefts. Childhood and adolescence are critical periods with respect to exposures, particularly stressors that can affect neurological development. For example, development of psychiatric disorders can occur as the result of stressors during adolescence and young adulthood. Complications related to psychiatric conditions, such as bruxism, decreased engagement in oral care, substance abuse, and social impairments, can increase one's risk of diminished oral health later in life.

Researchers also believe that these exposures may exhibit a dose-response effect where more frequent exposures may ultimately lead to protective or deleterious effects. When repeated exposures to stressors are experienced by individuals and populations, this concept is often cited as allostatic load. Increased allostatic load may influence the occurrence of diseases through both biological and psychological phenomena. For example, high allostatic load is associated with the development of chronic diseases, such as diabetes. Complications related to chronic diseases, such as immune dysfunction and xerostomia from medications, can increase one's long-term risk of periodontitis, dental caries, and other oral diseases. Further, depression, anxiety, and other conditions that may develop as a consequence of sustained psychological stress can contribute to decreased engagement in preventive oral care, particularly if these conditions are untreated and occur on a chronic basis.

Exposures may also be protective. A key example of a protective exposure in oral health is water fluoridation to reduce dental caries. Non-biologic factors, such as supportive family structures or policies that support oral health attainment, can also be protective. For example, policies that limit sales of soft drinks in schools potentially reduce the exposure of children and adolescents to fermentable carbohydrates that can contribute to tooth decay and diabetes when consumed frequently.

In the 2000s, researchers began observing that common risk factors exist between multiple chronic health conditions. Oral health researchers began to extend the non-biological determinants of health to several oral conditions, including dental caries and periodontitis. A key focus in the impact of non-biological determinants of health involves the pediatric population, particularly given the long-term implications of poor oral health as children age. Larson and colleagues examined the impact of socio-economic status race, insurance status, and maternal health on children's overall health attainment and noted a strong linear correlation between multiple social risk factors and poor oral health (Larson et al., 2008).

Recent advantages in molecular biologically have allowed researchers to begin examining epigenetic phenomena where social and environmental exposures may ultimately modify gene expression without altering the sequence of DNA itself (Seo et al., 2015). Epigenetic phenomena usually occur through the modification of methyl groups in DNA (methylation), modification of proteins (histones) that support DNA and regulate transcription of genes, or modification of non-coding RNA that influence gene expression. Epigenetic changes may be facilitated by exposure to cigarette smoke, malnutrition, stress, inflammation, and other exposures. Researchers currently believe that these phenomena are implicated in processes that include tooth development, periodontal diseases, and oral cancer.

It is believed that epigenetic phenomena influencing disease states are largely reversible. Lifestyle changes, such as smoking cessation, improved nutrition, stress reduction, or resolution of inflammatory processes can prevent or reduce expression of genes involved in periodontal diseases, oral cancer, and other chronic diseases. However, modification of gene expression in parental genes by methylation (imprinting) is believed to be largely irreversible and can contribute to anomalies in craniofacial development. Hence, optimal nutrition and reduction of potentially harmful environmental exposures is critical to preventing developmental defects that can affect one's oral functioning throughout life.

13.4 Effects of Aging on the Oral Cavity

Humans typically develop 32 permanent teeth by completion of adolescence. An optimal dentition includes incisors, canines, and either premolar or molar occlusion. Maintenance of dental hard tissues involves a balance between ongoing deposition of mineral content in the enamel and the loss of enamel and dentin through the effects of physical attrition and dissolution by dietary and bacterial acids. The enamel is typically stronger than the underlying dentin due to its higher mineral content. However, the underlying dentin that comprises the bulk of a tooth's structure exhibits greater organic content and is more susceptible to decay by cariogenic bacteria.

13.4.1 Aging and Tooth Loss

Tooth loss generally increases with age secondary to past trauma, caries, fracturing of restored teeth, severe periodontitis, or the treatment of oral tumors. However, it can also occur through planned circumstances, such as the removal of 3rd molars (wisdom teeth) or the removal of pre-molars to support orthodontic treatment. The removal of teeth electively can impair oral functioning if additional teeth are lost later in life.

Generally, it is believed that the impact of edentulism is decreasing in developed countries due to the provision of comprehensive oral healthcare. However, individuals of lower socioeconomic status are more likely to experience this condition due to limited access to preventive oral care, sub-optimal nutrition, and other factors.

Further, individuals with systemic health conditions are at a higher risk of experiencing edentulism. For example, diabetics have an increased risk of periodontal disease progression and can experience tooth loss more quickly than non-diabetic patients with periodontitis. Patients with psychiatric conditions may experience fracturing of teeth and subsequent tooth loss due to bruxism (tooth grinding) commonly observed as oral complications of psychiatric conditions or medications used to treat them.

Edentulism typically affects one's overall physical and mental health. The ability to function without some or all teeth typically varies between individuals. However, alterations in the ability to masticate foods of higher consistency, such as meats and cruciferous vegetables, typically occurs when some or all principal teeth are lost. This alteration in functioning can lead to impaired digestion, malnutrition, an increased risk of infections, and altered reparative processes.

Edentulism may also exhibit psychological effects. Given that the teeth are integral for facial esthetics, their loss can lead to lower self-esteem, anxiety, and depression. Edentulism may impact the management of these conditions in individuals that are experiencing psychiatric co-morbidities. Further, individuals experiencing difficulty eating may experience a state of helplessness, particularly if they lose their appetite, have to change the types of foods they consume, or experience alterations in taste perception. Impaired nutrition can trigger or further accentuate physical and mental decline.

13.4.2 Effects of Aging on Periodontium

The periodontium is integral to maintaining the dentition and consists of the gums, supporting alveolar bone, and ligaments that attach the teeth to the bone. Teeth are typically surrounded by a 1–3 mm gingival sulcus. Destruction of the periodontium through inflammation or physical injury can increase sulcus depth and lead to periodontal pockets that are difficult to maintain. Such pockets are often the result of periodontitis, a condition where both the soft and hard tissue support of the teeth is lost.

Periodontitis is common in the aging population. The United States Centers for Disease Control estimate that 47.2% of adults 30 years of age and older have periodontitis; the prevalence of this condition increases to 70.1% for adults 65 years of age and older (US Centers for Disease Control, 2022). Periodontitis prevalence is greater in individuals of lower socioeconomic status, as well as men. Ongoing exposure to oral inflammation, such as the effects of cigarette smoke and impaired oral hygiene, contribute to the increased prevalence of this condition by age. Further, chronic diseases associated with aging, such as diabetes, increase one's risk of developing periodontitis and can also increase its severity.

Severe periodontitis may ultimately lead to partial or complete tooth loss. The risk of experiencing severe periodontitis is increased in conditions that cause inflammation or immune dysregulation, such as diabetes, smoking, or HIV. The teeth may become mobile as the bone and supporting gingival tissues are lost around the teeth, requiring extraction to prevent aspiration of the affected teeth into the lungs or entry into the alimentary canal.

13.4.3 Effects of Aging on Salivary Glands

The salivary glands provide protection and lubrication to the oral cavity. Enzymes in saliva control oral microrganisms and reduce the risk of caries, gingival inflammation, and fungal infections. The mineral content of saliva aids in the repair of enamel that may be damaged by bacterial and dietary acids. Saliva is also integral to digestion, providing enzymes that are necessary to digest macromolecules and facilitate taste. Alterations in taste can reduce one's desire to eat or result in a shift toward foods that contain high refined carbohydrate content and that can increase one's risk of dental caries. Further, saliva provides lubrication, allowing food to move more effectively through the upper alimentary canal. Individuals with xerostomia may also experience impairments in digestion, leading to malnutrition and associated complications. Altered nutrition is particularly a concern in older adults that have diabetes and other chronic diseases as it can compromise management of these conditions and result in physical decline. The psychological effects of diminished nutrition, impaired disease management, and ultimately altered quality of life can lead to depression, anxiety, or worsening of psychiatric disorders.

While saliva production typically does not decrease with age, diseases associated with aging can impair saliva secretion. Diabetes can lead to xerostomia (dry mouth) due to the osmotic actions of increased serum glucose. Medications used to treat many chronic diseases and psychiatric conditions can cause xerostomia. Further, immune conditions, such as Sjogren's syndrome and sarcoidosis, can result in the destruction of salivary gland tissue. Radiation therapy for head and neck cancer may also destroy salivary gland tissue and lead to xerostomia.

Decreased salivary flow increases the risk of oral diseases and may also lead to diminished quality of life. Older adults with chronic xerostomia and gingival recession secondary to periodontitis exhibit a higher risk of root caries. Such caries lesions often progress rapidly due to the increased collagen content of tooth roots, resulting in caries lesions that are difficult to restore and that may ultimately require extraction of the tooth. Root caries can also undermine teeth, resulting in fracturing of coronal tooth structure and aspiration of tooth tissue into the lungs or alimentary canal.

13.4.4 Effects of Aging on Oral Soft Tissues

Oral soft tissues are exposed to various chemical, microbial, and physical agents throughout life. Some oral soft tissue conditions related to physical agents, such as chronic mechanical trauma to the buccal mucosa or gingival tissues, typically exhibit little to no effect on oral health. However, lifetime exposure to alcohol, tobacco, and other chemical irritants can lead to dysplastic changes in oral tissues.

Oral cancer risk typically increases with age, particularly among individuals that were exposed to carcinogens early in life. Exposure to ultraviolet radiation from the sun or other sources increases the risk of developing squamous cell carcinoma of the lips. Although exposure to physical and chemical carcinogens has traditionally been associated with oral and pharyngeal cancers in older individuals, cancers associated with human papillomavirus infections are increasing observed in younger individuals. Routine vaccination against oncogenic serotypes of these viruses may reduce the incidence of oropharyngeal cancers in the older adult population during the coming decades.

The psychological sequelae of treatments for oral and pharyngeal cancers are a key concern for both patients and providers. Treatment of these lesions often involves surgery, radiation, chemotherapy, or combinations of these modalities. These treatments often result in damage to anatomical structures, impaired functioning, and potentially decreased quality of life. Patients receiving treatment for oral and pharyngeal cancers are at an increased risk of developing depression, particularly if their quality of life is affected. Additionally, mucositis, muscle fibrosis, and other physical complications of head and neck cancer treatment can precipitate functional decline, particularly if an individual's nutrition is impaired.

Oral soft tissues also loose elasticity with age. The buccal mucosa commonly collapses inwardly, increasing the risk of acute or chronic occlusal trauma. While chronic occlusal trauma to oral tissues rarely causes concerns, acute trauma to the buccal mucosa and other oral tissues can cause pain or infections that may interfere with nutrition, sleep, and other functions. Further, collapse of the oropharyngeal tissues may be a contributory factor in obstructive sleep apnea. Dentists are increasingly involved in the inter-disciplinary management of sleep apnea, including screening patients for this condition and fabricating oral appliances for patients that may not be able to tolerate continuous positive airway pressure (CPAP).

Edentulism may also lead to changes in the intra- and extra-oral soft tissues. Loss of teeth leads to impaired support for the cheeks, tongue, lips, and other oral soft tissues. Additionally, movement of any remaining teeth can also lead to alterations in soft tissue support. Oral soft tissues that are not supported appropriately may become traumatized, resulting in pain, infection, and impaired oral functioning. Further, individuals that experience more extensive tooth loss may experience "sinking" of the lips and premature aging of facial tissues, potentially resulting in psychological distress.

13.4.5 Effects of Aging on Masticatory Apparatus

The masticatory apparatus includes the temporomandibular joints (TMJ), maxilla, mandible, muscles of mastication, and associated ligaments. The TMJ has both hinging and gliding functions, with the mandible articulating at the base of the skull. A disc exists between the condylar heads of the mandible and the articular eminence at the skull's base. Four principal pairs of masticatory muscles guide movement of the jaw and allow it to function as a class III lever for mastication of food.

Like other joints, the TMJ can experience long-term wear. Many older adults will experience noises or some limited motion of the jaw due to long-term degradation of the articular disc. Many individuals do not experience any long-term disability from these conditions. However, degradation of the disc can cause limited jaw motion in individuals that experienced substantial trauma to the TMJ earlier in life or that experience long-term physical or psychiatric conditions that place strain on the joint. For example, individuals that experience bruxism secondary to anxiety disorders or sustained psychological stress may experience temporomandibular joint-related disability with age. Individuals that experience rheumatoid arthritis or joint inflammation secondary to other diseases can also experience degradation of the TMJ, impaired motion, and pain.

Masticatory muscle dysfunction may also impair jaw functioning. The masticatory and facial muscles typically lose tone with age, with this process being more accentuated in individuals with neuromuscular disorders or those taking medications that affect neuromuscular functioning. Decreased masticatory muscle tone can affect food mastication, leading to impaired nutrition and an increased risk of aspiration pneumonia.

Individuals experiencing psychiatric and other neurological disorders may also present with increased masticatory muscle tone and activity as both manifestations of their conditions and side effects of medications used to treat them. Hypertonicity of these muscles can result in bruxism, increased attrition of the teeth, and damage to the TMJ. Individuals with anxiety, depression, and other neurological conditions are more likely to experience bruxism and clenching of teeth, as well as orofacial pain. Acute and chronic orofacial pain, combined with changes in oral functioning and quality-of-life, can contribute to decompensation with respect to physical and psychiatric conditions.

13.4.6 Oral Health Outcomes of Centenarians

Evaluating the oral health status of centenarians provides an opportunity to examine factors that contribute to positive oral health outcomes for older adults. However, challenges associated with ascertaining lifetime exposures have limited researchers in precisely examining factors related to oral longevity. Historically, studies examining oral health outcomes of older adults have relied upon cross-sectional or case-control designs that examine associations between exposures and outcomes ascertained through interviews or surveys. Such studies are inherently influenced by information biases, such as errors in subjects recalling past exposures or errors related to interviewers ascertaining exposure- or outcome-related data. Some studies will include an objective clinical evaluation performed by trained and calibrated clinicians to reduce the subjectivity that may result when study participants are asked to self-report their own oral health status. However, most studies will still require ascertainment of exposure data through questionnaires or interviews, particularly as past exposure data for older adults may not be available through computerized medical records or biological specimen repositories.

Recent epidemiologic studies examining the oral health of centenarians suggest that this population largely self-reports satisfactory oral health. A cohort study of 162 Dutch centenarians by Beker and colleagues suggested that the majority of study participants experienced good oral health, with 76% reporting no oral discomfort, 65% reporting adequate mastication, and only 18% experiencing signs of xerostomia (Beker et al., 2019). Scoring with respect to these factors was similar between both edentulous and dentate centenarians, with 83% of participants experiencing complete edentulism mitigated by use of maxillary and mandibular complete dentures and 17% maintaining at least some of their natural dentition. A key limitation of this study is that it relied on self-reporting of oral health through interviews, with the potential bias that participants might reply with more positive or optimistic responses based on generational values of cooperating with healthcare personnel. Additionally, this study is subject to selection bias in that it examined a cohort of cognitively healthy centenarians, limiting its generalization to the greater centenarian population.

Given that centenarians reporting high levels of oral health may exhibit health behaviors that support higher levels of oral health attainment, researchers are particularly interested in patterns of oral health attainment within their families. Kaufman and colleagues examined edentulism rates, the presence of oral disease symptoms, and oral health-sustaining behavior among 73 centenarians in the New England Centenarian Study (NECS), 467 centenarian offspring, and 251 offspring birth cohort referent subjects (Kaufman et al., 2014). The authors noted that 36.5% of centenarians exhibited edentulism relative to 46% of their birth cohort members that were surveyed between the ages of 65–74 years of age. Additionally, the authors noted that members of the centenarian offspring birth cohort were 2.7 times more likely to experience edentulism than the offspring of centenarians. Although Kaufman and colleagues suggest that low edentulism rates and high self-reported oral health levels observed in centenarians and their offspring may also be associated with lower rates of cardiovascular diseases and diabetes, they do not specifically examine the role of diet, health care utilization, and other health behaviors in supporting this relationship.

While studies suggest that centenarians generally report good oral health, some researchers suggest that this population exhibits unique concerns that present challenges for oral care professionals and other caretakers. In a clinical and health behavior survey of 55 centenarians in Germany, Sekundo and colleagues noted that this population exhibited decreased engagement in preventive oral care, including dental visits (Sekundo et al., 2020). Further, they noted that while 98.2% of their study participants received assistance with their activities of daily living, only 12.7% received assistance with their oral care. While majority of participants in this study population expressed wishing to receive dental care, 63.7% exhibited decreased or limited capacity to participate in comprehensive dental care. Further evaluation of these barriers and strategies for mitigating them is integral to ensuring that older adults can access preventive oral healthcare and basic dental treatment services regardless of their cognition, systemic health, or living situation.

13.4.7 Supporting the Oral Health of an Aging Population

Facilitation of optimal oral health outcomes for an aging population occurs through four principal activities that may overlap:

- Public Health (Epidemiologic Surveillance, Program Management, and Policy Development)
- Clinical Practice (Direct Preventive and Treatment Service Provision in Health Centers, Private Practices, Hospitals, and Institutional Environments)
- Research
- Education

13.4.8 Role of Public Health Professionals

Public health professionals play a key role in supporting optimal oral health outcomes throughout the human lifespan. Epidemiologists conduct population-level oral health assessments and epidemiologic studies to ascertain trends with respect to oral disease occurrence, health behaviors, resource allocation, and oral care access. Data from these analyses assist government agencies, institutions, and other stakeholders in planning programs and allocating resources to address current and emerging issues. Data also assist government officials and other stakeholders with the development of policies that may address such issues as the incorporation of adult oral healthcare services into public insurance programs, the independent practice of dental hygienists in long-term care facilities, and funding of post-graduate geriatric dentistry programs for providers.

Public health professionals in local, state, and federal organizations also design, implement, and evaluate programs that address needs identified through population-level assessments and epidemiologic analyses. Ongoing program evaluation is a critical activity in that it helps to validate the continued operation of programs and demonstrate their impact to stakeholders. This process typically begins before a program is initiated and solicits the involvement of community stakeholders in addition to epidemiologists and other public health professionals. Over time, these stakeholders will identify areas that require modification in the program, including obsolete activities or new foci. In some cases, data may suggest the elimination of a program or establish the basis for developing a new one.

Public health professionals in the non-governmental sector also play key roles in program and policy development. Non-governmental and academic organizations may conduct population health assessments and research that government organizations are not able to perform due to resource limitations, political roadblocks, and other factors. Organizations performing such work typically have liaisons that work with governmental agencies to foster alliances, educate agency stakeholders about emerging issues, and develop strategies to work with them to address issues of interest. For example, the charitable arm of a state dental association may obtain data from its members regarding trends related to edentulous patients that may not be able to afford dentures. The dental asssociation's policy analyst and government relations specialist would educate legislators and agency stakeholders regarding this issue and collaborate to develop programs, such as a denture access grant for patients being seen at the state's dental school, to enable low-income patients to receive needed prostheses.

Despite the program's scope and size, ongoing evaluation would be an important component of this effort. The state dental association would establish a panel of stakeholders from multiple entities, including the dental school, clinicians, and the state public health agency, to guide ongoing evaluation of the program. An epidemiologist specializing in program evaluation might be recruited from a university to aid stakeholders in developing a data collection and analysis plan, including identifying short-, intermediate-, and long-term impacts. For example, metrics that might be considered could include cost-savings with respect to systemic health outcomes prevented by improving patients' nutrition and changes in quality of life following prosthesis delivery. In this case, early development of a data collection and analysis plan is imperative to ensure that desired data are available and proper evaluation instruments are selected to measure the impacts of interest.

Professional organizations also play a key role in developing position statements and guidelines that influence both public health activities and clinical practice. Professional organizations often track emerging issues through insight provided by their members and policy analysts that they may employ. When such issues are identified, organizational leaders collectively develop and approve statements that educate the public and other stakeholders regarding the profession or organization's position on the issue. Such statements may solely serve as an affirmation of awareness of an issue or acknowledgement that the issue will be evaluated more extensively within a given period. More straightforward issues may solely be addressed through a direct position statement. Urgent issues without definitive solutions or more complex issues related to the provision of clinical care are typically addressed by working groups tasked to develop clinical guidelines. Such groups typically incorporate subject-matter experts from interdisciplinary fields and from sectors that include academic, governmental, and private organizations.

Policy statements formulated by professional organizations often have broad impact in public health, clinical, legal, governmental, and business settings. Such statements can be held as "standards of care" by hospitals, third party payers, professional boards, and juries. Further, statements and guidelines suggesting the necessity of treatments or procedures may be used to justify training, credentialing, or reimbursing providers to offer a particular diagnostic procedure or intervention. For example, research suggesting the effectiveness of non-surgical periodontal treatment in managing blood glucose levels in diabetics with periodontitis may lead third-party payers to increase the number of periodontal maintenance sessions covered by dental insurance plans.

13.4.9 Current State of Clinical Public Health Activities

Historically, activities of the public health establishment have overlapped with professionals providing direct clinical services. Many local health departments have maintained clinics that provide preventive and basic dental services, with a particular focus on children and uninsured adults. The services offered by these clinics are often limited to prevention and disease elimination. Some public health dental clinics may not have resources to support comprehensive oral care that includes crowns, root canal therapy, removable prostheses, and other treatments designed to maintain teeth.

In recent years, there has been a movement for local health departments to focus on epidemiologic analyses and policy development to support "health system design" as opposed to direct provision of clinical services. While some local health agencies may continue to provide clinical services, many of these activities have been transitioned to public-private collaborations with universities, hospitals, non-profit groups, and other organizations.

A key advantage of this transition is that private organizations may have pre-existing programs that provide a greater scope of services or may be able to obtain resources to offer comprehensive oral care to individuals of all ages, including older adults. Partnerships with community health centers and other non-profit clinics are particularly valuable in that these organizations often maintain cultural knowledge and influence within underserved populations, allowing for focused health education and messaging related to preventive care. Further, many of these organizations apply a life-course approach to care provision, allowing them to support oral health development from an early age.

Universities may collaborate with some local health agencies to provide clinical services. A key advantage of this strategy is that health professions students are introduced to underserved populations and opportunities to serve these populations. Further, students and post-graduate residents are introduced to technical skills, such as mobile dentistry, that can be applied to provide care in schools, long-term care facilities, and other non-traditional settings. Additionally, the importance of oral health development across the human lifespan is reinforced, particularly when students work with individuals ranging from infants to older adults.

Federal, state, and local public health agencies may collaborate with private providers. For example, private providers enrolled in the United States' Medicaid program may serve communities where increased emergency room visits for non-traumatic oral conditions have been ascertained. The state Medicaid and public health agencies, in addition to the respective hospitals, may collaborate with the providers through a care coordination program so that these individuals are linked to comprehensive oral healthcare services.

13.4.10 Mechanisms for Providing Clinical Care for the Aging Population

Private dental practices are the predominant venue for providing comprehensive oral healthcare in the United States and other countries. Such practices can be solo-provider offices, large groups with multiple providers, as well as clinics run by healthcare systems. The latter include hospitals, academic medical centers, as well as non-profit medical clinics.

A key limitation for these clinics is that many are supported through insurance reimbursements. Patients without dental insurance or without insurance plans accepted by the practice are typically required to pay directly for the services rendered. Increasingly, some private providers have moved to "fee-for-service" practice models and do not accept insurance, requiring patients to pay for services directly regardless of insurance coverage. These practice models can present a barrier to uninsured patients or those that are on fixed incomes.

In the United States and some other countries, clinics run by hospitals, academic institutions, and non-profit groups typically accept public insurance programs and offer a range of clinical services in one setting. Such clinics are ideal for patients with complex dental and medical conditions due to the multi-disciplinary approaches and resources typically seen in such settings. Some institutions may also offer reduced fees or no-cost treatment for non-insured individuals. However, traveling to clinics may be difficult for individuals with physical limitations or that do not have access to transportation.

Portable and mobile dental clinics have aided in reducing some barriers to oral care for the aging population in recent years. These mechanisms provide access to oral healthcare for individuals that are homebound or that live in long-term care facilities. Such clinics may operate as extensions of a private or institutional "brick-and-mortar" dental practice, or may operate as "stand alone" programs. Portable dentistry typically entails moving specially designed dental equipment into a home or facility and removing it when the services are complete. Mobile dentistry typically employs vehicles that have been converted into a dental clinic and providing services within the vehicle's operatories.

There exists considerable variation in the services provided by mobile or portable dental clinics. Facilities that host vehicle-based dental operatories are typically able to provide a broader scope of services paralleling those provided in brick-and-mortar dental offices. The services provided by portable dental operations are typically limited by the equipment that is provided. Some portable dental clinics provide a range of comprehensive services, while others provide basic dental care that may include preventive dental care, non-complicated extractions, and simple dental restorations. Individuals seen in both portable and mobile dental clinics that require extensive dental restorations or dento-alveolar surgery procedures may require treatment in brick-and-mortar facilities.

Tele-dentistry has been valuable in increasing access to dental care for home- and institution-bound individuals in recent years. In synchronous tele-dentistry encounters, a dentist based at a remote location typically evaluates a patient with the assistance of a trained tele-presenter through a video and audio link. The trained tele-presenter may be another oral health professional (such as a registered dental hygienist), or may also be an allied clinician (such as a registered nurse). In cases where an individual is home-bound, the attending dentist can instruct family members or other persons assisting the patient on how to provide feedback regarding the texture, feel, and other characteristics of lesions or conditions being evaluated.

At a minimum, synchronous encounters can allow the dentist to evaluate a patient and determine if arrangements need to be made for an in-person visit. Brick-and-mortar dentists can use tele-dentistry as a mechanism to conduct treatment planning conferences with other healthcare providers and family members that may be involved in a patient's oral healthcare. Additionally, these encounters can be used to conduct post-operative assessments, non-surgical disease management, and patient education, reducing the need for short-duration office visits.

Asynchronous tele-dentistry encounters can aid in enhancing communication between providers and enhancing access to direct clinical services. Dentists and other clinicians can evaluate patients, record data, obtain laboratory or imaging studies, and then submit the data to other providers for review. Asynchronous tele-dentistry is particularly advantageous to providers in rural areas where access to specialists may be limited, allowing patients to access some specialty services (such as TMD evaluations and oral pathology) without traveling.

Both synchronous and asynchronous encounters allow for the remote supervision of dental hygienists. The use of tele-dentistry for supervision of hygienists can allow them to provide preventive oral care services at remote sites, long-term care facilities, schools, and institutions without physically having a dentist on site. In a basic application of this model, the dental hygienist would obtain radiographs and collect dental evaluation data for an off-site dentist to review. The dentist may also meet with the patient and dental hygienist through a synchronous encounter to review collected data and further assess the patient with the dental hygienist serving as tele-presenter.

The use of tele-dentistry for remote supervision of dental hygienists is typically regulated by licensure boards and may not be possible in all jurisdictions. When remote supervision is possible, some jurisdictions may require a patient to receive a preliminary in-person examination from a dentist before subsequent assessments may be performed through tele-dentistry. While tele-dentistry is currently limited to supporting preventive and non-surgical periodontal care delivered by registered dental hygienists, its application does increase access to these services in populations that may otherwise be at risk for oral decline.

13.4.11 The Role of Research in Supporting Oral Health for Aging Populations

Research is a key activity that supports oral health attainment across the human lifespan. Oral health research can be focused on the basic biomedical sciences, social sciences, health policy, clinical practice, or health services.

Public health practice often overlaps with research. Epidemiologic analyses often provide valuable insight regarding the impact of oral health conditions on the aging population and factors that may reduce this population's risk of experiencing oral health conditions. Further, program evaluation analyses often provide insight regarding the potential effectiveness of preventive, therapeutic, or educational interventions. Knowledge from these insights can be applied to design randomized control trials to further evaluate the effectiveness of interventions.

A key area of epidemiologic research involves evaluating the systemic effects of oral inflammation. Epidemiologic research within the past 20 years has suggested a relationship between oral inflammation and several health conditions associated with aging, including cardiovascular and neurodegenerative conditions. The increasing use of comprehensive electronic health records may allow epidemiologists to further examine these associations and determine any causal relationships that may exist.

13.4.12 Medical Education's Role in Workforce Development and Interdisciplinary Care

Medical education facilitates interprofessional practice and the removal of barriers to coordinated care. The aging population is often affected by conditions that influence the safe provision of medical and dental care. Existing and new health care providers must be well-versed in interprofessional collaboration to ensure that information is shared between members of a patient's care team so that care may be provided in a coordinated manner. Interprofessional collaboration is integral to facilitating early detection of chronic health conditions, such as hypertension and diabetes, that are often screened for during oral healthcare appointments. Further, interprofessional collaboration plays a key role in preventing adverse events, such as drug interactions that may result from polypharmacy.

Pre-professional oral healthcare training programs have incorporated collaborations between medical and nursing schools to facilitate referrals for hypertension management, interprofessional diabetes care, behavioral healthcare, and management of acute pain. An underlying theme in interprofessional practice is supporting individuals in establishing both medical and dental "homes" for ongoing preventive care. Many individuals utilize oral healthcare services more than primary medical care services. Given that dentists may detect early signs of hypertension, diabetes, and other systemic health conditions, they play a key role in reinforcing messaging related to primary care.

Primary care providers may also encounter individuals that do not have a dental home and that may also present with oral manifestations of systemic diseases. Increasingly, primary medical providers are developing referral pathways to dentists for patients ranging from infants to older adults. While care coordination is more common in institutional clinics and other large practices, private providers are increasingly aware that this approach is integral to maximizing both physical, mental, and oral longevity for patients across the human lifespan.

13.4.13 Program and Treatment Planning for the Aging Population

Planning clinical and public health interventions for the aging population can be challenging due to inherent variation in individual needs and ability to engage in care or programming. In 2013, Pretty and colleagues developed the Seattle Care Pathways, a tool for guiding both individual- and population-level interventions for older adults (Pretty et al., 2014). Interventions are linked to five levels of cognitive and physical dependency that are correlated with Canadian Study of Health and Aging Frailty Scores.

While the Seattle Care Pathways are focused on older adults, they may be applied across the human lifespan. Clinicians and social workers can apply the Seattle Care Pathways to discuss future changes in dependency that might occur in younger individuals with chronic health conditions and assist them in developing short-, moderate-, and long-term oral healthcare plans. Public health professionals can use the dependency levels in the Seattle Care Pathways to identify focus areas for epidemiologic research, policy development, and program implementation.

A lack of dependency is the first level in the Seattle Care Pathways. Non-dependent individuals are those that receive regular exercise and have high levels of physical and mental fitness with respect to their age range. Non-dependent individuals can receive the full scope of oral healthcare services, including complex oral and maxillofacial surgery or prosthodontic procedures. Population-level interventions for non-dependent individuals would focus on encouraging individuals to maintain their oral and overall wellness.

Pre-dependent individuals are those with chronic health conditions that are well-controlled and are not exerting an influence on an individual's oral health. Patients in this category can typically receive the full scope of oral healthcare services with modifications as necessary. Clinicians and public health professionals should educate pre-dependent individuals regarding any potential changes in dependency that could occur in the future and how these changes might affect their oral health and processes for oral care delivery.

Low dependency is the third dependency level in the Seattle Care Pathways. Individuals exhibiting this level of dependency have chronic health conditions that do affect their oral health. These individuals typically do not require assistance in attending dental appointments or performing oral homecare. However, both patients and providers should be aware of moderate- and long-term changes in dependency that might occur and tailor oral healthcare treatment plans accordingly. Additionally, collaboration with allied health professionals may be necessary to address oral complications of systemic diseases. Preventive and population-level care should focus on supporting individuals in maintaining their dentitions and reducing future need for surgical interventions, such as tooth extractions or advanced restorative dentistry treatment.

Individuals with medium dependency are those with systemic diseases that affect their oral health and ability to perform oral homecare. These individuals may receive assistance in attending dental appointments and performing oral homecare. Individuals unable to attend oral healthcare appointments in traditional settings may be candidates for portable oral healthcare delivered in their homes or institutional settings. Key interventions in this population would entail preventive dental care, including examinations for early detection of dental caries, gingival diseases, and oral soft tissue lesions. Restorative dentistry may focus on simple interventions to control tooth decay and maintain teeth, such as placing silver diamine fluoride on caries lesions and restoring them with glass ionomer material. More extensive procedures, such as surgical tooth extractions and biopsies, would be conducted within a dental office or surgical center.

Individuals exhibiting medium dependency typically are not ideal candidates for dental implants or advanced restorative dental procedures. Missing teeth are typically replaced using simple removable prostheses. In some cases, dental implants may be considered to aid in the retention of complete dentures for individuals with severe bone loss in their jaws.

High dependency is the fifth dependency level in the Seattle Care Pathways. Individuals exhibiting high dependency are those with multiple systemic health conditions that affect their oral health. These individuals cannot leave their home or care facility and typically rely on providers with portable equipment for oral healthcare. Provision of preventive and palliative oral healthcare is a key focus in this population. High dependency individuals may receive dental examinations for early detection of oral diseases and preventive dental care to reduce the need for more advanced interventions. Silver diamine fluoride may be applied to reduce progression of caries lesions, particularly in individuals that exhibit limited cooperation.

Active caries lesions may also be treated using hand instruments and restored using glass ionomer restorative materials. Advanced procedures, such as tooth extractions, would not be performed unless necessary to eliminate pain or address an infection.

13.5 Summary

The basis for optimal oral health attainment in late adulthood begins during the prenatal period and is modified throughout life. Although the anatomy and physiology of tissues of the oral cavity can be negatively modified by various physical, chemical, environmental, and psychosocial stimuli, these tissues do exhibit resiliency and are amenable to interventions that reinforce optimal functioning. While centenarians generally report favorable levels of oral health attainment, they may experience functional limitations and limited caretaker support that impede their engagement in preventive oral care. Further research is required to ascertain exposures, health behaviors, and other factors that influence oral health attainment in centenarians. The development and implementation of strategies to ensure that all older adults – including centenarians – achieve optimal oral health outcomes relies on a multidisciplinary effort and interprofessional collaboration between clinicians, researchers, public health professionals, policy makers, and other stakeholders.

References

Beker, N., van der Maarel-Wierink, C. D., de Baat, C., et al. (2019). Self-reported oral health in the Dutch 100-plus study of cognitively healthy centenarians: An observational cohort study. *BMC Geriatrics, 19*, 355. https://doi.org/10.1186/s12877-019-1358-x

FDI World Dental Federation. FDI's definition of oral health. https://fdiworlddental.org/fdis-definition-oral-health. Accessed 13 Nov 2022.

Glick, M., et al. (2016). A new definition for oral health developed by the FDI World dental federation opens the door to a universal definition of oral health. *Journal of the American Dental Association (Chicago, IL), 147*, 915–917.

Kaufman, L. B., Setiono, T. K., Doros, G., Andersen, S., Silliman, R. A., Friedman, P. K., & Perls, T. T. (2014). An oral health study of centenarians and children of centenarians. *Journal of the American Geriatrics Society, 62*(6), 1168–1173. https://doi.org/10.1111/jgs.12842. Epub 2014 Jun 2. PMID: 24889721; PMCID: PMC4057979.

Larson, K., Russ, S. A., Crall, J. J., & Halfon, N. (2008). Influence of multiple social risks on children's health. *Pediatrics, 121*, 337–344.

Pretty, I. A., Ellwood, R. P., Lo, E. C., MacEntee, M. I., Müller, F., Rooney, E., Murray Thomson, W., Van der Putten, G. J., Ghezzi, E. M., Walls, A., & Wolff, M. S. (2014). The Seattle care pathway for securing oral health in older patients. *Gerodontology, 31*(Suppl 1), 77–87. https://doi.org/10.1111/ger.12098. PMID: 24446984.

Sekundo, C., Langowski, E., Kilian, S., & Frese, C. (2020). Oral health and functional capacity of centenarians. *Scientific Reports, 10*, 22215. https://doi.org/10.1038/s41598-020-78842-w

Seo, J. Y., Park, Y. J., Young-Ah, Y., Hwang, J. Y., Lee, I. B., Cho, B. H., Son, H. H., & Seo, D. G. (2015 Feb). Epigenetics: General characteristics and implications for oral health. *Restorative Dentistry and Endodontics, 40*(1), 14–22.

US Centers for Disease Control. Oral Health – Periodontal Disease. https://www.cdc.gov/oral-health/conditions/periodontal-disease.html. Accessed 18 Nov 2022.

Young, T. K. (2004). *Population health: Concepts and methods* (pp. 156–157). Oxford University Press.

Chapter 14
Contributions to Longevity and Well-being from Nature

Antoinette V. Shappell, Kelly A. Burnett, and Sean H. Gartland

Key Take Away Points

1. In addition to genetics, factors such as stress, physical activity, religion/ spirituality, social connectedness and our environment impact longevity andwell-being.
2. Natural environments are more restorative cognitively, psychologically, and physiologically compared to urban or artificial environments.
3. Nature-based activities promote ways to manage stress, engage in physical activity, socially connect with others and experience spirituality, all of which are important for longevity.
4. Natural environments promote the engagement in nature-based activities which have many health and well-being benefits.

A. V. Shappell (✉)
Department of Veterans Affairs, Patient Care Services, Washington, DC, USA

Georgetown University School of Medicine, Washington, DC, USA

George Washington University School of Medicine and Health Sciences, Washington, DC, USA

Uniformed Services University of the Health Sciences, Bethesda, MD, USA
e-mail: Antoinette.Shappell@va.gov

K. A. Burnett
Department of Veterans Affairs, Patient Care Services, Washington, DC, USA

S. H. Gartland
Department of Veterans Affairs Capt. James A. Lovell Federal Healthcare Center, North Chicago, IL, USA

R. E. Kheirbek, M. D. Llorente (eds.), *Current Perspectives on Centenarians*, International Perspectives on Aging 36,
https://doi.org/10.1007/978-3-031-30915-1_14

14.1 Introduction

Aging is a complex process with a host of variables impacting longevity. The Danish twin study, published in 1996, studied 2872 twin pairs born between 1870 and 1900 and found that the heritability of extreme longevity was 0.26 in men and 0.23 in women. As a result of this landmark study, many concluded that only about 25% of the average person's lifespan is dictated by our genes, whereas the other 75% is dictated by our lifestyle (Herskind et al., 1996). This statistic leaves one questioning "what characteristics and habits create a healthy lifestyle that promotes longevity?"

Undoubtably, the environment in which we live plays a role in our well-being. The connection of nature to human health and well-being has been studied for years. There are many notable correlations and benefits of spending time in nature including healthy ageing. The Biophilia Hypothesis postulates that human beings have an innate tendency to seek connections with nature and positively respond to natural environments for adaptation reasons, because nature is the environment in which they evolved (Kellert & Wilson, 1993). There are many ways to connect with nature ranging from enjoying panoramic views of the outdoors to listening and appreciating natural sounds to hiking the earth's terrain to cultivating plants for nutrition. Connecting with nature is beneficial for attaining and maintenance of general well-being as well as restoring well-being during times of illness or chronic disease states. This chapter will highlight the connection between time spent in nature and longevity.

14.2 Illustrative Vignette

Ms. M, a 103yo widowed Italian woman has lived her life on the Italian island of Sardinia. She was the youngest in a sibship of seven and grew up on her parent's coastal property. She completed elementary school education and was married at the age of 17. She raised her five children and later helped to raise her grandchildren. Her husband, who was a farmer, passed away 2 years ago at the age of 104.

She eats small meals, mostly consisting of vegetables, that are locally grown on her family's estate and meat on occasion. She lives with her youngest daughter and granddaughter. Her only medical problem is hypercholesteremia. She had an appendectomy at age twenty-one. Ms. M never smoked tobacco and only occasionally drinks alcohol, usually red wine on celebratory occasions. She has no history of any illicit drug use.

Mrs. M is a devout Catholic and still attends weekly mass. She spends her days tending to her herb garden and knitting on her patio while appreciating natural scenery. She spends her evenings playing cards with family and taking short walks in her coastal village with friends.

14.3 Longevity and Well-being

The Danish Twin Study highlighted the significance of non-heritable factors for longevity. Stress, lifestyle, religion/ spirituality, social connectedness and the environment all impact longevity and well-being. Natural environments are more restorative cognitively, psychologically, and physiologically compared to urban or artificial environments. Additionally, natural environments promote the engagement in nature-based activities which have many health and well-being benefits.

14.3.1 Stress & Longevity and Well-being

Stress, particularly chronic stress, is linked with accelerated aging. Life adversity and stress can modulate the rate of cellular aging. Although stress is an inevitable part of life, the knowledge of its impact on aging leads one to believe that restoring well-being or managing stress well may curtail the aging process thus yielding to longevity. Aging of centenarians has been shown to be slowed down by good adaptability, which allows for a positive and effective response to stress throughout their whole lives (Tafaro et al., 2009). The ability to adapt to adversity and thereby manage stress successfully is key to extraordinary ageing. In a study of 263 centenarians, Buettner found that the world's longest-lived people experience stress but have daily routines to shed or cope with stress (Buettner & Skemp, 2016). Natural environments are rich in characteristics necessary for restorative experiences and the body of literature connecting the healing power of nature-based activities for the health and well-being of the elderly is growing (Gagliardi & Piccinini, 2019).

14.3.2 Physical Activity & Longevity and Well-being

Maintaining a physically active lifestyle for the benefit of human health has been written about throughout the medical literature for decades. Researchers have hypothesized about the various types of physical activity, how much time and how frequently one needs to engage in physical activity for optimal health and wellness. The U.S. Department of Health and Human Services' guidelines for physical activity recommend 150 minutes of moderate-intensity activity per week or 75 minutes of more vigorous exercise per week (U.S. Department of Health and Human Services, 2018).

While exercise is important for health, well-being and longevity, researchers at Johns Hopkins emphasize that even minimal amounts of exercise make a difference (Ahmed et al., 2013). More recently, a study of older adults demonstrated the benefits associated with participating in any leisure time physical activity for reducing mortality risk including cardiovascular and cancer mortality (Watts et al., 2022).

This is further supported by research done by Dan Buettner, in collaboration with National Geographic and National Institute on Aging. Together, they used epidemiological data, statistics and birth certificates and found five demographically confirmed, geographically defined areas with the highest percentage of centenarians. He coined the term, Blue Zones, for these five areas around the globe. Buettner and his team explored these areas and subsequently published the common evidenced based denominators that they believed to slow the aging process (Buettner & Skemp, 2016). Among commonalities seen in the Blue Zones was "moving naturally." They learned that centenarians were not necessarily running marathons or frequent members of fitness centers but rather lived in environments that prompted them to move regularly without cognitively thinking about moving (Buettner & Skemp, 2016).

14.3.3 Religion/ Spirituality & Longevity and Well-being

A connection between religion, spirituality, aging and health has been recognized and reviewed for years (Zimmer et al., 2016; Koenig, 2012). There is wide breadth of literature citing benefits of religiosity and/ or spirituality (r/s) with cardiovascular conditions (Abu et al., 2018; Powell et al., 2003), mental health (Vitorino et al., 2018) and cognition (Agli et al., 2015). Moreover, adults who were religious/ spiritual showed lower cortisol responses to laboratory stressors suggesting that spiritual and/or religious individuals may experience a protective effect against the neuroendocrine consequences of stress (Tartaro et al., 2005) which impacts overall well-being.

Research has linked (r/s) with longevity (McCullough et al., 2000; Powell et al., 2003; Chida et al., 2009) and reveals that attending faith-based services four times per month will add four to 14 years of life expectancy (Musick et al., 2004). A study of 16 centenarians in the Midwest region of the United States, found that spirituality served as a critical component in the everyday lives of the participants, while providing a framework for helping older adults make sense of having lived a very long life (Manning et al., 2012). Religion, and more broadly, spirituality provides different perspectives and meaning for people but also provides a social network. This is further supported by interviews conducted on centenarians as part of a qualitative study as their findings indicated that spirituality is a key factor of support, an important resource in late life, and contains aspect of continuity over the life course for participants (Manning et al., 2012). In a larger study of 263 centenarians, all but five belonged to some faith-based community (Buettner & Skemp, 2016).

14.3.4 Social Connectedness & Longevity and Well-being

Naturally, humans are social beings. Social relationships, similar to physical activity and movement, are important/ vital for health and well-being. Loneliness is an emotional response to social isolation. Both loneliness and social isolation have been correlated with an increase in mortality (Holt-Lunstad, 2018, Steptoe et al., 2013). Studies have found that loneliness, social isolation and lack of social relationships are linked to cardiovascular disease (Golaszewski et al., 2022; Holt-Lunstad and Smith, 2016) and behaviors such as smoking, alcohol and drug use (Farmer et al., 2022; Cubbin et al., 2008), all of which negatively impact mortality. Strong social relationships, however, can increase the likelihood of survival by as much as 50% relative to individuals whose relationships are weaker (Holt-Lunstad et al., 2010). This is consistent with findings that highly satisfying relationships correlate with improved physical health, decreased stress, healthier lifestyle choices and longevity (Waldinger, 2015). In his study of centenarians, Buettner notes that one of the common denominators among centenarians is putting loved ones first. His work revealed that successful centenarians are more likely to commit to a life partner, invest in their children with time and love and are more likely to live with or near their families (Buettner & Skemp, 2016).

14.3.5 Environment & Longevity and Well-being

When considering environmental factors on longevity, the chapter would be incomplete without highlighting the impact of pollution on well-being and longevity. The 2017 *Lancet* Commission on pollution and health reviewed data from the Global Burden of Diseases, Injuries and Risk Factors Study (GBD) 2015 and found that pollution was responsible for an estimated nine million deaths or 16% of all deaths globally (Landrigan et al., 2018). This statistic makes pollution the world's largest environmental risk factor for disease and premature death.

Are Longevity & Well-being Connected with Nature?

14.3.6 Stress & Nature

> I go to nature to be soothed and healed, and to have my senses put in order. –John Burroughs.

> The physician heals, Nature makes well. –Aristotle.

Ulrich, a pioneer in exploring the restorative benefits of nature, conducted a study that reviewed the rates of patients recovering from gallbladder surgeries in relationship to their views from their hospital windows. He found that those patients with a natural view of a garden and trees spent fewer days in the hospital, requested less pain medication and had more positive attitudes when compared to those patients who had a view of a brick wall (Ulrich, 1984). Nearly four decades later, photos of nature are commonly seen in hospitals and clinics and healing gardens have been strategically placed at hospitals, providing a place for both patients and staff to relax, recover and rejuvenate while appreciating the beauty.

Soon after publishing a comparison of surgical recovery rates with patient window views, Ulrich proposed the Stress Recovery Theory (SRT). This is a psycho-evolutionary theory that proposes that engagement with natural environments promote the recovery or restoration from excessively arousing states, both psychologically and physiologically. This is done by activation of the parasympathetic nervous system. (Ulrich et al., 1991). He emphasized a decline in attention, and performance in general, as a consequence of stress. To investigate his hypothesis, Ulrich tested the psychological benefits of natural environments by exposing 120 subjects to view a 10-minute stressful film of workplace accidents. Then, he exposed the subjects to another 10-minute film of one of six different recovery environments which were videos of various natural and urban settings. A battery of physiological measures was recorded. Subjects also gave self-ratings of their affective states. The results of Ulrich's experiment were then compared between groups exposed to films of natural versus urban settings for their recovery environments. Overall, those subjects who viewed the natural recovery environments consistently demonstrated positive changes in the physiological activity levels recorded, had a shift towards a more positively toned emotional state and these changes were also accompanied by sustained attention/intake. His findings were consistent with his predictions of restorative influences of nature thereby supporting the psycho-evolutionary theory.

Rachel and Stephen Kaplan (1989, 1995) published their Attention Restoration Theory (ART), another psychological restoration theory, which is centered more on restoration of cognition. It suggests that mental fatigue and concentration can be improved by spending time in or looking at nature. Mental fatigue may be the result of prolonged periods of concentration but also from energy used for "directed attention" also known as "voluntary attention" which was described by William James in 1892. One can maintain focus by both directing their attention to a particular task and by simultaneously inhibiting all potential incoming distractions. A common example to illustrate directed attention is when one may direct their attention to their computer when working while also inhibiting or blocking incoming distractions such as traffic from outside their office window. Directed attention fatigue is more common in busy, crowded urban areas. Prolonged mental effort leads to "directed attention fatigue" and often has devastating impacts. ART conjectured that people respond to nature and natural environments with "fascination" or "involuntary or effortless" attention which allows for "resting" of the brain. According to ART, contact with nature and spending time in natural environments is thought to improve cognitive function by replenishing "directed attention."

Both Stress Recovery & Attention Recovery theories share an evolutionary approach and are supported by the Biophilia Theory. They both describe the health benefits of contact with nature and postulate that natural environments make us smarter, improve our moods and are more restorative than urban or artificial environments. In ART, "mental fatigue" is what drives an individual to a restorative place whereas "physiologic stress" is the driver for restoration in SRT. Another difference between the theories is in the timing of the benefit. Whereas SRT proposes that time in nature immediately makes people happier and decreases stress levels,

ART posits that after our brains have restored from being fascinated by nature, we can then perform cognitive tasks better and more efficiently. Nonetheless, they both support that nature is good for managing stress and general wellbeing. Since Ulrich and the Kaplans published their respective research findings, there has been an increase of research citing the many health and well-being benefits of engaging with nature (Cameron et al., 2020; Pritchard et al., 2020) which set the stage for healthy ageing.

14.3.7 Nature-Based Activities & Well-being and Longevity

Shinrin-yoku (SY), also known as the Japanese art of "forest bathing," is an activity that centers on engaging with nature. The term was coined in 1982 by the Japanese Ministry of Agriculture, Forestry and Fisheries. "Shinrin" means "forest" and "yoku" means "bath" and it literally means to soak in the forest through our five senses. Although it originated in Japan, it has gained popularity around the world including in the United States. The activity is based on Shinto and Buddhist practices and does not require any training or specific techniques. Forest bathing can be done alone, in groups or even with a guide. It can be as simple as walking in a natural environment while being mindful of one's surroundings but may also include experiencing nature through other senses such as listening to, touching and smelling flowers and leaves. To experience the sense of taste, many will drink foraged tea in the forest. Research supports that forest walks, a nature-based activity, when compared with urban walks yielded lower concentrations of the stress hormone cortisol, decreased amygdala activation, lower pulse rate, lower blood pressure, greater parasympathetic nerve activity and lower sympathetic nerve activity (Lee et al., 2011; Park et al., 2010; Sudimac et al., 2022).

More recently, forest bathing has been studied among elderly with chronic illnesses. Elderly with chronic obstructive pulmonary disease (COPD) who participated in a leisure forest bathing trip were compared to a control group who visited an urban area. The group who engaged in forest bathing was found to have decreased levels of perforin and granzyme B expressions, accompanied by decreased levels of pro-inflammatory cytokines and stress hormones as well as improved moods as assessed by the profile of mood states (POMS) (Jia et al., 2016). These results among forest bathers were consistent with reduction of inflammation and stress levels. Another group studied forest bathing in elderly patients with chronic heart failure (CHF) as an adjunctive therapy and compared outcomes to patients who were in an urban control area. The group who engaged in forest bathing showed a significant reduction in brain natriuretic peptide (BNP) in comparison to the group who spent time in an urban area as well as their own baseline levels. The forest bathing group also had lower levels of cardiovascular disease related pathologic factors and improved emotional mood state, as measured by POMS, demonstrating that forest bathing had a beneficial effect on CHF patients and may be an effective adjunctive therapy for cardiovascular disorders (Mao et al., 2017). These studies are examples of how nature-based activities can improve health and well-being during times of illness.

Farming, an occupation which includes both growing crops and raising livestock, has been associated with exceptional longevity. Specifically, the occupation as a farmer at age 40 in the year 1930 was a predictor for male longevity (Gavrilov, 2015), which is consistent with studies showing that farming and having a farm background has had positive effects on late-life survival (Preston, 1998; Gavrilova, 2007). On a smaller scale, gardening is an activity that also gives the opportunity to immerse oneself in nature while reaping many health benefits. According to Buettner, many centenarians share the common hobby of gardening (Buettner, 2008). The pastime includes growing and caring for plants, cultivating food crops for home consumption and the growing of ornamental plants for aesthetic purposes. The activity of gardening is unique because it combines physical activity and allows for the exposure of vitamin D in the outdoors and communal gardens allow for the opportunity to engage in social interaction. Chalmin-Pui and colleagues electronically distributed a questionnaire within the United Kingdom and their data revealed that more frequent gardening (i.e. 2–3 times per week) corresponded to reductions in perceived stress, increased subjective well-being and increased self-reported physical activity levels. Their results are novel in that they observed a 'dose' effect with the perceived health benefits increasing in line with frequency of gardening activities (Chalmin-Pui et al., 2021). Another study conducted a field experiment comparing cortisol levels and self-reported moods in subjects after performing a stressful cognitive test. They found that thirty minutes of outdoor gardening led to restored positive moods and significantly lower salivary cortisol levels, when compared to those who engaged in thirty minutes of reading after the stressful task. The authors concluded that their results provided evidence that gardening, a nature-based activity, can promote neuroendocrine and affective restoration or relief from acute stress (Van Den Berg & Custers, 2011).

In addition to being a pastime of many centenarians, the therapeutic benefits of gardening gave rise to horticulture therapy in the nineteenth century. The word horticulture is derived from the Latin hortus, "garden," and colere, "to cultivate" and it is the art and science of cultivating plants in gardens for the purpose of human healing and rehabilitation by stimulating the five senses. Initially, documented as having positive benefits on those suffering from mental illness, it has also demonstrated to aid in healing of those who are suffering from physical and cognitive illness (Zhao et al., 2022). Horticulture therapy has also shown therapeutic value in older adults by improving physical function and quality of life, reducing BMI, improving cognitive function and enhancing a positive mood (Chan et al., 2017; Wang et al., 2022). Participation in horticulture activities also significantly improved the happiness, satisfaction, well-being and sleep quality of the elderly while also significantly increasing mucosal immunity proteins (Shen et al., 2022).

In conclusion, people exposed to chronic stress age more rapidly. However, regular exposure to nature and participation in nature-based activities can attenuate a stress response, and may enhance one's ability to adapt to adversity, a characteristic commonly seen among centenarians. The use of natural environments for pastime activities to maintain well-being as well as to restore health during times of illness is well recognized among elderly and centenarians. Time in nature is associated with lower blood pressure, heart rate, cortisol levels, improved cognition and positive affective states. Biomarkers of cardiovascular disorders, immunity, inflammation, stress levels, sleep quality and mood in elderly with chronic illnesses can also benefit from engagement with nature. Such measures are favorable and conducive to both well-being and longevity and, therefore, should be taken into consideration when understanding variables such as adaptability among centenarians.

14.3.8 Active Lifestyle & Nature

> Movement is a medicine for creating change in a person's physical, emotional, and mental states. –Carol Welch.

> Exercise and temperance can preserve something of our early strength even in old age. –Cicero.

In recent years, attention has also been given to the benefits of exercising while in "green spaces" or natural environments associated with vegetation and other natural elements (Taylor & Hochuli, 2017). "Green exercise" is a term that was first used in 2003 to describe the potential synergistic benefit to health that occurs when exercising while being exposed to nature (Pretty, J 2003). Studies suggest that people who exercise outdoors will exercise for longer periods of time and more energetically that those who only exercise indoors (Ceci & Hassmen, 1991; Focht, 2009). Moreover, there is evidence that people who use parks and other natural spaces are three times more likely to achieve recommended levels of physical activity (Giles-Corti et al., 2005).

Research supports that the availability of parks, trails and nature can positively affect people's attitudes toward being active and encourage physical activity (Wolf, 2008). One group of researchers found that participants tended to walk faster outdoors compared to when walking indoors while paradoxically reporting a lower rating of perceived exertion while outdoors (Focht, 2009). Left to interpretation, one may conclude that physical movement may feel as though it needs less effort than when in a natural environment. Therefore, it is not surprising that the longest living people in the world live in environments that promote an active lifestyle through natural movement.

In summary, an active lifestyle has been noted to be a common factor among centenarians. Whether engaging in an exercise program or moving naturally, doing so in natural environments appear to have superior benefits in comparison to doing so indoors.

14.3.9 *Religion/ Spirituality & Nature*

In all things of nature there is something of the marvelous. –Aristotle

On Earth there is no Heaven but there are pieces of it. –Jules Renard

Spirituality is an abstract topic, but the word is derived from the Latin "spiritus" which means "breadth of life." Spirituality has been defined as the human motivation to discover and connect with the sacred (Pargament, 1999). A present-day definition of spirituality by Kamitsis and Francis is "an individual's inner experience and/ or belief system, that gives meaning to existence, and subsequently allows one to transcend beyond the present context" (Kamitsis & Francis, 2013). Transcendence is thought to be at the core of spirituality (Buck, 2006). The word transcendence is derived from the Latin prefix "trans" meaning "beyond" and the word "scandare" meaning "to climb" so by definition, "achieving transcendence" means to rise above or climb beyond limitations. The very essence of nature seems to elicit a relatively unique emotional and spiritual experience (Ashley, 2007). Nature can be perceived as boundless and powerful while also invoking curiosity, thereby instilling many emotions, including a sense of awe (Ballew & Omoto, 2018). Commonly, positive nature experiences invoke a feeling of transcendence (Dustin et al., 2009) suggesting that time spent in nature is linked to spirituality (Marsh, 2008; Naor & Mayseless, 2019). While Naor and Mayseless (2019) were studying Nature Based Therapy (NBT) and its therapeutic effect, they note the positive effects of spirituality as a tangential finding. They found that nature was reportedly experienced as "an actual and tangible experience of the spiritual in physical form—nature as an embodiment of spirituality." Their findings illustrate the connection between the spiritual experience of a natural setting and the outdoors' significant therapeutic effects. Leisure and recreational activities in outdoor natural settings may also be associated with spiritual experiences (Heintzman, 2015). For example, human interaction with nature through gardening offers the development of spiritual well-being (Naor & Mayseless, 2019). A review of the practice of Shinrin-yoku or forest bathing found that this practice may also enhance or actualize human spirituality (Hansen & Jones, 2020). Therefore, it is not surprising that spirituality experienced in the outdoors, can add years to healthy longevity by decreasing stress and feelings of connectedness to something bigger than oneself.

In summary, both religion and spirituality are linked to longevity and well-being. Experiencing nature can be a spiritual experience as time spent in nature may facilitate feelings of transcendence. Notably, the vast majority of centenarians studied report being religious or spiritual.

14.3.10 Social Connectedness & Nature

> Perhaps the secret of living well is not in having all the answers but in pursuing unanswerable questions in good company. –Rachel Naomi Remen

> People experience the life-changing force of healing relationships when something powerful comes out of one and touches something good in another. –Larry Crabb

The benefits of spending time in nature include improved mood and well-being and decreased anxiety and stress (Kaplan, 1995; Gerdes et al., 2022; Hartig et al., 2003; Ulrich et al., 1991, White 2019). Such factors increase the likelihood that people will connect and engage with others. The well-being benefit of green space may rely on improved social interaction (Maas et al., 2009). Izenstark and Ebata demonstrated this by inviting mother and daughter dyads to spend 20 minutes walking through a nature area and 20 minutes walking in a shopping mall (Izenstark & Ebata, 2017). Results revealed that the nature walk was perceived as more fun, interesting, relaxing and also contributed to great cohesion between the mother and daughter. This study reinforces how an outdoor activity in nature can strengthen family relations. Another group of researchers in Singapore studied how relationships between social cohesion, nature experiences and nature connection could interrelate and vary across different types of urban green spaces. Oh and colleagues found that people who had more frequent garden visits, identified strongly as a part of nature, enjoyed being in nature and are also those who perceived stronger social cohesion (Oh et al., 2022).

Viewing gardens and taking part in gardening was associated with improved well-being, increased physical activity and reduced social isolation (Howarth et al., 2020). In Willcox's studies of centenarians in Okinawa, Japan, he noted that gardening is a common hobby of residents, and many maintain small personal gardens well into old age. Willcox found that positive health effects are derived from the social benefits of gardening. He further describes how Okinawans value the concept of social connectedness, or "yuimaru", and how bringing and sharing their produce at a local market serves as a venue for this connection with others (Willcox et al., 2002). In addition to such local or farmers' markets, community gardens, are another form of exposure and connection to natural environments. Community gardens, where people of different families garden side by side or communally, also provide opportunity to engage and socially connect with others thereby potentially contributing to community bonding and building a sense of community (Guitart et al., 2012).

In summary, social connectedness is positively correlated with longevity and nature-based activities especially gardening facilitate a means for fostering social relationships.

14.3.11 Natural Environment

> Live in the sunshine, swim the sea, drink the wild air. – Ralph Waldo Emerson

> If human civilization is going to invade the waters of the earth, then let it be first of all to carry a message of respect – Jacques Yves Cousteau, Philippe Diole (1972) "The whale, mighty monarch of the sea"

There are many different types of pollutants or unwanted waste, linked to various diseases in humans. Pollution can be found in air, land and water. Fortunately, the harmful effects of pollution can be countered to some degree with nature. Green space has been linked with increased longevity in Japan. (Takano et al., 2002). Trees, for example, provide a significant number of benefits including improving both air and water pollution, mitigating heat by lowering temperatures, shielding people from UV rays as well as providing natural beauty. Moreover, trees and vegetation decrease air temperatures which has an indirect benefit of reducing energy needs for cooling which in turn increases pollutant emissions. Reduction in air temperature also make conditions for smog less favorable.

Green space has been shown to provide air quality benefits which is particularly important for human health. Specifically, trees, remarkably help to reduce air pollution. They are effective at filtering atmospheric pollutants such as sulfur dioxide and nitrogen dioxide through their leaves and also removing particulate matter from the air. Particulate Matter (PM), also known as particle pollution in air, has been linked to adverse health effects. Examples of PM include but are not limited to smog, smoke, dust, bacteria, viruses, fungi, mold and allergens.

In regard to water pollution, the primary benefit of trees is that the rain can be intercepted by their leaves and gradually released by evaporation or transpiration rather than landing on buildings or other urban surfaces, picking up pollutants and then carrying them to streams and other bodies of water. This significantly reduces storm water pollution.

In summary, one's environment plays a role in their health and a natural environment has many advantages and can minimize the impact of pollution, which can be detrimental to well-being and longevity.

14.4 Conclusion

Health, well-being and longevity are linked to stress management, levels of physical activity, religion/ spirituality, social connectedness and our environment. All these factors can be positively influenced by spending time in nature.

14.5 Chapter Summary

Aside from genetics, longevity is influenced by many variables to include stress management, levels of physical activity, religiousness/ spirituality, social connectedness and the environment in which we live. Nature has many restorative properties which help us to recover from stress which may in turn curtail the aging process. Health and well-being benefit from both spirituality and social relationships while experiencing nature has been shown to improve one's health and well-being. Experiences in nature through nature-based activities such as gardening and forest bathing decrease stress, promote movement, have facilitated both social relationships and spirituality further supporting and perhaps synergistically promoting health and well-being.

Multiple Choice Questions

1. How are natural environments restorative?
   - A. Cognitively
   - B. Psychologically
   - C. Physiologically
   - D. All of the above

   CORRECT ANSWER: D
2. Nature based activities promote ways to
   - A. Manage stress
   - B. Engage in physical activity
   - C. Socially connect with others and experience spirituality
   - D. All of the above

   CORRECT ANSWER: D
3. Both Stress Restoration & Attention Recovery theories:
   - A. Postulate that time in nature can be stressful.
   - B. Describe the health and well-being benefits of contact with nature.
   - C. Support the importance of social connectedness.
   - D. Describe the importance of regular physical activity.

   CORRECT ANSWER: B
4. Spirituality can be described as having components of:
   - A. Motivation to connect with the sacred
   - B. Rising above limitations
   - C. Connectedness to something bigger
   - D. All of the above

   CORRECT ANSWER: D.

References

Abu, H. O., Ulbricht, C., Ding, E., Allison, J. J., Salmoirago-Blotcher, E., Goldberg, R. J., & Kiefe, C. I. (2018). Association of religiosity and spirituality with quality of life in patients with cardiovascular disease: A systematic review. *Quality of Life Research, 27*(11), 2777–2797. https://doi.org/10.1007/s11136-018-1906-4. Epub 2018 Jun 11. PMID: 29948601; PMCID: PMC6196107.

Agli, O., Bailly, N., & Ferrand, C. (2015). Spirituality and religion in older adults with dementia: A systematic review. *International Psychogeriatrics, 27*(5), 715–725. https://doi.org/10.1017/S1041610214001665. Epub 2014 Aug 26.

Ahmed, H. A., Blaha, M. J., Nasir, K., et al. (2013). Low-risk lifestyle, coronary calcium, cardiovascular events, and mortality: Results from MESA. *American Journal of Epidemiology, 178*(1), 12–21. https://doi.org/10.1093/aje/kws453

Ashley, P. (2007). Toward an understanding and definition of wilderness spirituality. *Australian Geographer, 38*(1), 53–69. https://doi.org/10.1080/00049180601175865

Ballew, M. T., & Omoto, A. M. (2018). Absorption: How nature experience promote awe and other positive emotions. *Ecopsychology*, 26–35. https://doi.org/10.1089/eco.2017.0044

Buck, H. G. (2006). Spirituality: Concept analysis and model development. *Holistic Nursing Practice, 20*(6), 288–292.

Buettner, D. (2008). *The blue zones: Lessons for living longer from the people who've lived the longest*. National Geographic Society.

Buettner, D., & Skemp, S. (2016). Blue zones: Lessons from the World's longest lived. *American Journal of Lifestyle Medicine, 10*(5), 318–321. https://doi.org/10.1177/1559827616637066. PMID: 30202288; PMCID: PMC6125071.

Cameron, R. W., Brindley, P., Mears, M., McEwan, K., Ferguson, F., Sheffield, D., et al. (2020). Where the wild things are! Do urban green spaces with greater avian biodiversity promote more positive emotions in humans? *Urban Ecosystem, 23*(2), 301–317.

Ceci, R., & Hassmen, P. (1991). Self-monitored exercise at three different RPE intensities in treadmill vs field running. *Medicine and Science in Sports and Exercise, 23*(6), 732–738.

Chalmin-Pui, L. S., Griffiths, A., Roe, J., et al. (2021). Why garden? – Attitudes and the perceived health benefits of home gardening. *Cities, 112*, 103118, ISSN 0264–2751. https://doi.org/10.1016/j.cities.2021.103118

Chan, H. Y., Ho, R. C., Mahendran, R., Ng, K. S., Tam, W. W., Rawtaer, I., Tan, C. H., Larbi, A., Feng, L., Sia, A., Ng, M. K., Gan, G. L., & Kua, E. H. (2017). Effects of horticultural therapy on elderly' health: Protocol of a randomized controlled trial. *BMC Geriatrics, 17*(1), 192. https://doi.org/10.1186/s12877-017-0588-z. PMID: 28851276; PMCID: PMC5576101.

Chida, Y., Steptoe, A., & Powell, L. H. (2009). Religiosity/spirituality and mortality: A systematic quantitative review. *Psychotherapy and Psychosomatics, 78*(2), 81–90.

Cubbin, C., Egerter, S., Braveman, P., & Pedregon, V. (2008). Where we live matters for our health: Neighborhoods and health. In *Issue brief 3. Neighborhoods and health* (p. 11). Robert Wood Johnson Foundation.

Dustin, D. L., Bricker, K. S., & Schwab, K. A. (2009). People and nature: Toward an ecological model of health promotion. *Leisure Sciences, 32*(1), 3–14.

Farmer, A. Y., Wang, Y., Peterson, N. A., Borys, S., & Hallcom, D. K. (2022). Social isolation profiles and older adult substance use: A latent profile analysis. *The Journals of Gerontology. Series B, Psychological Sciences and Social Sciences, 77*(5), 919–929. https://doi.org/10.1093/geronb/gbab078. PMID: 33959768.

Focht, B. C. (2009). Brief walks in outdoor and laboratory environments: Effects on affective responses, enjoyment, and intentions to walk for exercise. *Research Quarterly for Exercise and Sport, 80*(3), 611–620.

Gagliardi, C., & Piccinini, F. (2019). The use of nature - based activities for the Well-being of older people: An integrative literature review. *Archives of Gerontology and Geriatrics, 83*, 315–327. https://doi.org/10.1016/j.archger.2019.05.012. Epub 2019 May 14. PMID: 31128876.

Gerdes, M. E., Aistis, L. A., Sachs, N. A., Williams, M., Roberts, J. D., & Rosenberg Goldstein, R. E. (2022). Reducing Anxiety with Nature and Gardening (RANG): Evaluating the Impacts of Gardening and Outdoor Activities on Anxiety among U.S. Adults during the COVID-19 Pandemic. *International Journal of Environmental Research and Public Health, 19*(9), 5121. https://doi.org/10.3390/ijerph19095121. PMID: 35564513; PMCID: PMC9100102.

Giles-Corti, B., Broomhall, M. H., Knuiman, M., et al. (2005). Increasing walking: How important is distance to, attractiveness, and size of public open space? *American Journal of Preventive Medicine, 28*(2 suppl 2), 169–176.

Golaszewski, N. M., LaCroix, A. Z., Godino, J. G., et al. (2022). Evaluation of social isolation, loneliness, and cardiovascular disease among older women in the US. *JAMA Network Open, 5*(2), e2146461. https://doi.org/10.1001/jamanetworkopen.2021.46461

Guitart, D., Pickering, C., & Byrne, J. (2012). Past results and future directions in urban community gardens research. *Urban Forestry & Urban Greening, 11*, 364–373. https://doi.org/10.1016/j.ufug.2012.06.007

Hansen, M. M., & Jones, R. (2020). The interrelationship of Shinrin-Yoku and spirituality: A scoping review. *Journal of Alternative and Complementary Medicine, 26*(12), 1093–1104. https://doi.org/10.1089/acm.2020.0193. Epub 2020 Sep 15. PMID: 32931299.

Hartig, T., Evans, G. W., Jamner, L., Davis, D., & Gärling, T. (2003). Tracking restoration in natural and urban field settings. *Journal of Environmental Psychology, 23*, 109–123.

Heintzman, P. (2015). Leisure and spirituality biblical, historical, and contemporary perspectives. Baker Academic.

Herskind, A. M., McGue, M., Holm, N. V., Sorensen, T. I. A., Harvlad, B., & Vaupel, J. W. (1996). The heritability of human longevity: A population-based study of 2,872 Danish twin pairs born 1870-1900. *Human Genetics, 96*, 319–323.

Holt-Lunstad, J. (2018). Why social relationships are important for physical health: A systems approach to understanding and modifying risk and protection. *Annual Review of Psychology, 4*(69), 437–458. https://doi.org/10.1146/annurev-psych-122216-011902. Epub 2017 Oct 16. PMID: 29035688

Holt-Lunstad, J., Smith, T. B., & Layton, J. B. (2010). Social relationships and mortality risk: A meta-analytic review. *PLoS Medicine, 7*, e1000316.

Holt-Lunstad, J., & Smith, T. B. (2016). Loneliness and social isolation as risk factors for CVD: implications for evidence-based patient care and scientific inquiry. *Heart, 102*, 987–989.

Howarth, M., Brettle, A., Hardman, M., & Maden, M. (2020). What is the evidence for the impact of gardens and gardening on health and well-being: A scoping review and evidence-based logic model to guide healthcare strategy decision making on the use of gardening approaches as a social prescription. *BMJ Open, 10*(7), e036923. https://doi.org/10.1136/bmjopen-2020-036923

Izenstark, D., & Ebata, A. (2017). The effects of the natural environment on attention and family cohesion: An experimental study. *Children, Youth and Environments, 27*(2), 93–109.

James, W. (1892). *Psychology: The briefer course*. Holt.

Jia, B. B., Yang, Z. X., Mao, G. X., Lyu, Y. D., Wen, X. L., Xu, W. H., Lyu, X. L., Cao, Y. B., & Wang, G. F. (2016). Health effect of forest bathing trip on elderly patients with chronic obstructive pulmonary disease. *Biomedical and Environmental Sciences, 29*(3), 212–218. https://doi.org/10.3967/bes2016.026. PMID: 27109132.

Kamitsis, I., & Francis, A. (2013). Spirituality mediates the relationships between engagement with nature and psychological wellbeing. *Journal of Environmental Psychology, 36*, 136–143. https://doi.org/10.1016/j.jenvp.2013.07.013

Kaplan, S. (1995). The restorative benefits of nature: Toward an integrative framework. *Journal of Environmental Psychology, 15*, 169–182.

Kaplan, R., & Kaplan, S. (1989). *The experience of nature. A psychological perspective*. Cambridge University Press.

Kellert, S. R., & Wilson, E. O. (1993). *The biophilia hypothesis*. Island Press.

Koenig, H. G. (2012). Religion, spirituality, and health: The research and clinical implications. *ISRN Psychiatry, 16*(2012), 278730. https://doi.org/10.5402/2012/278730. PMID: 23762764; PMCID: PMC3671693.

Landrigan, P. J., Fuller, R., Acosta, N. J. R., et al. (2018). The *lancet* commission on pollution and health. *Lancet, 391*, 462–512.

Lee, J., Park, B. J., Tsunetsugu, Y., et al. (2011). Effect of forest bathing on physiological and psychological responses in young Japanese male subjects. *Public Health, 125*(2), 93–100.

Maas, J., van Dillen, S. M., Verheij, R. A., & Groenewegen, P. P. (2009). Social contacts as a possible mechanisms behind the relation between green space and health. *Health & Place, 15*, 586–595.

Manning, L. K., Leek, J. A., & Radina, M. E. (2012). Making sense of extreme longevity: explorations into the spiritual lives of centenarians. *Journal of Religion, Spirituality and Aging, 24*(4), 345–359. https://doi.org/10.1080/15528030.2012.706737. Epub 2012 Sep 27. PMID: 23139646; PMCID: PMC3489187.

Mao, G., Cao, Y., Wang, B., Wang, S., Chen, Z., Wang, J., Xing, W., Ren, X., Lv, X., Dong, J., Chen, S., Chen, X., Wang, G., & Yan, J. (2017). The salutary influence of Forest bathing on elderly patients with chronic heart failure. *International Journal of Environmental Research and Public Health, 14*(4), 368. https://doi.org/10.3390/ijerph14040368. PMID: 28362327; PMCID: PMC5409569.

Marsh, P. E. (2008). Backcountry adventure as spiritual development: A means-end study. *Journal of Experiential Education, 30*(3), 290–293.

McCullough, M. E., Hoyt, W. T., Larson, D. B., Koenig, H. G., & Thoresen, C. (2000). Religious involvement and mortality: A meta-analytic review. *Health Psychology, 19*(3), 211–222.

Musick, M. A., House, J. S., & Williams, D. R. (2004). Attendance at religious services and mortality in a national sample. *Journal of Health and Social Behavior, 45*(2), 198–213. https://doi.org/10.1177/002214650404500206. PMID: 15305760.

Naor, L., & Mayseless, O. (2019). The therapeutic value of experiencing spirituality in nature. *Spirituality in Clinical Practice.*

Oh R, Zhang Y, Nghiem L et al. (2022). Connection to nature and time spent in gardens predicts social cohesion. *Urban Forestry and Urban Greeening*. https://doi.org/10.1016/j.ufug.2022.127655

Pargament, K. I. (1999). The psychology of religion and spirituality? Yes and no. *The International Journal for the Psychology of Religion, 9*, 3–16.

Park, B. J., Tsunetsugu, Y., Kasetani, et al. (2010). The physiological effects of *Shinrin-yoku* (taking in the forest atmosphere or forest bathing): Evidence from field experiments in 24 forests across Japan. *Environmental Health Preventive Medicine, 15*, 18–26.

Powell, L. H., Shahabi, L., & Thoresen, C. E. (2003). Religion and spirituality. Linkages to physical health. *American Psychology, 58*(1), 36–52. https://doi.org/10.1037/0003-066x.58.1.36. PMID: 12674817.

Pretty, J., Griffin, M., Sellens, M., & Pretty, C. *Green exercise: Complementary roles of nature, exercise and diet in physical and emotional Well-being and implications for public health policy*. University of Essex; CES Occasional Paper 2003–1.

Pritchard, A., Richardson, M., Sheffield, D., & McEwan, K. (2020). The relationship between nature connectedness and eudaimonic Well-being: A meta-analysis. *Journal of Happiness Studies, 21*(3), 1145–1167. https://doi.org/10.1007/s10902-019-00118-6

Shen, J. L., Hung, B. L., & Fang, S. H. (2022). Horticulture therapy affected the mental status, sleep quality, and salivary markers of mucosal immunity in an elderly population. *Scientific Reports, 12*(1), 10246. https://doi.org/10.1038/s41598-022-14534-x. PMID: 35715581; PMCID: PMC9205955.

Steptoe, A., Shankar, A., Demakakos, P., & Wardle, J. (2013). Social isolation, loneliness, and all-cause mortality in older men and women. *Proceedings of the National Academy of Sciences of the United States of America, 110*, 5797–5801.

Sudimac, S., Sale, V. & Kühn, S. (2022). How nature nurtures: Amygdala activity decreases as the result of a one-hour walk in nature. *Molecular Psychiatry*. https://doi.org/10.1038/s41380-022-01720-6.

Tafaro, L., Tombolillo, M. T., Brükner, N., Troisi, G., Cicconetti, P., Motta, M., Cardillo, E., Bennati, E., & Marigliano, V. (2009). Stress in centenarians. *Archives of Gerontology and Geriatrics, 48*(3), 353–355. https://doi.org/10.1016/j.archger.2008.03.001. Epub 2008 Apr 23. PMID: 18433899.

Takano, T., Nakamura, N., & Watanabe, M. (2002). Urban residential environments and senior citizens' longevity in megacity areas: The importance of walkable green spaces. *Journal of Epidemiology Common Health, 56*, 913–918.

Tartaro, J., Luecken, L. J., & Gunn, H. E. (2005). Exploring heart and soul: Effects of religiosity/spirituality and gender on blood pressure and cortisol stress responses. *Journal of Health Psychology, 10*(6), 753–766. https://doi.org/10.1177/1359105305057311. PMID: 16176954.

Taylor, L., & Hochuli, D. F. (2017). Defining greenspace: multiple uses across multiple disciplines. *Landscape and Urban Planning, 158*, 25–38. https://doi.org/10.1016/j.landurbplan.2016.09.024

U.S. Department of Health and Human Services. (2018). Physical Activity Guidelines for Americans, 2nd edition. Retrieved from https://health.gov/paguidelines/second-edition/pdf/Physical_Activity_Guidelines_2nd_edition.pdf

Ulrich, R. S. (1984). View through a window may influence recovery from surgery. *Science, 224*(4647), 420–421.

Ulrich, R. S., Simons, R. F., Losito, B. D., et al. (1991). Stress recovery during exposure to natural and urban environments. *Journal of Enviornmental Psychology, 11*, 201–230.

Van Den Berg, A. E., & Custers, M. H. (2011). Gardening promotes neuroendocrine and affective restoration from stress. *Journal of Health Psychology, 16*(1), 3–11. https://doi.org/10.1177/1359105310365577. Epub 2010 Jun 3. PMID: 20522508.

Vitorino, L. M., Lucchetti, G., Leão, F. C., Vallada, H., & Peres, M. F. P. (2018). The association between spirituality and religiousness and mental health. *Scientific Reports, 8*(1), 17233. https://doi.org/10.1038/s41598-018-35380-w. PMID: 30467362; PMCID: PMC6250706.

Waldinger, R. (2015). What makes a good life? Lessons from the longest study on happiness. TED Talks. https://www.ted.com/talks/robert_waldinger_what_makes_a_good_life_lessons_from_the_longest_study_on_happiness

Wang, Z., Zhang, Y., Lu, S., Tan, L., Guo, W., Lown, M., Hu, X., & Liu, J. (2022). Horticultural therapy for general health in the older adults: A systematic review and meta-analysis. *PLoS One, 17*(2), e0263598. https://doi.org/10.1371/journal.pone.0263598. PMID: 35143551; PMCID: PMC8830630.

Watts, E. L., Matthews, C. E., Freeman, J. R., Gorzelitz, J. S., Hong, H. G., Liao, L. M., McClain, K. M., Saint-Maurice, P. F., Shiroma, E. J., & Moore, S. C. (2022). Association of leisure time physical activity types and risks of all-cause, cardiovascular, and cancer mortality among older adults. *JAMA Network Open, 5*(8), e2228510. https://doi.org/10.1001/jamanetworkopen.2022.28510. PMID: 36001316; PMCID: PMC9403775.

Willcox, B. J., Willcox, D. C., & Suzuki, M. (2002). The healing web: Yuimaru in Okinawa. In *The Okinawa program: How the world's longest-lived people achieve everlasting health--and how you can too* (pp. 279–280). essay). Three Rivers Press.

Wolf, K. L. (2008). City trees, nature and physical activity: A research review. *Arborist News, 17*(1), 22–24.

Zhao, Y., Liu, Y., & Wang, Z. (2022). Effectiveness of horticultural therapy in people with dementia: A quantitative systematic review. *Journal of Clinical Nursing, 31*(13–14), 1983–1997. https://doi.org/10.1111/jocn.15204. Epub 2020 Feb 20. PMID: 32017241.

Zimmer, Z., Jagger, C., Chiu, C. T., Ofstedal, M. B., Rojo, F., & Saito, Y. (2016). Spirituality, religiosity, aging and health in global perspective: A review. *SSM Population Health, 10*(2), 373–381. https://doi.org/10.1016/j.ssmph.2016.04.009. PMID: 29349154; PMCID: PMC5758000.

Chapter 15
Supercentenarians

Maithri Kondapaka and Raya Elfadel Kheirbek

Key Take Away Points

1. Supercentenarians are rare.
2. Supercentenarians are "experts" at delaying chronic disease and disability.
3. Global collaboration is crucial for assembling a validated database of supercentenarians.
4. There is no consensus on the trajectory of mortality in extreme age.

Illustrative Vignette

Jeanne Louise Calment was born in Arles, France in 1875. During her long life, spanning approximately 122 years, she witnessed two World Wars, the 1918 Spanish Flu Pandemic, the advent of aviation, and the evolution of human communication from the telegraph to the internet. When asked about her exceptional longevity she stated, "I'm starting to think I must be a phenomenon." (Jeune et al., 2010*)*

15.1 Supercentenarians and the Compression of Morbidity

A supercentenarian is defined as any individual greater than the age of 110. These rare and exceptional individuals embody the concept of "compression of morbidity". First described in 1980 by James Fries, the "compression of morbidity" hypothesis posits that if the onset of infirmity can be delayed, then the lifetime burden of illness can be compressed into a period of time closer to the end of life (Fries, 2000).

M. Kondapaka · R. E. Kheirbek (✉)
University of Maryland School of Medicine, Baltimore, MD, USA
e-mail: rkheirbek@som.umaryland.edu

R. E. Kheirbek, M. D. Llorente (eds.), *Current Perspectives on Centenarians*, International Perspectives on Aging 36,
https://doi.org/10.1007/978-3-031-30915-1_15

Individuals at the extremes of age can be divided into three conceptual categories: survivors, delayers, and escapers. Survivors are those individuals who develop chronic illness before the age of 80, while delayers are those individuals who develop chronic illness after the age of 80. Escapers, on the other hand, are individuals who live to 100 years of age and beyond without developing common chronic illnesses (Evert et al., 2003).

Several studies have demonstrated that at the extremes of age not only does the overall incidence of so called "age-related diseases" decrease, but the onset of such diseases is delayed (Akushevich et al., 2012; Evert et al., 2003; Hitt et al., 1999).

Akushevich et al. in their 2012 study identified two specific patterns regarding the incidence of age-related disease. The incidence of some diseases initially increases with age, but eventually plateaus or declines. These include heart failure, myocardial infarction, stroke, renal disease, colon cancer, Parkinson's Disease, and Alzheimer's Disease. The incidence of other diseases declines continually with age or after a short period of increase. These include COPD, asthma, emphysema, diabetes, prostate cancer, and female breast cancer (Akushevich et al., 2012).

Evert et al. in their 2003 study observed that approximately 50% of their 424 subjects (aged 97–119 years) reached the age of 100 without developing heart disease, stroke, or non-skin cancer (Evert et al., 2003). An additional third of these individuals delayed the onset of these diseases until or after the age of 80 (Evert et al., 2003). In a larger 2012 study conducted by Andersen et al. which included a broader profile of diseases (including COPD, diabetes, hypertension, osteoporosis, thyroid disease, and dementia), 15% of the subjects reached the age of 100 without developing common age-related diseases (Andersen et al., 2012).

Although autopsy data is limited, there are anecdotal case studies which support these observational findings. One such study, conducted on a deceased centenarian woman from Okinawa, not only noted an absence of significant coronary artery disease, stroke, and cancer, but also showed little evidence of major organ damage, although there was evidence of amyloid deposition in multiple organ systems (Bernstein et al., 2004).

The development of cancer at advanced age has been of particular interest. Numerous demographic, epidemiologic, and autopsy studies demonstrate that the incidence of cancer peaks between the ages of 85–90 and subsequently plateaus or even declines as patients approach ages close to 100 and above. Mortality due to cancer and rates of metastatic disease follow a similar trajectory. This pattern is observed among various cancers including esophageal, stomach, colon, pancreatic, lung, bladder, uterine, ovarian, and renal cancer as well as blood cancers such as leukemia, multiple myeloma, and non-Hodgkin lymphoma (Bonafè et al., 2002; DeSantis et al., 2019; Hashim et al., 2020; Miyaishi et al., 2000; Nolen et al., 2017; Pavlidis et al., 2012; Smith, 1996; Stanta et al., 1997).

Not only is the onset of chronic disease delayed, but for many centenarians, functional status is also preserved for a longer period of time with many individuals remaining independent well into their nineties. (Hitt et al., 1999; Silver et al., 2001).

15.2 Supercentenarians Versus Centenarians

But how do supercentenarians fare? Living to the extremes of age is not without its challenges, as supercentenarians often face significant blindness, hearing loss, poor dentition, thin skin, sarcopenia, and poor orientation (though long-term memory may be preserved) (Coles, 2004). However, observational studies involving supercentenarians show that individuals greater than the age of 110 also markedly delay or escape the onset of age-related disease, physical impairment, and cognitive decline (Andersen et al., 2012; Schoenhofen et al., 2006). Oftentimes, they did so to a greater degree when compared to centenarians or even semi-supercentenarians. Not only did supercentenarians have decreased incidence of age-related disease, but they also displayed the greatest delay in onset of disease. Compared to centenarians, there is a greater proportion of "escapers" in the supercentenarian population compared to "survivors" (Andersen et al., 2012). In general, supercentenarians spend a smaller percentage of their lives with disease such that their health span is nearly equivalent to their life span (Andersen et al., 2012).

In some studies, most supercentenarians did not develop clinically significant disease until the average age of 105–109, although limited autopsy studies confirm the presence of subclinical disease burden (Andersen et al., 2012; Willcox et al., 2008a). Cataracts, osteoarthritis, and fractures tended to be the most common ailments, while heart disease, stroke, cancer, and diabetes, which still occur to some degree in younger centenarians, were rare or not evident among supercentenarians (Schoenhofen et al., 2006; Willcox et al., 2008a).

Remarkably, supercentenarians have been noted to maintain their independence, on average, until the age of 105 thus delaying disability for 5–10 years longer than their centenarian counterparts (Willcox et al., 2008a; Willcox et al., 2008b). In an observational study conducted by Schoenhofen et al., of the 32 supercentenarians included, 41% required minimal assistance or were completely independent (Schoenhofen et al., 2006). However, it should be noted that once decline occurred, it occured rapidly (Andersen et al., 2012; Willcox et al., 2008a). Indeed, a precise cause of death can only be determined for a minority of supercentenarians. In many cases, death can only be attributed to a general, global deterioration in an individual's health which suggests that senescence itself can be a cause of death at extreme age (Mesle & Vallin, 2021).

Aging is a complex phenomenon. The exceptional longevity enjoyed by centenarians and supercentenarians is the result of multiple immunologic, genetic, and environmental factors. Distinct changes in the profile of the immune system, the make up of the gut microbiota, the methylation of DNA, and the activity of telomerase are observed in individuals greater than 100 of age, each likely contributing to extreme longevity (Arosa et al., 2017; Biagi et al., 2016; Daunay et al., 2022; Fagnoni et al., 1996; Franceschi et al., 1995; Hashimoto et al., 2019; Martínez De Toda et al., 2020; Miyaji et al., 2000; Sansoni et al., 1993; Santoro et al., 2021; Tedone et al., 2019; Wang et al., 2022).

15.3 How Many Supercentenarians Are There?

It is generally accepted that supercentenarians are rare. The rate of occurrence is estimated to be between 1 in 871,600 to 1 in five million (Perls, 2023; Santos-Lozano et al., 2015).

Per a 2022 report written by Young, as of January 26th, 2022, there were 23 living supercentenarians greater than 113 years of age accounted for by the Gerontology Research Group (GRG) (Young, 2022). Young does emphasize, however, that the list maintained by the GRG does not account for *all* living supercentenarians, but only those whose claims were validated. Worldwide, there are estimated to be about 800–1000 supercentenarians (Young, 2022).

Providing a true estimate of supercentenarians is challenging because as age increases, the quantity and quality of data allowing for validation of age decreases (Centenarians, 2010). To illustrate, in the year 2010, the decennial US Census estimated that there were 330 supercentenarians living in the United States alone (Centenarians, 2010). By comparison, the GRG, in their annual report, were only able to validate 85 supercentenarians *worldwide* in 2010 through the efforts of its international team (Young et al., 2010b). Indeed, the rate of validation decreases as the extremes of age are reached. It is estimated that at least 65% of cases claiming an age of 110–111 are invalid, a percentage that increases to 98% for ages >115 and to essentially 100% for ages >120 (Young et al., 2010a).

While a portion of invalid claims may be the result of administrative errors, some may be due to the deliberate misrepresentation of age for publicity, for social entitlement fraud, or for inclusion in or exclusion from military service and/or employment. Some claims of extreme age may also occur in cultural, social, or religious settings where individuals of advanced age, both living and deceased, are revered (Young et al., 2010a).

However, the greater the age, the greater the scrutiny. For claims exceeding 115 years of age especially, rigorous investigation is required to validate the individual's age (Young et al., 2010a). The investigation begins with the birth registration (and death registration if the individual is deceased) (Young et al., 2010a; Poulain, 2010). Supporting documents are then collected. These include passports, marriage certificates, military/electoral/tax registers, employment/education records, census reports, etc. (Poulain, 2010). Validation additionally requires the investigator to reconstruct a timeline of life events (graduation, marriage, birth of children, death, etc.) not only for the supercentenarian in question, but also for his/her parents and siblings (Young et al., 2010a; Poulain, 2010). This is to ensure there is no mistaken identity. This is to also ensure that the individual's birth date not only makes sense in relation to that of their parents and siblings, but also makes sense in relation to the dates of other notable life events (Young et al., 2010a; Poulain, 2010). Ultimately, identification should be unequivocal and unambiguous.

While the vast of majority of claims are invalid, there is also a secondary problem: there are valid claims that go unaccounted for (Coles, 2004). This is driven by several factors: (1) Data protection laws vary from country to country. This makes it challenging to obtain and validate documents with personal identifiable information.

(2) Individuals and/or their families may not be aware of or have no incentive or interest to participate in supercentenarian identification efforts. (3)There are many countries for which validated data is not yet available. Notably, the two most populous countries, China and India, are not listed in either the IDL or GRG, along with many countries in Southeast Asia, Africa, and the Middle East (Coles, 2004).

There are currently two major databases which maintain a list of validated supercentenarians, both living and deceased. Each list is updated periodically and is maintained through the collaborative efforts of an international team of demographers, researchers, and dedicated amateurs (Young et al., 2010b).

There are a number of ongoing studies that rely on and contribute to these repositories such as The New England Centenarian Study, The Georgia Centenarian Study, The Okinawa Centenarian Study, and The Ashkenazi Jewish Centenarian Study (Young et al., 2010a).

15.4 The International Database on Longevity (IDL)

The International Database on Longevity or IDL was founded in 2010 by Jean-Marie Robine (National Institute for Health and Medical Research, Montpellier, France), Jacque Vallin (French Institute for Demographic Studies, Paris, France) and James Vaupel (Max Planck Institute for Demographic Research, Rostock, Germany) (Contributors [Internet], 2023).

The IDL was initially established to collect demographic data on validated supercentenarians in order to measure mortality at the extremes of age. The database was later expanded to include semi-supercentenarians as well (105–110). The IDL currently has records on over >18,000 validated supercentenarians and semi-supercentenarians from 13 countries (11 European countries, the United States, and Japan). Age is validated according to the established protocols of the country of origin. Identifying information transmitted to the IDL is kept confidential; however, deidentified information regarding sex, date of birth, date of death, place of birth, and place of death are provided for research purposes. The IDL also provides metadata which elucidates the data source and data collection process for each record (IDL International Database on Longevity [Internet], 2023). The ultimate goal of the IDL is to "make reliable demographic data on the oldest-old accessible to the research community" (Cournil et al., 2010).

15.5 The Gerontology Research Group (GRG)

The Gerontology Research Group or GRG was founded in 1990 by L. Stephen Coles and Stephen M. Kaye. Based in Los Angeles, California, the GRG has collaborators from around the globe (About the Gerontology Research Group (GRG) [Internet], 2023).

The GRG includes records from over 30 countries and, as of 2015, had the records of over 1700 validated supercentenarians. Like the IDL, the GRG provides basic demographic information such as sex, date of birth, date of death, place of birth, and place of death for deceased supercentenarians on their list; however, unlike the IDL, the GRG also provides the name of the individual as well as an annual list of currently living supercentenarians (Coles, 2004; GRG World Supercentenarian Rankings List [Internet], 2023).

The GRG's aim is to support ongoing research into healthy aging and longevity with a mission to "slow and ultimately reverse age related decline" (Home - GRG Mission and Statute [Internet], 2023).

15.6 Life Expectancy, Life Span, and Mortality

Life expectancy is defined as the average number of additional years an individual is expected to live. It is influenced by multiple factors including year of birth, current age, sex, race, and geography (Bezy, 2023). Life expectancy is most commonly expressed as life expectancy at birth, although it can be calculated at any year of life.

Life expectancy is a hypothetical measure calculated using life tables. A life table, which is also referred to as a mortality or actuarial table, is a statistical device which shows the probability of an individual living to or dying at a certain age (Bell & Miller, 2005). There are two types of life tables which are commonly used. A cohort life table shows the mortality rates over the lifetime of a population born in the same year (or within the same time frame). A period life table shows the mortality rates for a population only at a specific period of time, typically spanning 1–3 years (Bell & Miller, 2005). The probabilities are derived from census and vital statistics data which provide estimates on the size of the population as well as the number of deaths (Bezy, 2023; Bell & Miller, 2005).Mortality data in supercentenarians is difficult to obtain given the challenges of identifying and verifying individuals who belong to this group. The GRG and IDL therefore provide invaluable data on the mortality of validated supercentenarians. However, the trajectory of mortality in supercentenarians remains the subject of ongoing debate. Some studies suggest that mortality rate declines and eventually plateaus after the age of 105 (Barbi et al., 2018). Statistical analysis of the data present in the IDL suggests that after the age of 110, human mortality remains constant with an annual probability of death equal to 50% with a corresponding life expectancy of 1.4 years (Gampe, 2010; Gampe, 2021). This assertion is not supported by other investigators who speculate that the mortality deceleration seen at ages above 105 is the result of either poor data quality or heterogeneity in the sample population. One other consideration is that the mortality deceleration does not occur at 110 years of age, but at higher and not yet observed ages (Gavrilov & Gavrilova, 2011; Gavrilova et al., 2017).

The presence or absence of mortality deceleration is important because it has implications on a much broader question: What is the maximum human lifespan?

Unlike life expectancy, life span refers to the longest period of time over which the life of an individual within a species may extend. However, there is no consensus on whether there is a fixed limit or whether this limit has already been reached.

Jeanne Louise Calment holds the record for the oldest validated supercentenarian. At her death in 1997, she was 122 years and 164 days. To this day, her record remains unbroken (Jeune et al., 2010). This has been taken as evidence that human longevity is reaching its biological limit, a limit which cannot be surpassed without significant scientific advancement (Dong et al., 2016; Finch et al., 2014; Vijg & Le Bourg, 2017). Those in this camp believe that though life expectancy has increased steadily over the past century, it cannot continue to increase indefinitely due to genetic, biologic, and environmental constraints (Coles, 2004; Vijg & Le Bourg, 2017). In one controversial study, Dong et al. proposed that the maximum human lifespan was around 115 years of age with cases that exceeded this limit treated as outliers. This was inferred from a recent plateau in the maximum reported age of death after the mid-1990s (Dong et al., 2016; Geddes, 2016); however, the statistical analysis underpinning this study was disputed (de Beer et al., 2017; Lenart & Vaupel, 2017; Oeppen & Vaupel, 2002; Rozing et al., 2017).

There are those, however, who hold that the maximum human lifespan has not yet been achieved. Given the rising numbers of centenarians, the steady increase in life expectancy since the nineteenth century, and the deceleration of mortality at extreme ages, some researchers conclude that there is no reason to suspect that the ceiling has been reached or that this ceiling is fixed. The plateau in mortality is a prime piece of evidence as the mortality rate would be expected to reach close to 100% if the maximum age had been reached (de Beer et al., 2017; Lenart & Vaupel, 2017; Oeppen & Vaupel, 2002).

15.7 Case Studies

15.7.1 Jeanne Louise Calment

Jeanne Louise Calment holds the record for the oldest validated supercentenarian. Born on February 21st, 1875, in Arles, France, Calment reached the unrivaled age of 122 years, 5 months, and 14 days at the time of her death on August, 4th 1997 (Jeune et al., 2010; Jeanne Calment, 122, World's Oldest Person (and Woman) Ever [Internet], 2023).

Jean-Marie Robine, a demographer from Montpellier, and Michael Allard, a doctor from Paris, worked closely for several years with Calment's personal doctor, Victor L'ebre and local archivist, Caroline Boyer, to document Calment's long life and to verify her age. Using the well-kept archives in Arles, Robine and Boyer, were able to assemble 23 documents detailing the birth, marriage, and death of Calment and her closest relatives including her parents and siblings (Jeune et al., 2010). Beginning in 1876, Calment is listed in no less than 16 local census documents.

The documents were then examined by impartial experts who ultimately found only minor errors in the records thus allowing Calment to be dubbed “la doyenne de l’humanite” (the elder of humankind) (Jeune et al., 2010).

Born to a wealthy shipbuilder in 1875, Calment was the youngest of 4 children, of which only two survived to adulthood. She attended school between the ages of 7 and 16. In 1896, at the age of 21, she married her second cousin and affluent merchant, Fernand Calment, with whom she later had one daughter, Yvonne, in 1898. She enjoyed an active lifestyle in which she pursued many hobbies including piano, painting, opera, tennis, and hunting. After the untimely death of her daughter in 1934, she raised her grandson, Frederic, who unfortunately died at the age of 36 in 1963. This was preceded by her husband’s death in 1942 at the age of 73 (Jeanne Calment, 122, World's Oldest Person (and Woman) Ever [Internet], 2023).

In 1965, at the age of 90, Calment agreed to sell her house to lawyer, Andre-Francois Raffrey, on the condition that he would make an annual payment to her in exchange for ownership of her house at the time of her death. Calment would ultimately outlive Raffrey, who died in 1995, nearly 30 years after the initial agreement was made (Jeune et al., 2010; Jeanne Calment, 122, World's Oldest Person (and Woman) Ever [Internet], 2023).

Calment enjoyed excellent health throughout the course of her life. She reportedly took up fencing at the age of 85 and continued to ride her bike at the age of 100. She lived independently until she was 110 years old, after which she moved into a retirement home (Jeanne Calment, 122, World's Oldest Person (and Woman) Ever [Internet], 2023). At 115, she suffered a broken hip and successfully underwent surgery although she was confined to a wheelchair thereafter (Jeune et al., 2010; Jeanne Calment, 122, World's Oldest Person (and Woman) Ever [Internet], 2023). Nevertheless, she was said to have enjoyed a glass of port and a cigarette daily. Towards the end of her life, she was nearly blind and very hard of hearing, but she did not suffer from serious illness nor did she display signs of significant dementia. She continued to give interviews and made media appearances until her 122nd birthday. She was fond of saying “I’ve never had more than one wrinkle, and I’m sitting on it”. When asked about the secret to longevity she advised the following: “Always keep your sense of humor. That’s what I attribute my long life to. I think I’ll die laughing.” (Jeune et al., 2010)

15.7.2 Jiroemon Kimura

Jiroemon Kimura, who holds the record as the world’s oldest man, was born as Kinjiro Miyake on April 19th, 1897 in a village called Kami-Ukawa in the Kyoto Prefecture of Japan. At the time of his death on June 12th, 2013 he was 116 years and 54 days old (Gondo et al., 2017).

Kimura's case was first verified by GRG correspondents, Hamish Todd and Ken Matsuoka, in conjunction with the Japanese Ministry of Health, Labor, and Welfare. It was later confirmed by the Supercentenarian Research Foundation and Gondo et al. in their 2017 paper published in Experimental Gerontology where they describe using both official and unofficial documents to reconstruct the timeline of Kimura's life. Official documents include school and employment records along with specialized government records which record all members of the family (KOSEKI and JYOSEKI) as well as their current place of residence (JYUMIN HYO) (Gondo et al., 2017). Unofficial documents include interviews and newspaper articles written about Kimura (Gondo et al., 2017).

Born to a family of farmers, Kimura was the fifth of 8 total children (Gondo et al., 2017). He attended school until the age of 14, before graduating in 1911. He later joined the local postal service and, in 1914, attended a specialized school in Kyoto for mail and telegraph delivery. He moved to occupied Korea for a brief period of time to care for his ailing brother during which time he worked for the Japanese Bureau of Communications. He subsequently returned to Japan at the end of 1920 and shortly after married Yae Kimura with whom he would have seven children between 1923–1943 (Gondo et al., 2017). As his father-in-law had no sons, he would assume the name Jiroeman Kimura in 1927 thus becoming the successor of the Kimura family (Gondo et al., 2017; Jiroemon Kimura, 116, World's Oldest Man Ever [Internet], 2023). Kimura would continue to work at the local post office until his retirement in 1962 at the age of 65 after which he continued to assist his son with farm work until he was well into his 90s (Gondo et al., 2017; Jiroemon Kimura, 116, World's Oldest Man Ever [Internet], 2023). In 1978, he and his wife began living with their eldest son's and eldest grandson's families. His wife died in 1979 at the age of 74. This was followed by the death of his son in 2000, the death of his grandson in 2005, and the death of his daughter-in-law in 2013. Towards the end of his life, he was cared for by his granddaughter-in-law, Eiko Kimura (Gondo et al., 2017; Jiroemon Kimura, 116, World's Oldest Man Ever [Internet], 2023).

Like Calment, Kimura enjoyed robust health throughout his life, as evidenced by his ability to do farm work even at 90. Though he spent the last part of his life mostly in bed, he never suffered from serious illness and could communicate clearly (Matsuyama, 2012). A man of routine, he would wake up early in the morning and read the newspaper with a magnifying glass even into his supercentenarian years while enjoying a breakfast of rice porridge and miso soup (McCurry, 2013). On his 116th birthday, then Japanese Prime Minister, Shinzo Abe, sent him a video message to celebrate. When asked about the secret to his longevity, Kimura stated "Maybe it's all thanks to the sun above me. I am always looking up towards the sky, that is how I am." (Oldest man in history Jiroemon Kimura dies at 116 [Internet], 2013)

Additional Resources

Gerontology Research Organization

Old Website: https://grg.org/
New Website: https://www.grg-supercentenarians.org/

International Database on Longevity:

Website: https://www.supercentenarians.org/en/ – Includes access to *Supercentenarians (2010)* and *Exceptional Lifespans (2021)*

Questions

1. Which one of the following poses a challenge to studying supercentenarians?
    A. Incorrect recording of age
    B. Lack of documents or official records to verify age
    C. Small population size
    D. Changing data protection rules affecting access to records
    E. All the above
2. Which of the following is NOT true?
    A. There are an estimated 800–1000 living supercentenarians worldwide.
    B. The incidence of cancer decreases with age after 85.
    C. The incidence of "survivors" is higher than the incidence of "escapers" at ages>110.
    D. The true cause of death is determined in only a minority of supercentenarians
    E. All are true.
3. Which of the following statements about the human lifespan is correct?
    A. Life expectancy = Life span
    B. There is consensus among the research community regarding the maximum lifespan of a human
    C. Life span is defined as the longest period of time an organism can live
    D. None of the above
    E. All the above

Answers:

1. E
2. C
3. C

References

About the Gerontology Research Group (GRG) [Internet]. (2023). Gerontology Research Group. [cited 2023 Jan 22]. Available from: https://grg.org/

Akushevich, I., Kravchenko, J., Ukraintseva, S., Arbeev, K., & Yashin, A. I. (2012). Age patterns of incidence of geriatric disease in the U.S. elderly population: Medicare-based analysis. *Journal of the American Geriatrics Society, 60*(2), 323–327. https://doi.org/10.1111/j.1532-5415.2011.03786.x. Epub 2012 Jan 27. PMID: 22283485; PMCID: PMC3288526.

Andersen, S. L., Sebastiani, P., Dworkis, D. A., Feldman, L., & Perls, T. T. (2012). Health span approximates life span among many supercentenarians: compression of morbidity at the approximate limit of life span. *Journals of Gerontology Series A: Biological Sciences and Medical, 67*(4), 395–405. https://doi.org/10.1093/gerona/glr223. Epub 2012 Jan 4. PMID: 22219514; PMCID: PMC3309876.

Arosa, F. A., Esgalhado, A. J., Padrão, C. A., & Cardoso, E. M. (2017). Divide, Conquer, and Sense: CD8+CD28- T Cells in Perspective. *Frontiers in Immunology, 7*, 665. https://doi.org/10.3389/fimmu.2016.00665. PMID: 28096804; PMCID: PMC5206803.

Barbi, E., Lagona, F., Marsili, M., Vaupel, J. W., & Wachter, K. W. (2018). The plateau of human mortality: Demography of longevity pioneers. *Science, 360*(6396), 1459–1461. https://doi.org/10.1126/science.aat3119. PMID: 29954979; PMCID: PMC6457902.

Bell FC, Miller ML. (2005). ACTUARIAL STUDY NO. 120 [Internet]. Life Tables for the United States Social Security Area 1900–2100. The United States Social Security Administration; [cited 2023 Jan 22]. Available from: https://www.ssa.gov/oact/NOTES/as120/TOC.html

Bernstein, A. M., Willcox, B. J., Tamaki, H., Kunishima, N., Suzuki, M., Willcox, D. C., Yoo, J. S., & Perls, T. T. (2004). First autopsy study of an Okinawan centenarian: Absence of many age-related diseases. *The Journals of Gerontology. Series A, Biological Sciences and Medical Sciences, 59*(11), 1195–1199. https://doi.org/10.1093/gerona/59.11.1195. PMID: 15602075.

Bezy JM. (2023). life expectancy [Internet]. Encyclopædia Britannica. Encyclopædia Britannica, Inc.; [cited 2023Jan22]. Available from: https://www.britannica.com/science/life-expectancy

Biagi, E., Franceschi, C., Rampelli, S., Severgnini, M., Ostan, R., Turroni, S., Consolandi, C., Quercia, S., Scurti, M., Monti, D., Capri, M., Brigidi, P., & Candela, M. (2016). Gut microbiota and extreme longevity. *Current Biology, 26*(11), 1480–1485. https://doi.org/10.1016/j.cub.2016.04.016. Epub 2016 May 12. PMID: 27185560.

Bonafè, M., Barbi, C., Storci, G., Salvioli, S., Capri, M., Olivieri, F., Valensin, S., Monti, D., Gonos, E. S., De Benedictis, G., & Franceschi, C. (2002). What studies on human longevity tell us about the risk for cancer in the oldest old: Data and hypotheses on the genetics and immunology of centenarians. *Experimental Gerontology, 37*(10–11), 1263–1271. https://doi.org/10.1016/s0531-5565(02)00137-7. PMID: 12470840.

Meyer J. Centenarians. (2010). [Internet]. United States Census Bureau; 2012 [cited 2023 Jan 22]. Available from: https://www.census.gov/content/dam/Census/library/publications/2012/dec/c2010sr-03.pdf

Coles, L. S. (2004). Demography of human supercentenarians. *The Journals of Gerontology. Series A, Biological Sciences and Medical Sciences, 59*(6), B579–B586. https://doi.org/10.1093/gerona/59.6.b579. PMID: 15215268.

Contributors [Internet]. (2023). International database on longevity. [cited 2023 Jan 22]. Available from: https://www.supercentenarians.org/en/home/contributors/

Cournil, A., Robine, J.-M., Maier, H., Gampe, J., & Vaupel, J. W. (2010). The international database on longevity: Structure and contents. In *Supercentenarians* (pp. 31–40). Springer.

Daunay, A., Hardy, L. M., Bouyacoub, Y., Sahbatou, M., Touvier, M., Blanché, H., Deleuze, J. F., & How-Kit, A. (2022). Centenarians consistently present a younger epigenetic age than their chronological age with four epigenetic clocks based on a small number of CpG sites. *Aging (Albany NY), 14*(19), 7718–7733. https://doi.org/10.18632/aging.204316. Epub 2022 Oct 3. PMID: 36202132; PMCID: PMC9596211.

de Beer, J., Bardoutsos, A., & Janssen, F. (2017). Maximum human lifespan may increase to 125 years. *Nature, 546*(7660), E16–E17. https://doi.org/10.1038/nature22792. PMID: 28658213.

DeSantis, C. E., Miller, K. D., Dale, W., Mohile, S. G., Cohen, H. J., Leach, C. R., Goding Sauer, A., Jemal, A., & Siegel, R. L. (2019). Cancer statistics for adults aged 85 years and older, 2019. *CA: a Cancer Journal for Clinicians, 69*(6), 452–467. https://doi.org/10.3322/caac.21577. Epub 2019 Aug 7. PMID: 31390062.

Dong, X., Milholland, B., & Vijg, J. (2016). Evidence for a limit to human lifespan. *Nature, 538*(7624), 257–259. https://doi.org/10.1038/nature19793. Epub 2016 Oct 5. PMID: 27706136.

Evert, J., Lawler, E., Bogan, H., & Perls, T. (2003). Morbidity profiles of centenarians: Survivors, delayers, and escapers. *The Journals of Gerontology. Series A, Biological Sciences and Medical Sciences, 58*(3), 232–237. https://doi.org/10.1093/gerona/58.3.m232. PMID: 12634289.

Fagnoni, F. F., Vescovini, R., Mazzola, M., Bologna, G., Nigro, E., Lavagetto, G., Franceschi, C., Passeri, M., & Sansoni, P. (1996). Expansion of cytotoxic CD8+ CD28- T cells in healthy ageing people, including centenarians. *Immunology, 88*(4), 501–507. https://doi.org/10.1046/j.1365-2567.1996.d01-689.x. PMID: 8881749; PMCID: PMC1456634.

Finch, C. E., Beltrán-Sánchez, H., & Crimmins, E. M. (2014). Uneven futures of human lifespans: reckonings from Gompertz mortality rates, climate change, and air pollution. *Gerontology, 60*(2), 183–188. https://doi.org/10.1159/000357672. Epub 2013 Dec 24. PMID: 24401556; PMCID: PMC4023560.

Franceschi, C., Monti, D., Sansoni, P., & Cossarizza, A. (1995). The immunology of exceptional individuals: The lesson of centenarians. *Immunology Today, 16*(1), 12–16. https://doi.org/10.1016/0167-5699(95)80064-6. PMID: 7880382.

Fries, J. F. (2000). Compression of morbidity in the elderly. *Vaccine, 18*(16), 1584–1589. https://doi.org/10.1016/s0264-410x(99)00490-9. PMID: 10689132.

Gampe, J. (2010). *Human mortality beyond age 110* (pp. 221–230). Supercentenarians. Springer.

Gampe, J. (2021). Mortality of supercentenarians: Estimates from the updated IDL. In *Exceptional Lifespans* (pp. 29–36). Springer.

Gavrilov, L. A., & Gavrilova, N. S. (2011). Mortality measurement at advanced ages: a study of the social security administration death master file. *North American Actuarial Journal, 15*(3), 432–447. https://doi.org/10.1080/10920277.2011.10597629. PMID: 22308064; PMCID: PMC3269912.

Gavrilova NS, Gavrilov LA, Krut'ko VN. (2017). Mortality trajectories at exceptionally high ages: a study of supercentenarians. Living 100 Monogr. 2017(1B). https://www.soa.org/Library/Monographs/Life/Living-To-100/2017/table-of-contents.aspx. Epub 2017 Jul 27. PMID: 29170764; PMCID: PMC5696798.

Geddes L. (2016). Humans may have already reached their maximum lifespan [Internet]. Scientific American. Scientific American; [cited 2023 Jan 22]. Available from: https://www.scientificamerican.com/article/humans-may-have-already-reached-their-maximum-lifespan/

Gondo, Y., Hirose, N., Yasumoto, S., Arai, Y., & Saito, Y. (2017). Age verification of the longest lived man in the world. *Experimental Gerontology, 99*, 7–17. https://doi.org/10.1016/j.exger.2017.08.030. Epub 2017 Aug 26. PMID: 28847724.

GRG World Supercentenarian Rankings List [Internet]. (2023). Gerontology Research Group. [cited 2023 Jan 22]. Available from: https://grg.org/WSRL/TableE.aspx

Hashim, D., Carioli, G., Malvezzi, M., Bertuccio, P., Waxman, S., Negri, E., La Vecchia, C., & Boffetta, P. (2020). Cancer mortality in the oldest old: a global overview. *Aging (Albany NY), 12*(17), 16744–16758. https://doi.org/10.18632/aging.103503. Epub 2020 Sep 3. PMID: 32882684; PMCID: PMC7521488.

Hashimoto, K., Kouno, T., Ikawa, T., Hayatsu, N., Miyajima, Y., Yabukami, H., Terooatea, T., Sasaki, T., Suzuki, T., Valentine, M., Pascarella, G., Okazaki, Y., Suzuki, H., Shin, J. W., Minoda, A., Taniuchi, I., Okano, H., Arai, Y., Hirose, N., & Carninci, P. (2019). Single-cell transcriptomics reveals expansion of cytotoxic CD4 T cells in supercentenarians. *Proceedings of the National Academy of Sciences USA, 116*(48), 24242–24251. https://doi.org/10.1073/pnas.1907883116. Epub 2019 Nov 12. PMID: 31719197; PMCID: PMC6883788.

Hitt, R., Young-Xu, Y., Silver, M., & Perls, T. (1999). Centenarians: The older you get, the healthier you have been. *Lancet, 354*(9179), 652. https://doi.org/10.1016/S0140-6736(99)01987-X. PMID: 10466675.

Home - GRG Mission and Statute [Internet]. (2023). Gerontology Research Group. [cited 2023 Jan 22]. Available from: https://www.grg-supercentenarians.org/

IDL International Database on Longevity [Internet]. (2023). International database on longevity . [cited 2023 Jan 22]. Available from: https://www.supercentenarians.org/en/

Jeanne Calment, 122, World's Oldest Person (and Woman) Ever [Internet]. (2023). Gerontology Research Group. [cited 2023 Jan 22]. Available from: https://grg.org/sc/scindex.html

Jeune, B., Robine, J.-M., Young, R., Desjardins, B., Skytthe, A., & Vaupel, J. W. (2010). Jeanne Calment and her successors. Biographical notes on the longest living humans. In *Supercentenarians* (pp. 282–323). Springer.

Jiroemon Kimura, 116, World's Oldest Man Ever [Internet]. (2023). Gerontology Research Group. [cited 2023 Jan 22]. Available from: https://grg.org/sc/scindex.html

Lenart, A., & Vaupel, J. W. (2017). Questionable evidence for a limit to human lifespan. *Nature, 546*(7660), E13–E14. https://doi.org/10.1038/nature22790. PMID: 28658239.

Martínez De Toda, I., Vida, C., García-Salmones, M., Alonso-Fernández, P., & De La Fuente, M. (2020). Immune function, oxidative, and inflammatory markers in Centenarians as potential predictors of survival and indicators of recovery after hospital admission. *The Journals of Gerontology. Series A, Biological Sciences and Medical Sciences, 75*(10), 1827–1833. https://doi.org/10.1093/gerona/glz250. PMID: 31628457.

Matsuyama K. (2012). Japanese 115-year-old becomes oldest man in history [Internet]. Bloomberg.com. Bloomberg; [cited 2023 Jan 22]. Available from: https://www.bloomberg.com/news/articles/2012-12-28/japanese-115-year-old-becomes-oldestman-in-recorded-history

McCurry J. (2013). World's oldest person Jiroemon Kimura 115, says rise with the Sun, read a paper [Internet]. The Guardian. Guardian News and Media; [cited 2023 Jan 22]. Available from: https://www.theguardian.com/world/2013/mar/07/world-oldest-person-jiroemon-kimura

Mesle, F., & Vallin, J. (2021). Causes of death at very old ages, including for supercentenarians. In *Exceptional Lifespans* (pp. 69–84). Springer.

Miyaishi, O., Ando, F., Matsuzawa, K., Kanawa, R., & Isobe, K. (2000). Cancer incidence in old age. *Mechanisms of Ageing and Development, 117*(1–3), 47–55. https://doi.org/10.1016/s0047-6374(00)00136-6. PMID: 10958922.

Miyaji, C., Watanabe, H., Toma, H., Akisaka, M., Tomiyama, K., Sato, Y., & Abo, T. (2000). Functional alteration of granulocytes, NK cells, and natural killer T cells in centenarians. *Human Immunology, 61*(9), 908–916. https://doi.org/10.1016/s0198-8859(00)00153-1. PMID: 11053634.

Nolen, S. C., Evans, M. A., Fischer, A., Corrada, M. M., Kawas, C. H., & Bota, D. A. (2017). Cancer-Incidence, prevalence and mortality in the oldest-old. A comprehensive review. *Mechanisms of Ageing and Development, 164*, 113–126. https://doi.org/10.1016/j.mad.2017.05.002. Epub 2017 May 11. PMID: 28502820; PMCID: PMC7788911.

Oeppen, J., & Vaupel, J. W. (2002). Demography. Broken limits to life expectancy. *Science, 296*(5570), 1029–1031. https://doi.org/10.1126/science.1069675. PMID: 12004104.

Oldest man in history Jiroemon Kimura dies at 116 [Internet]. (2013). BBC News. BBC; [cited 2023 Jan 22]. Available from: https://www.bbc.com/news/world-asia-22851848

Pavlidis, N., Stanta, G., & Audisio, R. A. (2012). Cancer prevalence and mortality in centenarians: A systematic review. *Critical Reviews in Oncology/Hematology, 83*(1), 145–152. https://doi.org/10.1016/j.critrevonc.2011.09.007. Epub 2011 Oct 22. PMID: 22024388.

Perls T. (2023). Centenarian Statistics [Internet]. Centenarian Statistics | New England Centenarian Study. [cited 2023 Jan 22]. Available from: https://www.bumc.bu.edu/centenarian/statistics/

Poulain, M. (2010). *On the age validation of supercentenarians* (pp. 3–30). Supercentenarians. Springer.

Rozing, M. P., Kirkwood, T. B. L., & Westendorp, R. G. J. (2017). Is there evidence for a limit to human lifespan? *Nature, 546*(7660), E11–E12. https://doi.org/10.1038/nature22788. PMID: 28658235.

Sansoni, P., Cossarizza, A., Brianti, V., Fagnoni, F., Snelli, G., Monti, D., Marcato, A., Passeri, G., Ortolani, C., Forti, E., et al. (1993). Lymphocyte subsets and natural killer cell activity in healthy old people and centenarians. *Blood, 82*(9), 2767–2773. PMID: 8219229.

Santoro, A., Bientinesi, E., & Monti, D. (2021). Immunosenescence and inflammaging in the aging process: Age-related diseases or longevity? *Ageing Research Reviews, 71*, 101422. https://doi.org/10.1016/j.arr.2021.101422. Epub 2021 Aug 13. PMID: 34391943.

Santos-Lozano, A., Sanchis-Gomar, F., Pareja-Galeano, H., Fiuza-Luces, C., Emanuele, E., Lucia, A., & Garatachea, N. (2015). Where are supercentenarians located? A worldwide demographic study. *Rejuvenation Research, 18*(1), 14–19. https://doi.org/10.1089/rej.2014.1609. PMID: 25386976.

Schoenhofen, E. A., Wyszynski, D. F., Andersen, S., Pennington, J., Young, R., Terry, D. F., & Perls, T. T. (2006). Characteristics of 32 supercentenarians. *Journal of the American Geriatrics Society, 54*(8), 1237–1240. https://doi.org/10.1111/j.1532-5415.2006.00826.x. PMID: 16913991; PMCID: PMC2895458.

Silver, M. H., Jilinskaia, E., & Perls, T. T. (2001). Cognitive functional status of age-confirmed centenarians in a population-based study. *The Journals of Gerontology. Series B, Psychological Sciences and Social Sciences, 56*(3), P134–P140. https://doi.org/10.1093/geronb/56.3.p134. PMID: 11316831.

Smith, D. W. (1996). Cancer mortality at very old ages. *Cancer, 77*(7), 1367–1372. https://doi.org/10.1002/(SICI)1097-0142(19960401)77:7<1367::AID-CNCR22>3.0.CO;2-Z. PMID: 8608517.

Stanta, G., Campagner, L., Cavallieri, F., & Giarelli, L. (1997). Cancer of the oldest old. What we have learned from autopsy studies. *Clinics in Geriatric Medicine, 13*(1), 55–68. PMID: 8995100.

Tedone, E., Huang, E., O'Hara, R., Batten, K., Ludlow, A. T., Lai, T. P., Arosio, B., Mari, D., Wright, W. E., & Shay, J. W. (2019). Telomere length and telomerase activity in T cells are biomarkers of high-performing centenarians. *Aging Cell, 18*(1), e12859. https://doi.org/10.1111/acel.12859. Epub 2018 Nov 28. PMID: 30488553; PMCID: PMC6351827.

Vijg, J., & Le Bourg, E. (2017). Aging and the inevitable limit to human life span. *Gerontology, 63*(5), 432–434. https://doi.org/10.1159/000477210. Epub 2017 May 17. PMID: 28511176.

Wang, Y., Dong, C., Han, Y., Gu, Z., & Sun, C. (2022). Immunosenescence, aging and successful aging. *Frontiers in Immunology, 13*, 942796. https://doi.org/10.3389/fimmu.2022.942796. PMID: 35983061; PMCID: PMC9379926.

Willcox, D. C., Willcox, B. J., Wang, N. C., He, Q., Rosenbaum, M., & Suzuki, M. (2008a). Life at the extreme limit: Phenotypic characteristics of supercentenarians in Okinawa. *The Journals of Gerontology. Series A, Biological Sciences and Medical Sciences, 63*(11), 1201–1208. https://doi.org/10.1093/gerona/63.11.1201. PMID: 19038835.

Willcox, B. J., Willcox, D. C., & Ferrucci, L. (2008b). Secrets of healthy aging and longevity from exceptional survivors around the globe: lessons from octogenarians to supercentenarians. *Journals of Gerontology Series A: Biological Sciences and Medical Science, 63*(11), 1181–1185. https://doi.org/10.1093/gerona/63.11.1181. PMID: 19038832; PMCID: PMC4986604.

Young, R. D. (2022). Validated living worldwide supercentenarians 113+, living and recently deceased: February 2022. *Rejuvenation Research, 25*(1), 46–48. https://doi.org/10.1089/rej.2022.0011. PMID: 35081749.

Young, R. D., Desjardins, B., McLaughlin, K., Poulain, M., & Perls, T. T. (2010a). Typologies of extreme longevity myths. *Curr Gerontol Geriatr Res, 2010*, 423087. https://doi.org/10.1155/2010/423087. Epub 2011 Mar 15. PMID: 21461047; PMCID: PMC3062986.

Young, R. D., Epstein, L., & Coles, L. S. (2010b). Validated worldwide supercentenarians, living and recently deceased. *Rejuvenation Research, 13*(1), 127–132. https://doi.org/10.1089/rej.2010.1033. PMID: 20230288.

Chapter 16
Implications of the Age-Friendly Healthcare Systems (AFHS) Movement on the Care of Centenarians

Anissa Nahabedian and Nicole Brandt

Key Take Away Points
1. Age Friendly Health Systems will help to improve the care of older adults and focus efforts on understanding "What Matters" to centenarians.
2. Aligning clinical, training, and research initiatives is critical to advancing the models of care when working with older adults.
3. AFHS help to promote the retooling of our current healthcare workforce but set the stage for our future workforce needs.

16.1 Introduction

Very old adults, ages 85 or older, represent the fastest growing population in most developed countries. (Boerner et al., 2018). Centenarians, the oldest old within this age segment, is expected to increase from approximately 441,000 in 2013 to 3.4 million in 2050. (United Nations, 2013). There are many unknowns when caring for this population, but it is important to note that centenarian hospitalizations cost 2.7 times more than the average hospital costs of the 85 plus population and 2.1 times the costs of the 65–84 population (Wier et al., 2010). Furthermore, these costs may be preventable as noted by a recent study reporting that approximately 29% of total hospitalization charges and 34% of all admissions hospitalizations are due to

A. Nahabedian · N. Brandt (✉)
The Peter Lamy Center on Drug Therapy and Aging, Baltimore, MD, USA

University of Maryland School of Pharmacy, Baltimore, MD, USA
e-mail: anahabedian@umaryland.edu; nbrandt@rx.umaryland.edu

R. E. Kheirbek, M. D. Llorente (eds.), *Current Perspectives on Centenarians*, International Perspectives on Aging 36,
https://doi.org/10.1007/978-3-031-30915-1_16

ambulatory care-sensitive conditions as primary diagnoses (Twersky & Davey, 2022) These statistics set the stage for opportunities to improve how we supply care to older adult.

16.1.1 Illustrative Vignette

Ms. Jenkins was a lively and independent centenarian who lived in a small senior community. She was known for her wit and wisdom and was loved by all who knew her. Despite her age, she remained active and engaged in her community. However, as she entered her 100th year, her health began to decline and she needed more support.

What Matters to Ms. Jenkins was to maintain her independence and continue to live in her own home. She cherished her daily routine of reading the newspaper, taking a walk in the park, and playing cards with her friends.

Medications became a challenge for Ms. Jenkins as she struggled to manage multiple prescriptions and keep track of her dosage. Her doctor and family worked together to simplify her medication regimen and ensure she was taking the right drugs at the right time.

Mentation was also a concern for Ms. Jenkins as she reported feeling forgetful and disoriented at times. Her doctor referred her for a cognitive evaluation and prescribed activities that would stimulate her mind, such as crossword puzzles and word games.

Mobility was a crucial aspect of Ms. Jenkins' well-being. She relied on a walker to get around and had trouble climbing stairs. To help her maintain her mobility, her family arranged for physical therapy and made modifications to her home to make it easier for her to navigate.

With the support of her doctor, family, and community, Ms. Jenkins was able to continue living in her own home and lead a fulfilling life. The 4 Ms framework of What Matters, Medications, Mentation, and Mobility played a critical role in ensuring her well-being and promoting healthy aging.

16.1.2 Age Friendly Health Systems

The John A. Hartford Foundation and the Institute for Healthcare Improvement built upon the work of the WHO (World Health Organization) to create Age-Friendly Health Systems (The John A. Hartford Foundation, 2023). Age Friendly Health Systems are those in which every older adult gets person centered care that helps to improve their quality of life. The framework guiding this initiative is the 4Ms. (Fig. 16.1) The "4 M's" (What Matters, Medication, Mentation and Mobility) initiative follows a set of evidence-based practices that prevents harm and aligns care with what matters to the older adult. Furthermore, it helps to guide clinicians to provide a more objective and concise way to care for older adults.

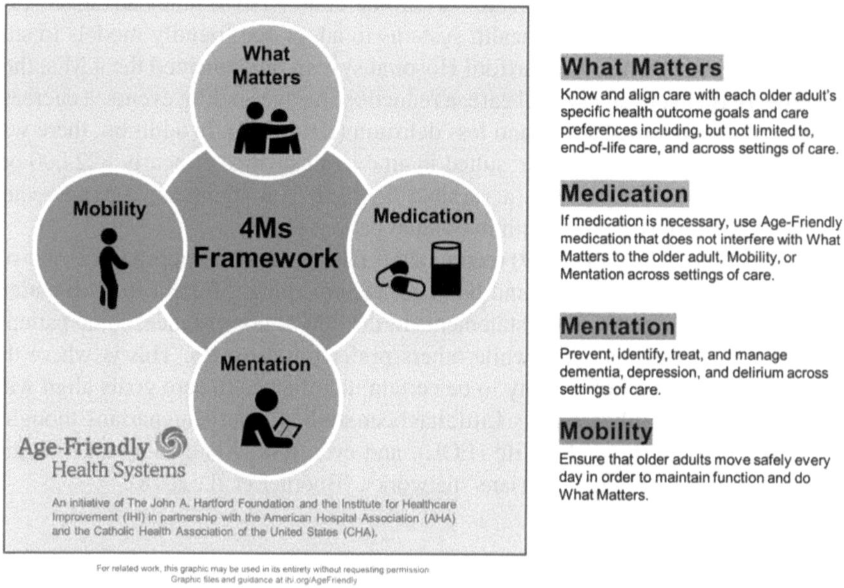

Fig. 16.1 The 4 M's Framework accessed at: https://institute.agefriendly.org/initiatives/age-friendly-org/

16.1.2.1 "What Matters"

The goal of "What Matters" is to generate conversations between healthcare providers and patients and to shift the conversation away from disease processes to focus on health goals and care preferences of the patient. An essential part of this is to professionally train the healthcare team and system to understand, document and act on "What Matters" to older adults. Documentation of the "What Matters" conversation can be recorded in the patient's electronic health record (EHR) or a white board template in a story board format that is in the patient's room that is easily accessible to all members of the healthcare team. Asking "What Matters" has been shown to lower inpatient utilization (54%), Intensive Care Unit (ICU) stays (80%) and increase hospice use (47.2%) as well as enhance patient satisfaction. (Agency for Healthcare Research & Quality (AHRQ), 2013).

Within an AFHS asking "What Matters" also allows each healthcare provider to align and provide care with the older adult's specific healthcare preferences and. "What Matters" to the older adult is the one of the crucial elements of the AFHS initiative and the basis for age-friendly care. This person-centered care approach goes beyond end-of-life care planning to include all elements important to the older adult that include health outcome goals, activities that matter most, medications, or family visits.

In addition to promoting holistic care, Matę et al., (2018) notes advanced care planning will be essential for health systems to adopt age friendly models to stay financially viable. When the Hartford Hospital system implemented the 4 M's, they saw a decrease in unwanted ICU care, a reduction in adverse drug events, a decrease in falls, fewer pressures sores, and less delirium (IHI, 2019). In addition, there was a decreased length of stay that resulted in an overall savings of nearly $22,000 per stay (IHI, 2019). While this is a variable figure, it is a significant savings when assessing the cost associated with individual patient care.

The Institute of Health (2019) recommends taking a systems approach to end-of-life planning noting that error and harm mean something different to each patient based on their "What Matters" statements in the 4 M's. For instance, some patients may want all measures taken while others prefer no measures. This is where the health system has an opportunity to be certain that the health care goals align with the patient's own healthcare goals. Little has been studied about centenarians'thoughts or plans regarding the end of life (EOL), and even less is known about how this topic is handled within centenarians' networks. (Boerner et al., 2018).

16.1.2.2 Mentation

Mentation, focuses on preventing, identifying, treating, and managing delirium, depression, and dementia across the continuum of care. It is a clinical syndrome that develops in older adults over a short period of time and is characterized by an acute alteration of attention, cognitive function and behavioral abnormalities caused by underlying medical conditions (Komici et al., 2022; Ramírez Echeverría et al., 2022). Risk factors for delirium include preexisting cognitive impairment, certain medications (i.e., High anticholinegic activity), uncontrolled pain, dehydration, constipation, fever, infection, depression, alcohol use, sleep deprivation, low blood oxygen levels, and immobility (National Institute on Aging, 2020; Komici et al., 2022; Ramírez Echeverría et al., 2022). The clinical manifestation of delirium can be subtle and pose diagnostic challenges for the hospital staff because it can present with a constellation of symptoms that may mimic or present like other illnesses.

The pathophysiology of delirium is complex and not usually due to a single underlying cause (Ramírez Echeverría et al., 2022). The most common predisposing factors are older age (≥ 70 years), dementia, and precipitant factors such as, functional disabilities, male gender, poor vision and hearing, and mild cognitive impairment (Ramírez Echeverría et al., 2022). Many medications can precipitate delirium, especially psychoactive medications, or anticholinergic drugs. Medication side effects account for up to 39% of delirium cases (Ramírez Echeverría et al., 2022). Assessment and early identification of mentation changes are critical. Delirium occurs in 25% of older adults after major surgery or acute illness and in 80% of older patients in the intensive care unit (ICU) (National Institute on Aging, 2020) and up to 70% of patients in a long-term care setting (Komici et al., 2022) Delirium can have a negative impact on the prognosis of people with acute illness, is an independent predictor of poor outcomes and is associated with a significant cost burden. Left untreated, delirium can result in significant cognitive dysfunction. That is why within AFHS inpatient and long-term care settings, delirium should be monitored with standardized screening tools (see resource list) as well as staff training which can promote early identification and treatment of delirium.

16.1.2.3 Medications

Older adults are the largest consumers of prescription and over the counter (OTC) medications which contributes to increased risk of adverse effects and hospitalizations. (Hamilton et al., 2011; Chui et al., 2017; Giardina et al., 2018). Kanaan et al. (2013) found that of identifiable ADEs during a 45 day follow up after hospitalization, 35% of ADEs were preventable and suggests the need for quality and safety to extend beyond a singular assessment tool (Kanaan et al., 2013). Intrinsic factors such as advanced age, frailty, and polypharmacy further contribute to greater risks in adverse outcomes (Zhou & Rupa, 2018). That is why system changes improve care transitions and focus on medications can help to reduce ADEs. (Guth et al., 2020).

A meta-analysis examining interventions to reduce ADRs in older adults found that pharmacist-led interventions reduced ADRs by 35% compared to 21% with non-pharmacist-led interventions.(Gray et al., 2018) Pharmacist involvement in medication management is associated with reduced ADRs, hospitalizations, and ED visits, as well as cost savings from discontinuing or switching to less costly drug therapy. (Cobb, 2014; Pellegrin et al., 2017). In addition to focusing on preventing adverse drug reactions, action is being taken to deprescribe medications, which refers to a process of medication withdrawal, supervised by a health care professional, with the goal of managing polypharmacy and improving outcomes in a systematic, proactive approach. (Reeve et al., 2015) Successfully deprescribing medications needs to be person centered and involve all members of the healthcare team. For instance, a patient's willingness to deprescribe medications has been found when: (1) patient/caregiver has interest in reducing the number of medications they are taking and (2) willingness to stop medicines they have been taking for a long time (Blum, 2023 Reeve, 2018). There are ongoing efforts looking at engaging pharmacists and aligning goals of care consistent with the AFHS (National Institute on Aging, 2021). Furthermore, global efforts are underway to establish Age Friendly Pharmacies due to the rapid growth of older adults and the need for services to address the medication related needs in the community (Chen et al., 2021; Interntional Pharmaceutical Federation Pharmacists (FIP), 2021).

16.1.2.4 Mobility

Mobility is defined as the ability or capacity to move which can be measured and evaluated in multiple ways. Research has shown us the importance of hospital-based mobility programs since hospitalized older patients spend greater than 80%

of their time lying in bed and less than 43 min per day walking, despite being ambulatory upon admission (Brown et al., 2009). Furthermore, lack of physical mobility in hospitalized older patients increases the risk for frailty and functional decline (Theou et al., 2016), further contributing to disability, morbidity, and mortality (Afilalo, 2011). Effectively promoting regular mobility in hospitalized older adults is a team effort that requires collaboration among disciplines, and a structured, organized, and purposeful approach. There are many resources available to aid in early mobility programs found at: https://browse.welch.jhmi.edu/early-mobility/web-resources.

Across all care settings, it is imperative that the healthcare team screens older to assess their highest level of mobility. For instance, staying mobile can buffer health challenges and negative perceptions of ability since older adults are able to remain socially engaged and active (Alidoust et al., 2019). The National Council on Aging (2021) promotes and supports programs for older adults to be engaged and exercise due to the positive impact on physical and mental well-being. Furthermore, the National Institutes on Aging -supported CAPABLE (Community Aging in Place, Advancing Better Living for Elders) home-based intervention program has been shown to be effective in increasing mobility, functionality, and the capacity to "age in place" for low-income older adults (Fields et al., 2022).

16.2 Impact of the AFHS Movement

The AFHS movement helps to frame out caring for centenarians. A recent study by Tinetti et al., (2021) evaluated the healthcare preferences of older adults who had multiple chronic conditions, a group frequently excluded from clinical trials due to coexisting conditions. The focus of this study was to examine what goals the older adult desire most, further noting that healthcare visits, testing, medication management, can be burdensome, time consuming and may conflict with what the patients are willing or able to do. The most common goals were related to activities around meals, spending time with friends, shopping and exercising. Other goals were related to decreasing medication, living with less pain, playing with grandchildren, and going to the park or gardening. Considering a patient's health conditions, function and health trajectory are all important aspects in providing holistic care. This model is not only person centered but has been shown to be economically advantageous. (Tabbush et al., 2019) (Table 16.1).

16.3 Preparing the Geriatric Workforce

As the population of older adults increases, the geriatric workforce continues to decrease (Rowe, 2021). According to the latest data outlined by the American Geriatrics Society (AGS) (2021) the number of older adults is quickly outpacing the

Table 16.1 The economic base for 4 M outcomes

4 M's	Economic Outcomes
What matters	Asking what matters and developing an integrated system to address it lowers inpatient utilization (54% decrease); ICU stays (80% decrease), while increasing hospice use (47.2%) and patient satisfaction (AHRQ, 2013)
Medication	Older adults suffering an adverse drug event have higher rates of morbidity, hospital admission and costs (Field et al., 2005) • 1500 hospitals in HEN 2.0 reduced 12,611 adverse drug events saving $78 million across 34 states (HRET, 2017)
Mentation	Depression in ambulatory care doubles the cost of care across the board (Unutzer, 2009) • 16:1 Return on Investment (ROI) on delirium detection and treatment programs (Rubin, 2013)
Mobility	Older adults who sustain a serious fall-related injury required an additional $13,316 in hospital operating cost and had an increased length of-stay (LOS) of 6.3 days compared to controls (Wong et al., 2011)

number of those who specialize in geriatrics. By 2025 it is estimated that there will be an increased need of 45% of geriatricians and yet there is not an increase in training programs to meet that need (AGS, 2021). (Figure X). According to Holveck and Wick (2018) with the looming geriatrician shortage other disciplines will have to help along with geriatricians to prevent disparities and address gaps in care. While all specialties will need to help, there appears to be insufficient curriculum in geriatric education. The authors found that those who do not specialize in geriatrics get very little formal geriatric training. For instance, an estimated 35% of pharmacy students reported that their didactic education failed to prepare them to care for older adults even though 93% of older adults live within five miles of a community pharmacy. (Holveck & Wick, 2018).

Additionally, there is a need for nurses and other healthcare practitioners in geriatrics to fill the gap as well as a need for more geriatric training. Few health professions are trained in geriatrics and report that less than 5% have any type of licensing for geriatrics care. Overall, 4% of social workers, 2.6% of advanced practice registered nurses and less than 1% of RN's and PA's and pharmacists are certified in geriatrics. (Flaherty & Bartels, 2019) Further stressing the need for innovation and collaboration for interprofessional work not only at an institutional level but also at a national level.

The American Geriatrics Society (2014) published a position statement on the essentiality of interdisciplinary teams to ensure quality geriatric care delivery. Interdisciplinary Team Training (IDT) is a well-developed model of care coordination effective in other specialties and improved health outcomes. IDT has been shown to improve continuity of care, enhance communication, offer better care transitions, improve medication adherence and avoidance of poly pharmacy, preservation of function and management of chronic illness (Fig. 16.2).

It is imperative to align efforts to improve the delivery of care (AFHS) as well as the training of our future workforce through Age Friendly Universities. At the University of Maryland, we have highlighted our efforts and the importance of partnership not only at a system level but a state level as well. (Schumacher et al., 2022)

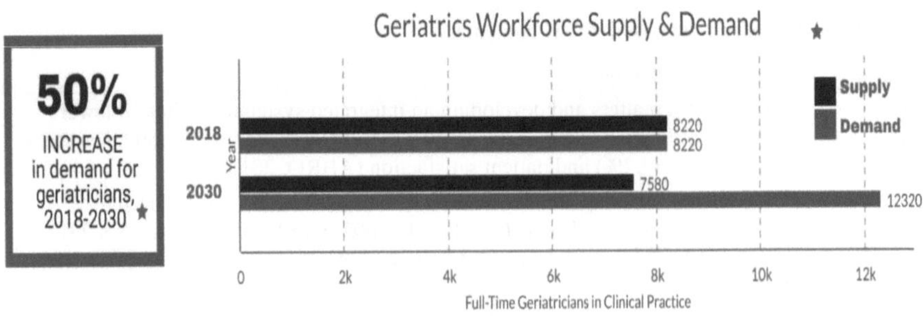

Fig. 16.2 Geriatrics Workforce Prediction. (AGS, 2021)

Within the United States there has been further alignment with national efforts through the Health Resources and Services Administration (HRSA) Geriatrics Workforce Enhancement Program (GWEP) which is vital to filling the need for expanding and improving the health care workforce. Clinical training could provide an increased focus on preparing clinicians to deliver care in an age-friendly manner across all types of clinical settings. The recommendations within the 17th report will promote broad changes within the health care system to advance age-friendly practices, train the health care workforce in age-friendly care, and improve the care of older adults, while also addressing the reduction of burnout and the promotion of wellness and resilience among health care providers. (HRSA, 2019).

16.4 Summary

As the aging population continues to grow, the demand for comprehensive, safe, and high-quality care continues to increase. Older adults typically have complex health needs and often experience multiple chronic medical conditions. That is why the 4Ms Framework of the Age-Friendly Health Systems initiative empowers hospitals and health care practices to provide older adults with care that is evidence based and aligned with what matters to them.

Multiple Choice Questions

1. ***The definition of age-friendly care includes (select all that apply)***
   (a) Follows an essential set of evidence-based practices
   (b) Causes no harm
   (c) Align care with What Matters to the older adult and their family or other caregivers.
   (d) Primary focus is to reduce hospital-based costs

2. ***The goal of "What Matters" is to:***
   (a) Ensure end-of-life planning
   (b) Generate conversations between healthcare providers and patients and focus on health goals and care preferences of the patient.
   (c) Make certain the patient takes responsibility for their care
   (d) Provide a data base to document medications
3. ***The following is true of delirium (select all that apply)***
   (a) Predisposing factors are older age
   (b) Typically has a single underlying cause and is easy to diagnose
   (c) Certain medications can precipitate delirium
   (d) Left untreated, delirium can result in significant cognitive dysfunction.

Answers

1. ***a,b,c***: *While age-friendly care can reduce hospital-based costs it is not the primary focus. The focus is safe, person-centered care.*
2. ***b.:*** The goal of "What Matters" is to generate conversations between healthcare providers and patients and to shift the conversation away from disease processes to focus on health goals and care preferences of the patient. An essential part of this is to professionally train the healthcare team and system to understand, document and act on "What Matters" to older adults.
3. **a,c,d:** The pathophysiology of delirium is complex and not usually due to a single underlying cause (Ramírez Echeverría et al., 2022). The most common predisposing factors are older age (≥ 70 years), dementia, and precipitant factors such as, functional disabilities, male gender, poor vision and hearing, and mild cognitive impairment (Ramírez Echeverría et al., 2022). Many medications can precipitate delirium, especially psychoactive medications, or anticholinergic drugs.

Resources

"What Matters"

Tools	Description	Reference to the Tool
Patient Priorities Care	Resources to support aligning care with what matters most to patients. The Specific Ask (Matters Most) Conversation Guide and the Patient Priorities identification conversation guide help identify the values, outcome goals, and care preferences for older adults with multiple chronic condition	Homepage - Patient Priorities Care
STEPS Forward	An online physician education module that guides physicians through how to discuss end-of-life decisions with patients and caregiver	End-of-Life Care: Facilitate Early Discussions with Patients I AMA STEPS Forward I AMA Ed Hub (ama-assn.org)

Mentation

Tools	Description	Reference to the Tool
Ultra-Brief 2-Item Screener (UB-2)	Delirium Screening	Ultra-Brief 2-Item Screener (UB-2)
Confusion Assessment Method (CAM)	Delirium Screening	The Confusion Assessment Method (CAM) | Hartford Institute for Geriatric Nursing (hign.org)
Confusion Assessment Method Intensive Care Unit (CAM-ICU)	Delirium Screening	Resource Downloads (icudelirium.org)

Medications

Tools	Description	Reference to the Tool
American Geriatrics Society (AGS) Beers Criteria	A reference list of medications to be avoided or used with caution for older adults.	https://doi.org/10.1111/jgs.15767
Screening Tool of Older Persons' Prescriptions (STOPP) & Screening Tool to Alert to Right Treatment (START)	Criteria to identify potentially inappropriate prescriptions (PIP) and potentially omitted prescriptions (POP)	https://www.ncbi.nlm.nih.gov/pmc/articles/PMC4339726/
US-FORTA (Fit fOR The Aged)	A list addressing the appropriateness of drugs for older people in the US depending on availability, usage, and expert rating	https://doi.org/10.1016/j.jamda.2019.07.023
Drugs Regimen Unassisted Grading (DRUGS) Scale	A method of assessing the ability of an older adult to manage their own medications based on identification, access, dosage and timing	https://doi.org/10.1016/j.amjopharm.2006.06.009
Medication Management Instrument for Deficiencies in the Elderly (MedMalDE)	A questionnaire to assess an older adult's medication adherence based on their knowledge, ability, and procurement	https://doi.org/10.1093/geront/46.5.661

Mobility

Tools	Description	Reference to the Tool
Timed Up & Go	Screen for mobility limitations	TUG_Test-print.pdf (cdc.gov)
Johns Hopkins-Highest Level of Mobility	Screen for mobility limitations	Activity and Mobility Promotion Tools, Resources and Research | Johns Hopkins Physical Medicine and Rehabilitation (hopkinsmedicine.org)

John A Hartford Foundations & WebMD released four videos exploring the 4Ms of age-friendly care to help older adults and family caregivers take control of their health as they age.

The four new videos at WebMD.com/AgeFriendly are:

- What Matters Is Most Important
- Medication: More Birthdays Often Means More Pills
- Mentation: Dementia vs. Normal Memory Loss
- Mobility: Getting Around and Preventing Falls

Institute for HealthCare Improvement: Resources exist to help build the business case for the AFHS initiative available at: https://www.ihi.org/Engage/Initiatives/Age-Friendly-Health-Systems/Pages/Resources.aspx.

References

Afilalo, J. (2011). Frailty in patients with cardiovascular disease: Why, when, and how to measure. *Current Cardiovascular Risk Reports, 5*, 467–472. https://doi.org/10.1007/s12170-011-0186-0

Agency for Healthcare Research and Quality. (2013). *2013 Annual Hospital-Acquired Condition Rate and Estimates of Cost Savings and Deaths Averted From 2010 to 2013*. https://www.ahrq.gov/sites/default/files/publications/files/hacrate2013_0.pdf

Alidoust, S., Bosman, C., & Holden, G. (2019). Planning for healthy aging: How the use of third places contributed to the social health of older adults. *Ageing and Society, 39*(7), 1459–1484. https://doi.org/10.1017/S0144686X18000065

American Geriatrics Society. (2014). Position statement on interdisciplinary team training in geriatrics: An essential component of quality health care for older adults. *Journal of the American Geriatrics Society, 62*(5), 961–965.

American Geriatrics Society. (2021). Workforce by the numbers. https://www.americangeriatrics.org/geriatrics-profession/about-geriatrics/geriatrics-workforce-numbers

Blum, K. (2023). *Survey: Most adults willing to stop medications if ok'd by doctors. Pharmacy practice news*. Survey: Most Adults Willing to Stop Medications If OK'd by Doctors - Pharmacy Practice News.

Boerner, K. K., Kim, Y., Rott, C., & Jopp, D. S. (2018). Centenarians' end-of-life thoughts and plans: Is their social network on the same page? *Journal of American Geriatrics Society, 66*(7), 1311–1317.

Brown, C. J., Redden, D. T., Flood, K. L., & Allman, R. M. (2009). The underrecognized epidemic of low mobility during hospitalization of older adults. *Journal of the American Geriatrics Society, 57*, 1660–1665. https://doi.org/10.1111/j.1532-5415.2009.02393.x

Centers for Disease Control and Prevention National Center for Injury Prevention and Control. (2017). Stopping elderly accidents, deaths and injuries. Assessment: Timed Up & Go (TUG). https://www.cdc.gov/steadi/pdf/TUG_Test-print.pd

Chen, S.-C., Lee, K.-H., Horng, D.-J., & Huang, P.-J. (2021). Integrating the public health Services model into age-friendly pharmacies: A Case study on the pharmacies in Taiwan. *Healthcare, 9*, 1589. https://doi.org/10.3390/healthcare9111589

Chui, M. A., Stone, J. A., & Holden, R. J. (2017). Improving over-the-counter medication safety for older adults: A study protocol for a demonstration and dissemination study. *Research Social Administrative Pharmacy, 13*(5), 930–937. https://doi.org/10.1016/j.sapharm.2016.11.006

Cobb, C. D. (2014). Optimizing medication use with a pharmacist-provided comprehensive medication management service for patients with psychiatric disorders. *Pharmacotherapy, 34*(12), 1336–1340. https://doi.org/10.1002/phar.1503
Fick, D. M., Inouye, S. K., Guess, J., Ngo, L. H., Jones, R. N., Saczynski, J. S., & Marcantonio, E. R. (2015). Preliminary development of an ultrabrief two-item bedside test for delirium. *Journal of Hospital Medicine., 10*(10), 645–650.
Field, T. S., Gilman, B. H., Subramanian, S., Fuller, J. C., Bates, D. W., & Gurwitz, J. H. (2005). The costs associated with adverse drug events among older adults in the ambulatory setting. *Medical Care, 43*(12), 1171–1176.
Fields, B., Yanes, C., Ennis, M., & Toto, P. (2022). Community aging in place, advancing better living for elders (CAPABLE) program: Understanding the potential involvement of care partners. *Health & Social Care in the Community, 30*(4), e1212–e1219. https://doi.org/10.1111/hsc.13529
Flaherty, E., & Bartels, S. (2019). Addressing the community-based geriatric healthcare workforce shortage by leveraging the potential of interprofessional teams. *Journal of American Geriatric Society, 67*(52), s400–s408.
Giardina, C., Cutroneo, P. M., Mocciaro, E., Russo, G. T., Mandraffino, G., Basile, G., Rapisarda, F., Ferrara, R., Spina, E., & Arcoraci, V. (2018). Adverse drug reactions in hospitalized patients: Results of the FORWARD (facilitation of reporting in hospital Ward) study. *Frontiers in Pharmacology, 9*, 350. https://doi.org/10.3389/fphar.2018.00350
Gray, S. L., Hart, L. A., Perera, S., Semla, T. P., Schmader, K. E., & Hanlon, J. T. (2018). Meta-analysis of interventions to reduce adverse drug reactions in older adults. *Journal of the American Geriatrics Society, 66*(2), 282–288. https://doi.org/10.1111/jgs.15195
Guth, A., Chou, J., Courtin, S. O., Ford, C., Hennawi, G., & Brandt, N. (2020). An interdisciplinary approach to implementing the age-friendly health system 4Ms in an ambulatory clinical pathway with a focus on medication safety. *Journal of Gerontological Nursing, 46*(10), 7–11.
Hamilton, H., Gallagher, P., Ryan, C., Byrne, S., & O'Mahony, D. (2011). Potentially inappropriate medications defined by STOPP criteria and the risk of adverse drug events in older hospitalized patients. *Archives of Internal Medicine, 171*(11), 1013–1019. https://doi.org/10.1001/archinternmed.2011.215
Health Research & Educational Trust (HRET). (2017). *Adverse drug events change package: 2017 update*. Health Research & Educational Trust. Accessed 27 Jan 2023, at www.hret-hiin.org.
Health Resources and Services Administration. (2022). Health workforce projections. Review Health Workforce Research | Bureau of Health Workforce (hrsa.gov)
Health Services & Resources Administration (HRSA). (2019). Preparing the current and future health care workforce for interprofessional practice in sustainable, age-friendly healthy systems. https://www.hrsa.gov/sites/default/files/hrsa/advisory-committees/community-based-linkages/reports/seventeenth-2019.pdf
Holveck, C. A., & Wick, J. Y. (2018). Addressing the shortage of geriatric specialists. *The Consultant Pharmacist, 33*(3), 130–138.
Institute for Healthcare Improvement. (2019). *"What Matters" to older adults: A tool kit for Health systems to design better care with older adults.* http://www.ihi.org/Engage/Initiatives/Age-Friendly-Health-Systems/Documents/IHI_Age_Friendly_What_Matters_to_Older_Adults_Toolkit.pdf
Institute for Healthcare Improvement. (2022). *What is an age-friendly health system?* http://www.ihi.org/Engage/Initiatives/Age-Friendly-Health-Systems/Pages/default.aspx
Interntional Pharmaceutical Federation Pharmacists (FIP). (2021). How pharmacies are helping to create age-friendly Communities. How pharmacies are helping to create AGE-FRIENDLY COMMUNITIES - FIP - International Pharmaceutical Federation Pharmacists in different cities around the world are helping to create age-friendly environments.
Johns Hopkins Medicine. (2023). *Johns hopkins highest level of mobility (JH-HLM) scale.* Activity and Mobility Promotion Tools, Resources and Research | Johns Hopkins Physical Medicine and Rehabilitation (hopkinsmedicine.org)

Kanaan, A. O., Donovan, J. L., Duchin, N. P., Field, T. S., Tjia, J., Cutrona, S. L., Gagne, S. J., Garber, L., Preusse, P., Harrold, L. R., & Gurwitz, J. H. (2013). Adverse drug events after hospital discharge in older adults: Types, severity, and involvement of beers criteria medications. *Journal of the American Geriatrics Society, 61*(11), 1894–1899. https://doi.org/10.1111/jgs.12504

Komici, K., Guerra, G., Addona, F., & Fantini, C. (2022). Delirium in nursing home residents: A narrative review. *Healthcare, 10*(1544), 1544. https://doi.org/10.3390/healthcare10081544

Mate, K. S., Berman, A., Laderman, M., Kabcenell, A., & Fulmer, T. (2018). Creating age-friendly health systems- A vision for better care of older adults. *Healthcare, 6*(1), 4–6.

National Insitute on Aging. (2020). Researchers test new approaches to prevent delirium in older adults. Researchers test new approaches to prevent delirium in older adults I National Institute on Aging (nih.gov)

National Institute on Aging. (2021). The dangers of polypharmacy and the case for deprescribing in older adults. The dangers of polypharmacy and the case for deprescribing in older adults I National Institute on Aging (nih.gov)

Pellegrin, K. L., Krenk, L., Oakes, S. J., Ciarleglio, A., Lynn, J., McInnis, T., Bairos, A. W., Gomez, L., McCrary, M. B., Hanlon, A. L., & Miyamura, J. (2017). Reductions in medication-related hospitalizations in older adults with medication management by hospital and community pharmacists: A quasi-experimental study. *Journal of the American Geriatrics Society, 65*(1), 212–219. https://doi.org/10.1111/jgs.14518.]

Ramírez Echeverría, M. D. L., Schoo, C., & Paul, M. (2022). Delirium. In *StatPearls*. StatPearls Publishing.

Reeve, E., Gnjidic, D., Long, J., & Hilmer, S. (2015). A systematic review of the emerging definition of "deprescribing" with network analysis: Implications for future research and clinical practice. *British Journal of Clinical Pharmacology, 80*(6), 1254–1268. https://doi.org/10.1111/bcp.12732

Rowe, J. W. (2021). The U.S. eldercare workforce is falling further behind. *Nature Aging, 1*, 327–329.

Schumacher, J., Brandt, N., Resnick, B., Nahabedian, A., Heavner, M., Netzer, G., Wilson, L., & Kheirbek, R. E. (2022). Merging an age friendly university with an age friendly health care system: Case study findings. *Innovation in Aging, 6*(Suppl 1), 568–569. https://doi.org/10.1093/geroni/igac059.2142

Tabbush, V., Pelton, L., Mate, K., & Duong, T. (2019). The business case for becoming an age-friendly health system. Accessed at: http://www.ihi.org/Engage/Initiatives/Age-Friendly-Health-Systems/Documents/IHI_Business_Case_for_ Becoming_Age_Friendly_Health_System.pdf

The John A Hartford Foundation. (2023). *Age-friendly care: It's about what matters to you*. Age--Friendly Care (johnahartford.org)

Theou O., Tan E. C., Bell J. S., Emery T., Robson L., Morley J. E., . . . Visvanathan R. (2016). Frailty levels in residential aged care facilities measured using the frailty index and FRAIL-NH scale. Journal of the American Geriatrics Society, 64, e207-e212. doi: https://doi.org/10.1111/jgs.14490.

Tinetti, M. E., Costello, D. M., Naik, A. D., Davenport, C. H., Bigos-Hernados, K., Van Liew, J. R., et al. (2021). Outcome goals and health care preferences of older adults with multiple chronic conditions. *JAMA Network Open, 4*(3), 1–15.

Twersky, S. E., & Davey, A. (2022). National hospitalization trends and the role of preventable hospitalizations among centenarians in the United States (2000-2009). *International Journal of Environmental Research and Public Health, 19*(2), 795. https://doi.org/10.3390/ijerph19020795

United Nations. (2013). World *population ageing*. WorldPopulationAgeingReport2013.pdf (un.org)

Wier, L. M., Pfuntner, A., Maeda, J., Stranges, E., Ryan, K., Jagadish, P., Collins, S. B., & Elixhauser, A. (2010). *HCUP facts and figures: Statistics on hospital-based care in the United States, 2009*. Agency for Healthcare Research and Quality.

Wong, C. A., Recktenwald, A. J., Jones, M. L., Waterman, B. M., Bollini, M. L., & Dunagan, W. C. (2011). The cost of serious fall-related injuries at three Midwestern hospitals. *Joint Commission Journal on Quality and Patient Safety, 37*(2), 81–87.

Zhou, L., & Rupa, A. P. (2018). Categorization and association analysis of risk factors for adverse drug events. *European Journal of Clinical Pharmacology, 74*(4), 389–404. https://doi.org/10.1007/s00228-017-2373-5

Index

R. E. Kheirbek, M. D. Llorente (eds.), *Current Perspectives on Centenarians*, International Perspectives on Aging 36,
https://doi.org/10.1007/978-3-031-30915-1

MIX
Papier aus verantwortungsvollen Quellen
Paper from responsible sources
FSC® C105338
www.fsc.org

If you have any concerns about our products,
you can contact us on
ProductSafety@springernature.com

In case Publisher is established outside the EU,
the EU authorized representative is:
Springer Nature Customer Service Center GmbH
Europaplatz 3, 69115 Heidelberg, Germany

Printed by Libri Plureos GmbH
in Hamburg, Germany